W9-CAG-155

Fundamentals of Hearing

Fundamentals of Hearing
An Introduction

William A. Yost
University of Florida

Donald W. Nielsen
Henry Ford Hospital, Detroit

Holt, Rinehart and Winston
New York   Chicago   San Francisco   Atlanta   Dallas
Montreal   Toronto   London   Sydney

Library of Congress Cataloging in Publication Data

Yost, William A
    Fundamentals of hearing.

    Includes bibliographical references and indexes.
    1. Hearing.   I. Nielsen, Donald W., joint author.
II. Title.
QP461.Y67   612'.85   76–54247

ISBN 0–03–016781–7

Design by Arthur Ritter

Copyright © 1977 by Holt, Rinehart and Winston
All rights reserved
Printed in the United States of America

    3   4   5   032   8   7   6   5

**To our colleagues
who were instrumental
in developing
our careers:**

G.R.J.		**W.D.F.**
D.E.R.	**D.C.T.**	**D.N.E.**
D.M.G.		**T.K.**

Preface

The field of audition has grown at a tremendous rate in the past three decades, with specialists generating a wealth of new knowledge about auditory processing. We believe this textbook will serve a need by making the fundamentals of this information available to those who are dependent on the basic facts of auditory function—students and professionals in such diverse fields as speech pathology, clinical audiology, psychology, medicine, engineering, biology, and physics.

In the 1940s and 1950s, Stevens and Davis, in their book *Hearing: Its Psychology and Physiology,* and Licklider and von Bekesy, in their chapters in S. S. Stevens' *Handbook of Experimental Psychology,* provided excellent introductions to audition. Since then only a few textbooks that attempt to cover audition at an introductory level have appeared.

Accordingly, *Fundamentals of Hearing: An Introduction* is intended to be an up-to-date textbook that outlines the *basics* of audition at an *introductory* level. We have attempted to introduce the beginning student to the concepts and terminology required to form a solid base for understanding auditory processing. We have avoided discussion of theories, models, or suppositions concerning auditory functioning except in situations in which such theories, models, or suppositions have become basic concepts of the study of audition. That is, we have tried to provide the fundamental ideas and facts of audition so that students can use this information to understand the theories, models, and suppositions found in advanced textbooks and in the many journal articles on audition.

We have tried to write the book in such a way that a student with little mathematical training (only the ability to solve a linear equation of the form $y = mx + b$ is required) and a minimum of training in physiology and anatomy should be able to read and profit from the contents of the book. Also, four appendixes covering sinusoids, logarithms, anatomy, and physiology are included to help the student extend the information contained in the fourteen chapters. In addition, the glossary of terms (combined with the subject index) contains definitions from various American National Standards Institute (ANSI) standards on acoustic terminology. These definitions have been thoroughly reviewed by ANSI and should therefore provide unambiguous terminology for the student.

We recognize the ambitious nature of this undertaking. Actually, it can be said that it is impossible to describe in fourteen short chapters such a wide field as audition, which has a rich history of mathematical, physical, physiological, and psychological content. The virtual impossibility becomes more evident with the constraint of writing for students who have little background in the supporting disciplines. Nevertheless, we have tried, aided by the fact that our collaboration, bringing together our differing knowledge in the field, has made this task more manageable.

The book has been kept short so that it may be used for a one-term course in hearing or as one of a few books in a course surveying sensory systems or in a course surveying the speech and hearing sciences. Thus we feel that the book can be used as a primary text or to supplement other material in the area of hearing science.

Although the primary aim of the book is to provide an introductory text in audition, we hope that the material included, especially that in the summaries, supplements, references, and glossary, will make the book one that any professional who needs facts about audition will want to have readily available. In other words, we have tried to make the book useful as a reference for introductory information about audition.

The book is divided into three sections, an overview chapter (Chapter 14), and four appendixes. The three sections (also indicated in the contents) are: The Stimulus: The Physics of Sound (Chapters 1–3); Auditory Anatomy and Physiology (Chapters 4–7); Psychophysics and Auditory Perception (Chapters 8–13). Each chapter concludes with a brief summary, followed by a "Supplement," a "grab-bag" of topics including in every case the relevant literature for the experiments mentioned in the chapter, as well as other sources that might help the student understand the chapter better or do additional work on a particular topic. Some supplements include as well a discussion of subject matter for the advanced student; in others we have rewritten statements in different ways to make sure that the limitations of the statements have been defined; or we have indicated that some new, but not firmly tested, ideas on a subject are currently being investigated.

The writing of a book of this scope requires a great deal of dedicated assistance from many people. We would like to acknowledge at least the following: Dianne Aquillo, Kathy Page, Debbie Green, and Patty Ohlman for their help in typing; Norman Green for his drafting assistance; and the staff of the Institute for Advanced Study of the Communication Processes at the University of Florida for their supporting help. We also are grateful to: Kim Duffey for typing; Sarah Crenshaw McQueen for artwork; Jane Burnham, Robert Turner,

and the rest of the staff of the Otological Research Laboratory of Henry Ford Hospital for their suggestions.

We also wish to thank the authors of journal articles and the publishers, all credited in the book and listed in full in the references, who graciously granted permission for use of diagrams and photographs. Since 1971, the students in the "Fundamentals of Hearing" classes at the University of Florida have helped to clarify the many ambiguities a textbook such as this can contain. We also wish to express our gratitude to the Deafness Research Foundation for its dedication to the support of research in hearing.

Dr. Ivan Hunter-Duvar and his technician, Richard Mount, at the Hospital for Sick Children, Toronto, have been very helpful in providing most of the superb photographs in this book. Their work formed an integral part of the planning and production of the book.

A book of this nature could not have been written without the dedicated assistance of some of our colleagues. The following provided thoughtful and most helpful critiques of the manuscript: Constantine Trahiotis, University of Illinois; Donald C. Teas, University of Florida; John F. Brandt, University of Kansas. Although their help was extremely important, the final work is our sole responsibility.

Special thanks are due Lee Yost, who helped edit the manuscript time and time again and was invaluable in demanding the clarity with which we hope the book is written. Finally, our love, appreciation, and thanks go to our families.

W.A.Y.

D.W.N.

Contents

Fundamentals of Hearing

CHAPTER 1
The World We Hear

Close your eyes and concentrate for a moment on all of the things happening around you. As you listen, you may notice a large and diverse group of activities. Your auditory system has enabled you to gain considerable information about your environment. You might be aware of a car moving down a distant street, a barking dog, the faint hum of a fan, the loud voice of a friend, the sound of your own breathing, the rustle of your clothes moving across your body. What you are experiencing are acoustic pressures.

These acoustic pressures constantly surround us. The human auditory system is remarkably sensitive to the countless number of objects that produce acoustic pressure. The pressures to which the auditory system is sensitive are called audible sounds. Scientists in the fields of auditory physiology and anatomy, psychoacoustics, and the related fields of

psychology, acoustical engineering, and medicine have attempted to understand the pressures to which the auditory system is sensitive and the way in which the various parts of the auditory system work to achieve this sensitivity.

To gain an appreciation of what we can hear and how our auditory system functions we require knowledge from many areas. Because of the auditory system's remarkable sensitivity, it is necessary to understand something about those objects that can produce acoustic pressure. It is also necessary to study the propagation of this pressure from the object to the auditory system. It is useful to know how other objects in the path of this pressure (such as the auditory system) are affected by the pressure and how those objects might alter the nature of the acoustic pressure. We need to understand the various parts of the auditory system (the field of anatomy) and how these parts work when acoustic pressure is present (the field of auditory physiology). We should also study the entire auditory system's sensitivity to acoustic pressure: that is, what pressures do we report as being "heard"?

In order to simplify our understanding of hearing, we will begin our discussion by assuming that there are three aspects of sound: *sound production, sound transmission,* and *sound analysis.* That is, a vibrating object produces sound, which is transmitted to an object, which then analyzes it. For instance, consider a tank of water with a plunger at one end and a rubber membrane at the other. The plunger is viewed as the sound-producing object, the water is the medium of sound transmission, and the membrane will provide some sound analysis. The water tank analogy was chosen because we can observe changes in all three parts of the system when sound is produced. Changes that occur in air are similar (but not identical) to those produced in water, but they are not easily observed. For instance, the motion of the plunger will produce waves or ripples in the tank. A similar motion in air will also produce waves or ripples in the air, but it is much easier to see the water waves than the air waves. We shall next describe how a plunger or any object can move in air in order to produce sound.

SOUND PRODUCTION

Sound may be defined in terms of either a psychological or a physical dimension. Let us first consider the physical definition: sound is a stimulus that has the capability for producing an audible sensation. Any object having the properties of *inertia* and *elasticity* may be set into vibration and hence may produce a sound. Thus *vibration* is the property of an object that makes sound production possible. If we "hear" the vibration, the sound is "audible." Vibration is the movement of an object

from one point in space to another point and usually back again to the first point. The fact that a force must be exerted on a body to make it move defines *inertia,* whereas the ability of the object after it is deformed or moved by this force to return to some starting or initial state defines *elasticity.* In practice, almost every object has inertia and elasticity; thus almost every object can be set into vibration and can produce sound.

There is no restriction on the type of vibration required to produce a sound. As long as an object moves from one point to another point and back again, it may produce a sound. The object may move regularly back and forth or completely at random; it may take years or fractions of a second for it to complete a vibratory cycle, or it may move only once or millions of times. All of these vibrations are capable of producing sound.

If our knowledge of vibration and sound production were limited to only general descriptions of vibration, the area of acoustics (the study of sound) would be very complicated. We would have no easy way of describing different vibrations and sounds. Fortunately there is a method of categorizing different vibrations. Joseph Fourier, a Frenchman who lived in the time of Napoleon I, described important theorems for the flow of heat; his analysis can be applied to the types of vibrations we have described. Fourier derived a theorem that specified that *any* vibration can be resolved into a sum of a particular type of vibrations, called *sinusoidal vibrations.* This sum of sinusoidal vibrations, called a *Fourier series,* can describe almost any arbitrary vibration. The derivation of these sinusoids is called *Fourier analysis.*

A sinusoid describes a particular relation between displacement and time, that is, a particular vibration (Appendix A contains a more detailed discussion of sinusoids). Figure 1.1 is a diagram of a sinusoid (also called a sine wave). Displacement simply means the dis-

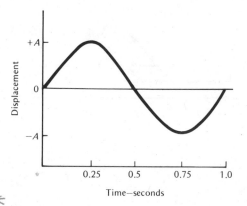

Figure 1.1 A sinusoidal relation between displacement and time. From the starting position at 0°, the peak amplitude is +A; the period is 1 second; the frequency is 1 Hz.

tance an object moves. A sine wave describes the regular back-and-forth motion of an object over a period of time. Notice that from the starting position (displacement $D = 0$) the motion goes upward to a maximum positive distance $(D = +A)$, then back to the starting position, then downward to a maximum negative distance $(D = -A)$, and finally back to the starting position. Theoretically, this back-and-forth vibration goes on forever, but since it repeats itself, we need to diagram only one complete transition of this motion.

Three properties (parameters) characterize a sinusoid: *frequency, starting phase,* and *amplitude*. Once we have specified the values of these three parameters, we have uniquely described a single sinusoid. Unless all three parameters are specified, there may be more than one sine wave in question. Since any vibration consists of a sum of several sinusoidal vibrations, then we can completely describe any vibration by specifying the amplitude, frequency, and starting phase of the various sinusoids that constitute the vibration. Any vibration consisting of more than one sinusoid is called a *complex vibration,* whereas a single sine wave is called a *simple vibration*. Since

vibrations are also called *waves* or *waveforms,* there can be simple and complex waveforms.

Generally, amplitude is a measure of displacement; frequency is a measure of how often per one unit of time the object moves back and forth (oscillates); and starting phase is a measure of the position of the object at the instant in time it begins to vibrate. The sinusoidal relation between displacement and time can be written in equation form:

$$D = A \sin (2\pi f t + \theta) \qquad (1.1)$$

where D is instantaneous amplitude, A a measure of maximum amplitude, f a measure of frequency, t a measure of time, and θ a measure of starting phase. (See Appendix A for a table of sine values.)

Equation (1.1) is an algebraic description of the waveform drawn in Figure 1.1. As can be seen in both representations of the sine wave, all three parameters (amplitude, frequency, and starting phase) are necessary to describe the sinusoidal relation. The parameters of the sine wave that we have been discussing refer to the physical description of the vibration. A large area of psychophysics is concerned with human perception of these parameters. That is, on a subjective basis, how does a person label the frequency, amplitude, and starting phase of a sinusoid? Generally we label changes in the amplitude of a sine wave as *loudness* and changes in frequency as *pitch*. We do not have a subjective term for starting phase since we are sensitive to changes in starting phases only under particular conditions. One of these conditions involves presenting to each ear a sine wave with a different starting phase. In this case changes in the difference of starting phase at the two ears result in changes in the perceived location of the stimulus in space. Thus for these conditions in which two ears are stimulated, changes in starting phase correspond to changes in the *locus of the stimulus*.

The relations of the physical descriptions to

the subjective descriptions of the parameters of the sine wave are somewhat complex. For instance, although changes in intensity are almost always perceived as loudness changes, variations in frequency (which are independent of intensity changes) can also result in perceived loudness changes. (Other interactions also occur; we shall treat these later in Chapter 13.) Because of these interactions between the physical and the subjective dimensions of the sine wave, we must be careful in describing the acoustical stimulus. In referring to the physical stimulus we should use only the terms "frequency," "amplitude," and "starting phase." In referring to how a human perceives the stimulus, we can use the subjective terms "pitch," "loudness," and (in some cases) "perceived location."

It is also important to mention that in many situations a human observer might not be able to describe the differences between two distinct physical stimuli, but he does know they are different. For this reason and since the subjective descriptions are not uniquely related to the physical dimensions, we shall use the physical parameters rather than the terms "pitch," "loudness," and "perceived location" throughout most of our discussion of hearing.

FREQUENCY

The frequency of a sinusoid is the number of cycles a sine wave completes per unit time; for instance, the number of times *per second* an object moves back and forth. The symbol "Hz" (standing for hertz) is used to denote this number. If there are 100 complete cycles in 1 second, then the sinusoid is said to have a frequency of 100 Hz. A complete *cycle* means that the sine wave begins and ends at the same point of displacement after having taken on all possible values of D. The sinusoid in Figure 1.1 has completed one cycle, but the vibration in Figure 1.2 has not. Notice that

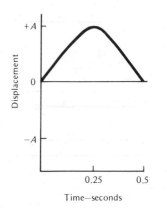

Figure 1.2 A vibration. This vibration is not, by itself, a sinusoid. It it were part of a sinusoid, its frequency would be 1 Hz.

since the sinusoid in Figure 1.1 completed its cycle in 1 second, its frequency is 1 Hz. The sinusoid in Figure 1.3 has completed five cycles in 1 second, and hence its frequency is 5 Hz. The frequency of the vibration in Figure 1.2

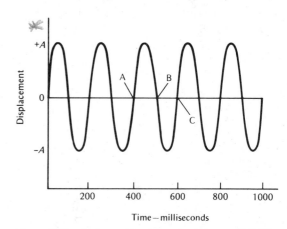

Figure 1.3 A sinusoid with a frequency of 5 Hz; the starting phase is 0°, the peak amplitude is $+A$. One period is between points A and C and not between points A and B or B and C.

would be 1 Hz, if it were part of a sinusoid, since it completed half its cycle in half a second; thus (if we had drawn a full cycle) it would have completed a full cycle in 1 second.

The amount of time a sinusoid takes to complete one cycle is called the _period_ of the sinusoid. Thus, the period of the sinusoid in Figure 1.1 is 1 second, and the period of the sinusoid in Figure 1.3 is ⅕ second. We usually express fractions of a second in terms of milliseconds (thousandths of a second, abbreviated ms). Thus the period of the sine wave in Figure 1.3 is 200 ms. Notice that although we defined the period in terms of one complete cycle, the period of a sinusoid may be found by determining the time between two identical points on the waveform. In Figure 1.3 the period may be determined, for instance, by finding the time between points A and C on the waveform. The time between points A and B equals only half a period. Notice point B is not exactly like point A (the sine wave is going up at points A and C and down at point B).

The frequency _f_ of a sinusoid is equal to 1 divided by the period _p_:

$$f = \frac{1}{p} \tag{1.2}$$

when _p_ is expressed in seconds. That is, frequency and period are reciprocally related. It is usually easiest to measure the period of a sine wave in seconds and then to derive its frequency by dividing the period into 1.

Either frequency or period may be used to describe the oscillation of a sinusoidal vibration. These two terms are also used to describe the repetition occurring in many nonsinusoidal vibrations. The only requirement of these vibrations is that they be periodic; that is, whatever pattern of vibration exists, it must be repeated. The complex vibration described in Figure 1.4 is periodic, although it is not a sinusoid. Its period is 500 ms since the time between two identical points (A and B, for instance) is 500 ms. Its frequency is 2 Hz because 2 Hz = 1/500 ms (1/0.5 second) or because the vibration went through one cycle (one pattern of vibration between points A

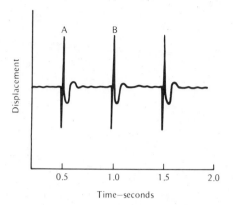

Figure 1.4 A complex periodic vibration that is not a sinusoid. The frequency of repetition is 2 Hz. The period is shown by the time indicated between points A and B (500 ms).

and B) in ½ second. For complex vibrations with a repetition rate we call the frequency of vibration _repetition frequency;_ for sinusoids we speak of sinusoidal frequency.

STARTING PHASE

The starting phase of a sinusoid corresponds to the amount of its displacement from zero at the instant in time the vibration begins. That is, the point in the displacement cycle at which the object begins to vibrate determines its starting phase. Although the starting phase may be discussed in terms of the starting displacement, it is usually defined in terms of time (period) or _degrees of angle_.

In terms of period, a sinusoid is said to start at zero phase, or to start "in phase," if at time equal to zero ($t = 0$) the displacement D equals zero. The sine wave in Figure 1.1 starts at zero phase. The sinusoid in Figure 1.5 starts at one-half of a period since, relative to zero starting phase (Figure 1.1), this sinusoid has begun one-half of a period later. In Figure 1.6 the starting phase is one-quarter of a period.

Since period is expressed in terms of seconds

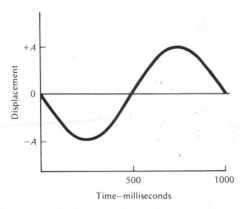

Figure 1.5 A sinusoid that begins at a 180° starting phase. Compare this sinusoid with the one in Figure 1.1, which begins at 0° starting phase.

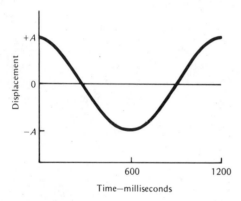

Figure 1.6 A sinusoid that begins at a 90° starting phase. Compare this sinusoid with those in Figures 1.1 and 1.5, which begin at different starting phases.

or milliseconds, the starting phase of a sinusoid can be defined in terms of time. Notice that the starting phase of a sinusoid, when expressed in time, is dependent on the frequency since period is related to frequency ($f = 1/p$). Both sinusoids in Figures 1.5 and 1.7 start at one-half of a period, but since their frequencies are different (by a factor of 4), the sine wave in Figure 1.5 starts at 500 ms relative to the zero starting-phase condition and the one in Figure 1.7 at 125 ms relative to zero starting-phase condition. Another way to calculate this difference in time is to observe that the

sinusoid in Figure 1.5 reaches the zero starting-phase position at 500 ms, whereas the sinusoid in Figure 1.7 reaches the zero starting-phase position at 125 ms.

Time is, therefore, not a totally convenient way to define starting phase since the frequency or period of the wave must also be

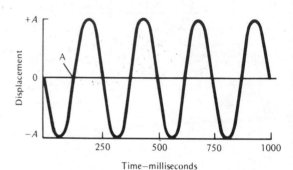

Figure 1.7 A sinusoid that begins at a 180° starting phase. Note that this sinusoid goes through 0° phase (point A) at 125 ms, while the sinusoid in Figure 1.5 goes through 0° phase at 500 ms. The sinusoids in Figures 1.5 and 1.7 both begin at 180° starting phase.

known. A better description of starting phase is the *phase angle,* which is independent of frequency. This definition stems from the fact that when a sinusoid has completed one cycle of vibration, it has traveled a complete circle (see Appendix A). Since there are 360 degrees in a circle, a sine wave has gone through 360° when it has completed one cycle, 180° when it has completed one-half of a cycle, 90° when it has completed one-quarter of a cycle, and so on. Thus degrees of circular angle can define the starting phase of a sinusoid. Both sinusoids in Figures 1.5 and 1.7 have a starting phase angle of 180°, those in Figures 1.1 and 1.3 start at a phase angle of 0°, and that in Figure 1.6 starts at a phase angle of 90°. If the wave begins when the displacement is positive, the starting phase must be between 0° and 180°, whereas if it begins at a negative displacement, the starting phase lies somewhere between 180° and 360°. Notice that although the sinusoids in Figures 1.5 and 1.7 have different frequencies, their starting phase in terms of phase angle is the same (180°).

Starting-phase angle is determined by noting the change in the starting displacement of a sinusoid relative to the 0° starting-phase condition shown in Figures 1.1 and 1.3. If, for instance, a sinusoid starts at maximum displacement at time equal to zero (see Fig. 1.6), then it has begun a quarter of a period later than the 0° starting-phase condition. Thus the starting phase is one-quarter of 360°, or 90°. Figure 1.8 shows a sinusoid divided into fractions of a period. The time or horizontal axis is divided

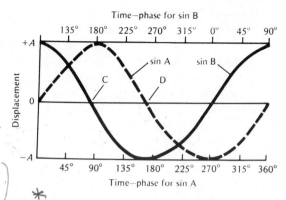

Figure 1.9 Two sinusoids of the same frequency. Sinusoid A starts at 0° starting phase and sinusoid B at 90° starting phase. This same 90° phase difference exists at time points C and D.

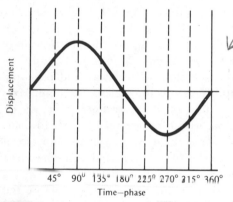

Figure 1.8 A sinusoid is divided into eight divisions of phase.

into eight equal divisions of phase. We can use this type of figure to determine starting phase. If the sinusoid starts at one of these eight positions, then the starting phase is shown on the horizontal axis.

Sometimes two sinusoids are said to be "out of phase" with one another. If the two are out of phase and have the same frequency, then they must have different starting phases. In Figure 1.9 sinusoid A is 90° out of phase with sinusoid B since sinusoid A starts at 0° phase and sinusoid B at 90° phase. However, since both sinusoids are of the same frequency, the phase difference between them could be deter-

mined at any two points along the time axis. At both points, C and D, for instance, the difference between the two waveforms is also one-quarter of a period, or 90° (360°/4).

If the two sinusoids are of different frequencies, as in Figure 1.10 (the frequencies differ by a factor of 2), then the relationship between the difference in starting phase is not as simple. The two sine waves in Figure 1.10 start

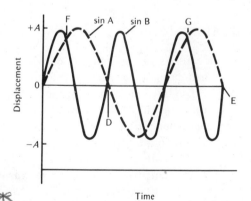

Figure 1.10 Two sinusoids (sin A, sin B) that differ in frequency by a factor of 2. The phase differences computed at different points (D, E, F, G) are not all the same, although the starting phases for both sinusoids are 0°. The phase difference at points D and E is 180°, while the phase difference at points F and G is 45°.

at the same phase. At points D and E sine wave A leads sine wave B; however, at points F and G sine wave B leads sine wave A.

In order to avoid confusing the phase difference computed at the start and that figured at some other points in time, we speak of *starting phases* and *instantaneous phases.* Starting phase is figured at time $t = 0$ (when the sine wave begins); instantaneous phase refers to the phase difference figured at any time point other than $t = 0$. Therefore, if two sinusoids have the same frequency, the starting-phase difference always equals the instantaneous phase difference. However, if the two sinusoids have different frequencies, starting phase will generally not equal instantaneous phase.

One last point should be made before we begin a discussion of amplitude. If a sine wave starts at a phase of 90°, it is called a *cosine* wave. Thus, the wave in Figure 1.6 could be considered a cosine wave. In terms of equation (1.1),

$$\cos x = \sin (90° - x)$$

where x is $2\pi f t$.

AMPLITUDE

Amplitude refers to the amount of vibratory displacement; that is, how far an object moves describes its amplitude. Sometimes intensity is used to describe this displacement or movement, but for our purposes we shall let amplitude refer to displacement and relate intensity to measures of pressure, power, and energy. The displacement of the sine wave varies with time. This time-varying displacement is called the *instantaneous amplitude* of the sine wave. Definitions of amplitude that do not vary with time include *peak amplitude, peak-to-peak amplitude,* and *root-mean-square (rms) amplitude.*

Peak amplitude refers to the maximum posi-

tive displacement the waveform achieves in one period. For a sine wave such as that in Figure 1.1, the peak amplitude is A. Peak-to-peak amplitude is the total distance from the maximum positive peak to the maximum negative displacement the waveform achieves in one period. For the sine wave in Figure 1.1 this is $2A$. The amplitude of nonsinusoidal (Fig. 1.4) waveforms can also be described in terms of peak or peak-to-peak amplitude.

Peak and peak-to-peak amplitudes appear to be adequate descriptions of the amplitude of sinusoids. However, for nonsinusoidal waveforms we might not wish to describe the amplitude with these values. For instance, the waveform in Figure 1.4 might have much larger peak and peak-to-peak amplitudes than the sinusoid in Figure 1.1. Yet over most of the period of the waveform in Figure 1.4 very little vibration occurs. Peak and peak-to-peak amplitudes are insufficient to summarize the amplitude of the waveform over an entire period. However, we might wish to compare the average amplitude of the waveform in Figure 1.4 over one period with the identical average amplitude of the sine wave in Figure 1.1. If we simply take the average of the instantaneous amplitudes over one period of a sine wave, we would always have zero average amplitude since half of the sine wave is positive and the other half is negative. If, however, we square each instantaneous amplitude, all of the negative numbers become positive. We could then compute the average of these squared instantaneous amplitudes, and then take the square root of this average. This result would not be zero. Such an averaging operation is called computing the root-mean-square, or rms, amplitude of a waveform. In equation form the rms amplitude A_{rms} may be expressed as:

$$A_{rms} = \sqrt{\frac{\sum\limits_{i=1}^{N} a_i^2}{N}} \tag{1.3}$$

where a_i is an instantaneous amplitude. The summing operation must be performed over one complete waveform period.

In the case of a sine wave the rms amplitude equals approximately 0.707 times the peak amplitude, or $0.707A$. When we talk about amplitude we will be using primarily the rms value since this technique enables us to compare simple and complex waveforms.

COMPLEX STIMULI

Although Fourier's theorem states that sinusoids are the basic vibrations, they are not the types of vibrations one experiences directly in everyday life. Most acoustic stimuli are complex stimuli, consisting of the sum of many sinusoids. As with sinusoidal stimuli there are various ways to describe a complex waveform. The waveforms drawn in Figures 1.1–1.10 are being defined in the *time domain*. The time-domain description relates the instantaneous amplitude of the complex (or simple) waveform to time. When the complex waveform is described in terms of the individual sinusoids that constitute the waveform, it is being described in the *frequency domain*. In the frequency-domain description the amplitude, frequency, and starting phase of each sinusoid in the complex wave must be determined.

Each sinusoid that is a constituent of a complex waveform is characterized by its frequency. Thus, when we say there are four sinusoids, we mean that four frequencies exist. The plot of the amplitude of each sinusoid as a function of its frequency is called the *amplitude spectrum*, whereas the plot of the starting phase of each sinusoid is called the *phase spectrum*. When the phase and amplitude spectra of a complex waveform are described, the waveform has been completely defined in the frequency domain.

Figure 1.11 demonstrates how a complex wave is portrayed in both the time and frequency domains. Figure 1.11a is a plot of the complex wave in only the time domain. Imagine that this wave consists of the sum of three sinusoids with frequencies of 200 Hz, 300 Hz, and 400 Hz. Figures 1.11b and 1.11c show the amplitude and phase spectra of these three sinusoids. To demonstrate that the frequency domain plots (Figs. 1.11b and 1.11c) are describing the same waveform as that in Figure 1.11a, the three sinusoids are drawn in the time domain in Figure 1.11d. In Figure 1.11e the amplitudes of the three sinusoids of Figure 1.11d have been summed at each successive point in time. As can be seen, this combined waveform looks exactly like that in Figure 1.11a.

Thus when we wish to ascertain the variation of a complex wave in time, we emphasize the waveform in the time domain. However, if the frequency content of the complex wave is important, we emphasize the amplitude and phase spectra. As was shown in Figure 1.11, it is not difficult to reconstruct the time-domain description of a wave from the amplitude and phase spectra, but deriving the frequency-domain spectra from the time-domain waveform requires the use of Fourier analysis. Although the technique of Fourier analysis will not be described in this book, we can diagram some more time-domain waveforms and their respective amplitude and phase spectra. First, however, two classes of spectra must be defined: *line spectra* and *continuous spectra*. A line spectrum describes a complex wave consisting of only a discrete number of sinusoids, whereas a continuous spectrum describes a wave in which all frequencies (a continuum) between certain limits are present.

In Figure 1.12 a few common complex stimuli and their time and frequency domain representations are shown. Figures 1.12b–e are line spectra, and Figures 1.12a and f are continuous spectra. For some line spectra (Figs. 1.12b–e) only integer multiples (1 times, 2 times, 3 times, and so on) of the lowest fre-

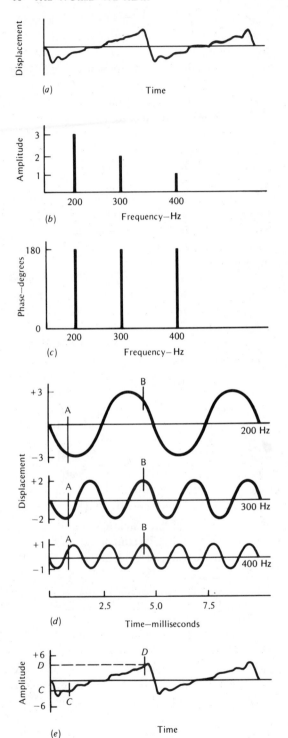

quency exist. For instance, in Figure 1.12c suppose that the lowest frequency is 100 Hz, then 200 Hz, 300 Hz, and so on are present (in the frequency domain). In this situation the lowest frequency present is called the *fundamental frequency*, and each higher multiple is called a *harmonic*. Thus, 100 Hz is the *fundamental frequency*, 200 Hz is the *second harmonic*, and 300 Hz is the *third harmonic*, and so forth. Many complex waves consist of a fundamental frequency and higher harmonics. A common example is the piano keyboard. Middle C has a fundamental frequency of 256 Hz and many higher harmonics, depending on the quality of the piano. Quite often the pitch we associate with a complex stimulus is the pitch of the fundamental frequency. Thus, middle C is a complex stimulus consisting of many sinusoids but with a fundamental frequency of 256 Hz.

Figure 1.12a demonstrates another interesting ramification of Fourier analysis: a sinusoid that is turned on and off is not a simple stimulus but consists of many sinusoids. The shorter in duration the sinusoid, the more noticeable these other sinusoids become. Perhaps you have heard the click that sometimes occurs when a tone is turned on and off. This click represents the ear's sensitivity to frequencies other than that of the switched sine wave that are present in the sinusoidal wave when it is turned on and off. The sinusoid sounds more like a tone and less like a click the longer it remains on. This is due to the

Figure 1.11 A complex waveform in the time domain (**1.11a**) and the frequency domain (amplitude spectrum, **1.11b**; phase spectrum, **1.11c**). The time domain representation of each sinusoid in the spectrum is in **1.11d**. Figure **1.11e** was constructed by adding together at each successive point in time (A, B) the amplitudes of the three sinusoids. Thus at point A, the summed amplitudes yield the amplitude *C;* at point B, the summed amplitudes yield the amplitude *D*.

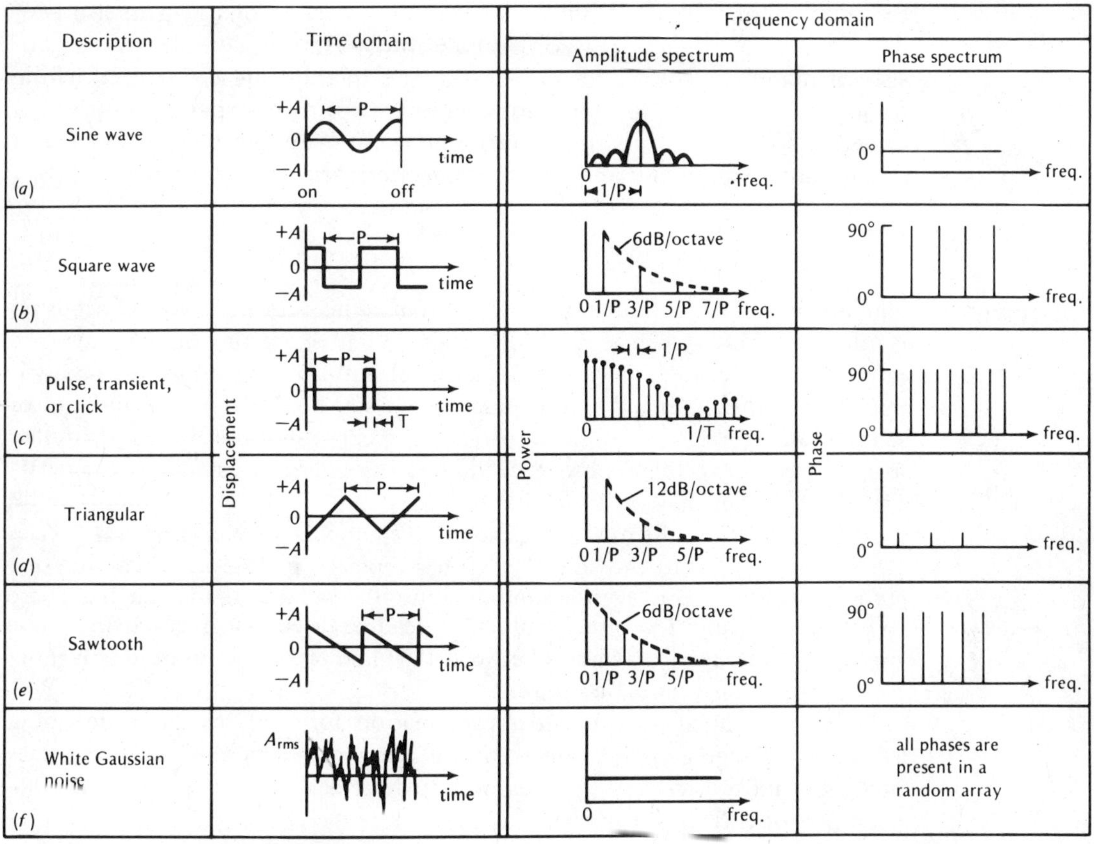

Description	Time domain	Frequency domain	
		Amplitude spectrum	Phase spectrum
(a) Sine wave	$+A$, 0, $-A$; on / off; P; time	0 $1/P$ freq.	$0°$ freq.
(b) Square wave	$+A$, 0, $-A$; P; time	6dB/octave; 0 1/P 3/P 5/P 7/P freq.	$90°$ ... $0°$ freq.
(c) Pulse, transient, or click	$+A$, 0, $-A$; P; T; time	1/P; 0 1/T freq.	$90°$ ... $0°$ freq.
(d) Triangular	$+A$, 0, $-A$; P; time	12dB/octave; 0 1/P 3/P 5/P freq.	$0°$ freq.
(e) Sawtooth	$+A$, 0, $-A$; P; time	6dB/octave; 0 1/P 3/P 5/P freq.	$90°$ ... $0°$ freq.
(f) White Gaussian noise	A_{rms}; time	0 freq.	all phases are present in a random array

(Left axis: Displacement; center axis: Power; right axis: Phase)

Figure 1.12 Time and frequency domain representations of a variety of different complex waveforms. In the frequency domain, both the amplitude and phase spectra are described. P refers to period; in **1.12c**, T refers to duration of the pulse. (See Chap. 3 for a definition of dB/octave.)

fact that if the sinusoid is on for longer and longer periods of time, the amplitudes of the other sinusoids become smaller and smaller relative to the amplitude at the frequency of the sinusoid. Thus we hear only the pure tone pitch corresponding to the frequency of the sine wave and not the clicking sound due to the presence of other frequencies. The auditory system's sensitivity to changes in the frequency domain as well as to those in the time domain underlies the necessity for describing an auditory stimulus in both domains.

Summary Any vibration is capable of producing an audible sound. Any vibration is equal to a sum of sinusoidal vibrations. A sinusoid (simple wave) has three physical parameters: amplitude (a measure of displacement in terms of peak, peak-to-peak, or rms amplitude), frequency (a measure of the number of vibrations per unit time), and starting phase (a measure of where the wave begins).] Joseph Fourier showed that a complex wave consists of many sinusoids and may be defined in the time domain or in the frequency domain by its amplitude and phase spectra. A spectrum may be a line or a continuous spectrum. Line spectra often reflect the presence of a fundamental frequency and its harmonic frequencies.

Supplement

Sound is a well-studied area of physics. From a theoretical viewpoint acoustics is often considered a "dead area" of physics. That is, the theories of sound are fairly well established, and so in the study of audition the stimulus (sound) is not an unknown event. Any introductory physics book covers the theories of sound. Roederer (1973) in *Introduction to the Physics and Psychophysics of Music* does an excellent job of introducing the physics of sound at a slightly higher level than that of this book.

At one time the unit used to describe the frequency of vibration was "cycles per second" (cps), but the "hertz" (Hz) has replaced it. We often describe one sinusoid as leading or lagging another sinusoid in phase. If the starting phase is between 0° and 180°, the sinusoid is leading a zero-degree starting-phase sinusoid; if the starting phase is between 180° and 360°, the sinusoid is lagging a zero-degree starting-phase sinusoid.

Equation (1.3) gives only an approximation for the rms amplitude of a vibration. The greater N becomes (that is, the more instantaneous amplitudes used), the more accurately equation (1.3) describes the rms amplitude. The definition of rms amplitude is:

$$A_{\text{rms}} = \sqrt{\frac{1}{p} \int_0^p x(t)^2 \, dt}$$

where $x(t)$ is the time-domain waveform and p is the period of repetition of the waveform. In this case the integral sign ($\int$) implies summing all possible values of instantaneous amplitudes (an infinite number) in one period of vibration.

Fourier analysis is a powerful mathematical tool. The last section of *Linear Circuits* by Scott (1964) offers basic coverage of the topic, yet even these chapters require a knowledge of differential and integral calculus. The areas concerning Fourier's theorem covered in this book provide a working idea of the concepts that underlie this area of applied mathematics.

The general equation showing Fourier's theorem for complex signals having a maximum frequency W and a duration T is

$$x(t) = \sum_{\text{K}=1}^{WT} a_K \cos \frac{2\pi}{T} Kt + b_K \sin \frac{2\pi}{T} Kt \qquad 0 \leqslant t \leqslant T$$

where $x(t)$ is the time-domain waveform, and a_K and b_K are the amplitudes of the cos and sin terms in the expression. If one knows the time-domain waveform $x(t)$, then a_K and b_K can be found by using integral calculus:

$$a_K = \frac{2}{T} \int_0^T x(t) \cos \frac{2\pi}{T} Kt \, dt$$

$$b_K = \frac{2}{T} \int_0^T x(t) \sin \frac{2\pi}{T} Kt \, dt$$

Thus, $x(t)$ is the time-domain representation of the waveform and

$$a_K \cos \frac{2\pi}{T} Kt + b_K \sin \frac{2\pi}{T} Kt$$

is the frequency-domain representation in Fourier's theorem.

Sometimes kHz or kilohertz is used to describe frequency. That is, 1500 Hz and 7000 Hz are sometimes listed as 1.5 kHz and 7 kHz.

CHAPTER 2
Sound Transmission

The Decibel

Interference

In everyday life we do not hear an object vibrate directly; rather we hear the effect of this vibrating object on the air as the vibration is transmitted to our ears. The vibration of an object causes waves to travel through the air to our ears, and we experience sound. Sound can travel through any elastic medium that has inertia. That is, sound can travel through air, water, steel, and so on, but not through a vacuum.

Since air is the medium of interest for most everyday situations, let us examine the transmission of sound through air. Air consists of molecules which are in constant random motion. When an object vibrates in air, the molecules *tend* to move in the direction the object moves rather than with their normal random motion. The air molecules next to the object move first and then pass this movement on to the adjacent molecules. The molecules themselves do not move from the object to the receiver; they only pass along a wave of motion.

In this trainlike progression (much like a row of dominoes) the motion of the air molecules is *propagated* (transferred) through the air toward the ear. When the air molecules next to the ear are moved by this motion, the eardrum (tympanic membrane) is vibrated by the molecules, and this eventually results in our experiencing audible sound.

Imagine that we photographed the air molecules when an object is vibrating. Figure 2.1 represents the picture we might see at that instant in time. The molecules appear to cluster at some points in space (this is called *condensation*), and they are further apart at other places (this is called *rarefaction*). The motion of the air molecule vibration would correspond to the direction of the arrows in Figure 2.1. That is, as the object pushes out, the air molecules *tend* to move away from the object; as the object moves back toward its starting point, the molecules have a tendency to begin moving back in the other direction. Thus the

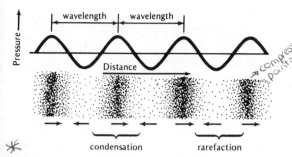

Figure 2.1 Diagram of what one might see if air molecules were photographed as a sound source vibrated. The rarefactions and condensations are shown, as well as the directions (arrows) in which the molecules were moving at the instant the picture was taken.

motion at a condensation tends to be away from the source, and the motion at a rarefaction tends to be toward the source. The distance between each successive condensation (or rarefaction) is the *wavelength* (λ) of the sound.

The water tank mentioned in Chapter 1 provides a convenient way to visualize the wave motion associated with a vibrating object. If we push water (like dropping a stone in a pool), waves are formed. The water waves are similar to the air waves associated with sound propagation. The crests of the wave are the condensations, the valleys are the rarefactions, and the distance between the adjacent waves is the wavelength. If you have ever watched a wave "move" through the water, you have observed that the water itself does not move but that the wave motion is passed along the water (propagated). A similar, but not identical, type of motion is associated with air molecules that are moved by a vibrating object. As the object vibrates, the sound wave moves through the air. The distance between successive identical points in the air motion is the wavelength, which is generally expressed in meters. The faster the object vibrates (high frequency), the closer together the rarefactions and condensations become, and thus the shorter the wavelength. The speed with which the wave motion is propagated through the medium (the *speed of sound*) also affects the wavelength. If the speed of sound is fast, then as the object vibrates, the first wave moves from the object and the second wave lags far behind. This causes the distance between successive rarefactions, and thus the wavelength, to be long. If the speed of sound is slow, the first wave travels a short distance before the second wave passes an identical spot, so the wavelength is short. Therefore both the frequency of vibration of the object and the speed of sound affect the wavelength. The equation relating wavelength (λ) in meters to the speed of sound (c) in meters per second and to the frequency (f) of vibration is:

$$\lambda = \frac{c}{f} \tag{2.1}$$

That is, wavelength is directly proportional to the speed of sound and inversely proportional to frequency of vibration.

The speed of sound in air is approximately 350 meters per second (m/s), although it can vary as a function of the temperature, density, and humidity of the air. The speed of sound is higher in a hot, humid area at sea level than in a cold, dry place at high altitude.

Let us examine what happens to frequency and amplitude of the vibration as sound is propagated from the source toward the ear. Figure 2.2 shows the relation between the sinusoidal vibration of the object and different measures of the motion of the air molecules. Remember that the object's vibration is diagramed as distance (displacement) versus time (Fig. 2.2a). Distance per unit time is a measure of velocity (for example, kilometers per hour); therefore, we can plot the object's vibration as velocity versus time, as shown in Figure 2.2b. Notice that the plot of velocity versus time has the same frequency as the plot of distance versus time but is 90° out of phase. This phase difference can be understood if we notice that at the beginning of the sinusoid the object is moving a great distance in a short period of time, and thus the velocity is high. As the object reaches its maximum distance, it must decelerate before it reverses direction; when this occurs, the velocity reaches zero. Thus, when the distance is smallest, the velocity is greatest, and when the distance is greatest, the velocity is smallest; hence the 90° phase relation between **Figures** 2.2a and 2.2b.

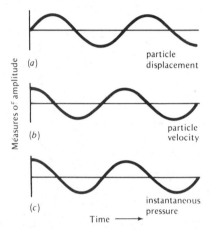

Figure 2.2 Three sinusoidal relations of a vibration. **2.2a**: object's displacement or particle displacement as a function of time; **2.2b**: velocity of this vibration as a function of time; **2.2c**: relationship between instantaneous pressure caused by the vibration and time.

The pressure p that a vibrating object exerts on an area is directly proportional to the vibrating object's velocity and inversely proportional to the area on which the vibrating object is pushing; that is,   .

$$p = \frac{MV}{tA} \qquad (2.2)$$

where M = mass, V = velocity, t = time and A = area. This equation describes the pressure one object can generate. We can therefore describe the air molecule pressure of the object if we let M equal the mass of an air molecule. Since the velocity changes as a function of time, the

pressure is an *instantaneous pressure;* that is, it varies as a function of time. This relation is shown in Figure 2.2c. We can compute the rms value of this instantaneous pressure in the same way we computed the rms value of displacement. The rms value of the instantaneous pressure can then be used to measure the pressure that the vibrating object can exert on some known area. Another way to define pressure is in terms of force:

$$p = \frac{F}{A} \qquad (2.3)$$

where p = pressure, F = force, and A = area. Pressure is thus equal to *force* per unit area. Any force has the capability of performing *work*. The pressure exerted on the eardrum is capable of providing *energy* (E) so that the eardrum can perform work. The amount of *power* (P) is proportional to the square of the pressure:

$$P = \frac{p^2}{d_a c} \qquad (2.4)$$

where d_a is the density of air, c the velocity of sound, and p^2 the square of pressure. The amount of work possible per unit of time is also referred to as the power (P):

$$P = \frac{E}{T} \qquad (2.5)$$

where T is time (how long the sound is being measured). Therefore the vibration can be described in terms of pressure, energy, or power. Each of these measures will have a different numerical value, but the relations do not affect the basic description of the sinusoidal vibration of the object. An object that vibrates with a frequency of 200 Hz might have a pressure of 1 dyne/cm², 2 joules of energy, or 10 watts of power, but its frequency remains 200 Hz (see Table 2.1). The term "intensity" is

Table 2.1   Units Used to Measure Quantities Related to Sound Intensities

Quantity	Units of Measurement
Force (F)	1 newton = 10^5 dynes
Potential difference (v)	volt (a pressurelike measure)
Pressure (p) [a]	1 newton/cm^2 = 10^5 dynes/cm^2 = 10^4 pascals
Energy (E) [b]	1 joule = 10^7 ergs = 10^7 dyne-cm = 1 newton-meter
Power (P) [c]	1 watt = 10^7 ergs/second = 1 joule/second
Sound intensity (I) [d]	watts/cm^2

[a] Pressure = force/area.
[b] Energy = force through distance.
[c] Power = energy/time.
[d] Sound intensity = energy/(time × area) = power/area.

often used to describe the amplitude of vibration when the measurement is of pressure, energy, or power.

THE DECIBEL

Our description of the intensity of a sound wave is still incomplete. If the ear were not as sensitive as it is, the foregoing definitions of pressure, energy, and power would be sufficient. Imagine that the smallest amount of power required to just detect a sound were measured; this amount could be called 1 unit of power. Now, imagine measuring the greatest amount of power required before the ear is destroyed. The range of powers from the smallest amount required to detect a sound to the largest amount tolerated before the ear is damaged is referred to as the *dynamic range of the auditory system*. If 1 unit of power represents the smallest power, then 1,000,000,000,-000,000 (10^{15}) units of power represents the greatest power. Thus, the auditory system has a dynamic range of 10^{15} units of power. This range is so large it is impossible to work with in practical situations (imagine trying to plot a function on graph paper from 1 to 10^{15} in 10-unit steps). It is advisable, therefore, to reduce the dynamic range to more easily handled numbers. One way to accomplish this

is to change the type of scale used to describe the dynamic range. The scale from 1 to 10^{15} is called an interval scale, since the difference (interval) between each successive number is a constant (in this case the difference is always one). For instance, the scale 2, 4, 6, 8, 10, . . . is an interval scale, with the interval being two. Another type of scale is the *ratio scale* in which the ratio between two successive numbers in the scale is a constant; the scale 2, 4, 8, 16, 32, . . . is a ratio scale in which the ratio between two successive numbers is 2/1. Another ratio scale is 10, 100, 1000, . . . , in which the ratio is 10/1. This last scale is the one used to reduce the numbers of the dynamic range of the auditory system to those more easily used.

Table 2.2 shows the relation between a

Table 2.2   Ratio Scale to Interval Scale

Ratio Scale (Y)		New Interval Scale (n)
10	(10^1)	1
100	(10^2)	2
1000	(10^3)	3
10,000	(10^4)	4
.	.	.
.	.	.
.	.	.
10, . . . n	(10^n)	n

ratio scale and an interval scale. Notice that the numbers in the ratio scale increase by the function 10^n, where $n = 1, 2, 3, \ldots$. The ratio scale numbers (Y) equal the number 10 raised to the new interval scale number (n):

$$Y = 10^n \qquad (2.6)$$

If the ratio scale number were known, the equation could be solved for the new interval scale number n. This solution involves the use of *logarithms* (see Appendix B). In terms of equation (2.6) the formula for n is $n = \log_{10} Y$, where $\log_{10}$ (or log, as used here) means the logarithm to the base 10. If we know the ratio scale number, we can find the new interval scale number by using a table of logarithms similar to that in Appendix B. Thus, from a table of logarithms, $\log 2 = 0.3$, or $10^{0.3} = 2$. Thus, the ratio scale number 2 corresponds to the new interval scale number 0.3.

Logarithms can be used to describe the dynamic range of the auditory system. The starting point is the logarithm of the ratio of two powers. This logarithm is labeled a *bel;* that is, a bel is $\log P_1/P_2$. Since a bel is not convenient to work with because it is too large an interval, the *decibel* (dB) is used. A decibel is one-tenth of a bel; thus the ratio of two powers expressed in decibels is $10 \log P_1/P_2$. If P_1 equals 10^{15} and P_2 equals 1 (which covers the dynamic range), then the dynamic range is as follows:

$$10 \log (10^{15}/1) = 10 \times \log 10^{15} = 10 \times 15 = 150 \text{ dB}$$

The dynamic range of the auditory system can now be described in terms of decibels, yielding a convenient range of numbers (150 dB). Notice that the original interval scale of powers ranging from 1 to 10^{15} has been reduced to a *new* interval scale of decibels ranging from 1 to 150 by transforming powers to decibels by use of logarithms.

Since $P = E/T$, the formula for energy in terms of decibels is

$$\text{decibel (dB)} = 10 \log \frac{P_1}{P_2} = 10 \log \frac{E_1/T}{E_2/T}$$

$$= 10 \log \frac{E_1}{E_2} \qquad (2.7)$$

Thus, the decibel can be the ratio of two powers *or* two energies. Since $P = p^2/k$, where $k = d_a c$, as described in equation (2.4), then the formula for decibels in terms of pressure (p) is:

$$\text{decibel (dB)} = 10 \log \frac{P_1}{P_2} = 10 \log \frac{p_1^2/k}{p_2^2/k}$$

$$= 10 \log \frac{p_1^2}{p_2^2} = 10 \log \left(\frac{p_1}{p_2}\right)^2 = 20 \log \frac{p_1}{p_2} \qquad (2.8)$$

Therefore, the decibel is *10 times the log of the ratio of two powers or energies* and *20 times the log of the ratio of two pressures.* Once intensity has been specified in terms of decibels, then the decibel has the same meaning regardless of whether it represents power, energy, or pressure. To convert from power, energy, or pressure to decibels or vice versa, we must keep in mind the units involved. Appendix B describes logarithms and demonstrates the rules used to convert from power, energy, or pressure to decibels and back again.

It is important to remember that the decibel is the *ratio of two quantities.* Because the decibel expresses how many units one intensity is above or below another intensity, it is meaningless to say that a sound has an intensity of 60 dB, since this statement does not indicate whether the intensity is 60 dB above the loudest pressure you can tolerate, 60 dB above the softest pressure you can hear, 60 dB above what your friend can hear, or anything else. In all cases the sound has a *relative* intensity of 60 dB, but each sound has a different *absolute* intensity. A decibel is a relative, not an absolute, measurement.

Two conventions are commonly used to define decibels in relative terms. Experiments conducted in the 1930s determined that a pressure of 0.0002 dyne/cm² was the smallest amount required for the average young adult to detect the presence of a 1000- to 4000-Hz sinusoid. When the decibel is expressed relative to 0.0002 dyne/cm², it is expressed in terms of *sound pressure level* (SPL). Hence, if intensity is expressed as 60 dB SPL, then the intensity is 60 dB above 0.0002 dyne/cm², or 20 micropascals (20 μPa). Another way to describe the decibel is in terms of *sensation level* (SL). Sensation level refers to the least intense sound that a particular person can detect in a particular experimental situation (for example, at a particular frequency). SPL is based on the reference of 0.0002 dyne/cm², whereas SL is based on the reference of the least pressure a particular person can detect in a specific experimental context. There are many other conventions used to define a reference level for the decibel; however, SPL and SL will be used exclusively throughout this book.

Two important facts must be obtained before determining the intensity of sound. First, we must know if the amplitude is measured in peak, peak-to-peak, or root-mean-square (rms) values. Second, if the intensity is expressed in decibels, we must know the reference used (SPL, SL, or some other reference value). Unless these two facts are specified, a statement such as "The music is 60 dB" contains no information about the intensity of the music, since no reference conditions are included.

INTERFERENCE

As sound travels through air it often encounters such objects as walls, floors, and people. How do these objects affect sound transmission? Broad areas of applied acoustics, such as architectural acoustics, are devoted to studying these effects. Our interests lie in understanding a few of these problems so that we can appreciate the changes that can occur in acoustic environments.

Consider a simple case of sound approaching and rebounding from a wall. Let us focus upon two of the possible results: (1) the wave coming off the wall can add to, or *reinforce,* the oncoming wave (Fig. 2.3), or (2) the wave coming off the wall can subtract, or *cancel,* the

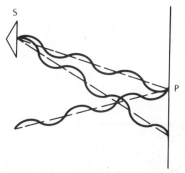

Figure 2.3 Speaker (S) creates sound waves that reflect off a wall at a point P. As the sound waves return, they can add to or cancel the effects of an oncoming sound wave.

oncoming wave. That is, the net result can be the summing of two sinusoids or the subtracting of two sinusoids. Thus a person sitting in front of the wall might hear a sound equal in intensity to the oncoming wave (no reflections), a more intense sound (in the case of reinforcement), or a less intense sound (cancellation). Figure 2.3 illustrates the sound coming from one point. If the sound is coming from several points or from a large area, then there are many possible reinforcements and cancellations. In addition to the wall, anything more dense than the air (the medium through which the sound is propagated) will reflect sound. Thus determining the intensity at any one place in a room becomes very complicated. The intensity determined at one point might be entirely different from that at another point. Notice that in Figure 2.3 the frequency is the same for all waves. If two waves of different frequency are reflected off a wall, complex interaction patterns may result.

As a consequence of these interactions, one frequency might be easier to hear than the other because its intensity is greater. Therefore the intensity of a sound may vary not only as a function of where in a room it is measured but also as a function of frequency.

In summary, we must be careful in assuming that the waveform arriving at some point in a room (the ear of a person, for instance) is identical to the waveform that leaves the source (a speaker). The two should be nearly the same *only if* the reflections off walls, floors, and objects are discounted and the distance from the source is calculated.

A continuous sinusoid played into a closed environment such as a room or a tube produces reflections, reinforcements, and cancellations that may result in what is called a *standing wave*. A standing wave generates *fixed areas* of cancellations and reinforcements within an enclosed environment. That is, there is not a wave that moves through the air, but rather a wave that is fixed in space but whose pressure at any one point in space is varying in time. The location of the reinforcements and cancellations depends on the interaction between the frequency of the sinusoid and the size of the environment. If the wavelength of the sinusoid is greater than the volume of the space or if it is extremely short in relation to the size of the space, a standing wave may not develop. Since wavelength and frequency are related, then the frequency region for which standing waves will exist may be approximated, given the size of the environment. If a space is 2 meters long, then the wavelength must be approximately 2 meters for a standing wave to develop. From the formula for wavelength (equation (2.1)) we can determine the frequency; we know that $\lambda = c/f$ and $c = 350$ m/s. Therefore

$$f = \frac{c}{\lambda} = \frac{350 \text{ m/s}}{2 \text{ m}} = 175 \text{ Hz}$$

Thus tones with frequencies slightly higher (shorter wavelengths) than approximately 175 Hz may produce standing waves in a 2-meter space.

As sound travels through space toward and to our ears, it encounters various obstacles, especially those associated with our auditory system. Many of these obstacles (for example, the eardrum) impede the transmission of the sound. This impedance can take one of two forms: a static *resistance* to the sound transmission, which absorbs the sound, or a *reactance*, which is a type of impedance that reduces the ability of the sound wave to oscillate at maximum efficiency. The term *impedance* is used to describe the combined effects of resistance and reactance. Thus the intensity of sound can be reduced when obstacles present an impedance to the transmission of sound. One property of impedance is that the extent to which the sound's intensity is reduced often depends on the frequency of the sound. Usually impedance is introduced when objects that are moved by the sound wave are in the path of the transmitted sound.

The intensity of sound also decreases as a function of distance. That is, the further we are from a sound source, the softer that sound becomes. Remember that sound radiates from a point such as that shown in Figure 2.4 and that the intensity of sound is inversely proportional to area over which it is measured. Sound actually radiates out in all three dimensions, that is, like a sphere. Since the surface area of a sphere is $4\pi r^2$, the intensity is proportional to one over the radius squared of the sphere. The radius of the sphere is the distance of the sound wave from its source. Therefore, the intensity I of a sound decreases by a factor of the square of the distance d, or

$$I = \frac{k}{d^2} \tag{2.9}$$

where k is a proportionality constant, the value of which does not depend on the dis-

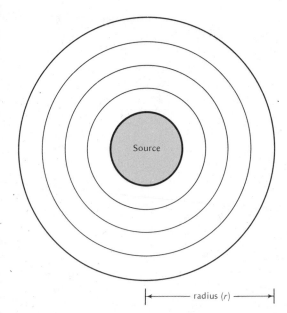

Figure 2.4 Sound waves moving out from a point source of sound. The distance the sound travels is the radius (*r*) of the circle. The intensity of the sound decreases by a factor of r^2.

tance of the sound from the source. This fact is often referred to as the *inverse-square law of intensity*. For instance, if one doubles the distance, the intensity decreases by a factor of 4, which is equivalent to 6 dB. The frequency of a wave does not change as the sound moves away from its source, but the intensity varies as described above. These relations hold only in a situation in which the sound encounters no obstacles.

An additional influence an object can exert on a sound wave is referred to as the *sound shadow*. The sound shadow can be viewed in the context of waves on the water (Fig. 2.5). Imagine throwing a pebble into the water and watching the waves radiate from the spot of impact. This is analogous to sound waves radiating from a sound source. A very large object in the water causes the waves to bounce off the object, as described previously (Fig. 2.5a); but a wave passes over a very small object with little change (Fig. 2.5b). A medium-

sized object produces some reflections from the object, but at some distance beyond the object the waves appear to have been unaffected. In fact, if we look carefully at this last situation, we notice that just past the medium-sized object there is an area where there are no waves at all. This area is referred to as the sound

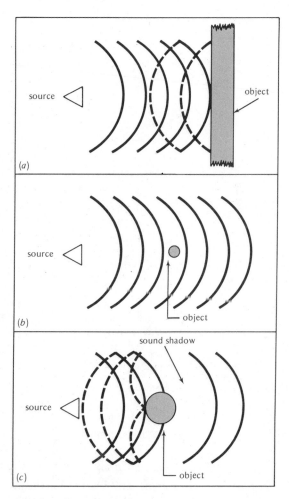

Figure 2.5 Simplified diagrams of sound waves passing objects. **2.5a:** Object larger than the wavelength: most of the wave is reflected. **2.5b:** Object much smaller than the wavelength: most of the wave passes the object. **2.5c:** Object close in size to the wavelength: sound shadow is produced beyond the object.

shadow (Fig. 2.5c). What is meant by "small," "medium," and "large" objects? These sizes are expressed in relation to the wavelength of the sound. If a sound has a wavelength of 2 meters, then a large object is one that is much larger than 2 meters, a small object is much smaller than 2 meters, and a medium-sized object is approximately 2 meters.

The relation between wavelength and object size accounts for the sound shadow. If an object is equal to or greater than the wavelength of the wave approaching it, then there will be an area on the other side of the object with few or no waves. That is, there is an area where the sound intensity has been reduced. This area of reduced wave motion will be at least as large as the wavelength of the oncoming sound. Thus, if a sound with a 2-meter wavelength (175 Hz) passes an object of approximately 2 meters, then approximately a 2-meter conical area of little or no sound will be produced on the other side of the object. The fact that the human head is an object that can produce a sound shadow has important implications for our ability to use our two ears. These implications will be encountered when the area of binaural (two-ear) hearing is discussed.

Summary Sound is propagated through the air from its vibrating source to a receiving object. The vibrating object causes a movement of air molecules that corresponds to the vibration of the object. The wavelength of vibration is a measure of the distance between successive points (rarefactions or condensations) in the sound wave. Sound intensity is measured in units of pressure, energy, or power. In audition the decibel is used to describe sound's intensity. The decibel is 10 times the logarithm of the ratio of two powers or energies and 20 times the logarithm of the ratio of two pressures. Sound waves can encounter various forms of interference as they travel. There can be cancellations and additions, standing waves can be formed, objects can create sound shadows in the sound wave field, and objects might introduce impedance to the transmission of sound. The intensity of sound decreases by a factor of the distance squared as it moves away from the sound source.

Supplement Most of the material covered in this chapter deals with aspects of architectural acoustics. An excellent reference is L. L. Beranek's (1954) book *Acoustics*. Roederer's (1973) *Introduction to the Physics and Psychophysics of Music* also provides some helpful illustrations concerning sound propagation.

Although we have used waves appearing in water as an analogy to wave motion in air, the reader should *not* assume that wave propagation is identical in the two media. Wave motion in water is significantly different from that in air. The analogies mentioned in this chapter are only simple comparisons.

Figure 2.2 describes the displacement, velocity, and pressure of the air molecules (or other objects) as they vibrate in air. The object's amplitude and frequency of vibration directly influence the air molecule's amplitude and frequency of vibration. Thus Figure 2.2 can be considered a description for either the object's or the air molecule's mode of vibration. The units of displacement, pressure, energy, and power can be found in a reference book of physical or chemical tables.

Impedance is usually identified by the symbol Z, resistance is symbolized by R, and reactance is symbolized by X; all are measured in ohms. Impedance is obtained by the following formula:

$$Z = \sqrt{R^2 + X^2} \tag{2.10}$$

The relationship between the frequency and area of space in which a standing wave might exist also depends on whether or not there are openings in the space. The pipes in an organ take advantage of standing waves to produce their relative pitches. The pitch is related to the length of the pipe; long pipes produce low frequencies, and short pipes produce high frequencies.

Technically, intensity refers to energy flux and thus only to power and energy. However, for convenience we will use intensity to refer to power, energy, *and* pressure throughout this book.

CHAPTER 3
Sound Analysis

Filters
Nonlinearities

FILTERS

What happens when a crystal glass is struck with a spoon? Often the glass rings at a high pitch. If water is put into the glass, it still might ring but at a lower pitch. Most objects have the ability to vibrate if they are struck or driven with the necessary force. The frequency at which the object rings or vibrates is called the object's *resonance frequency*. An empty glass has a higher resonance frequency than a full glass. Many different driving forces can cause an object to resonate; however, the ease with which one can cause the resonant vibration depends on how close the *driving frequency* is to the resonance frequency. A driving frequency equal to the object's resonance frequency is the best driving force with which to initiate the ringing. The farther the driving frequency from the resonance frequency, the smaller the *amplitude* of vibration of the object that is ringing or resonating. It is often possible for a small driving amplitude to cause an object to resonate with an amplitude

greater than that of the driving force. Thus a resonator can be used to amplify the intensity of a small amplitude driver. Of course, the greatest amplification occurs when the driver and the resonator have the same frequency.

In addition to possessing an amplification property, resonators can be used to determine the frequency of an object whose frequency is unknown. Imagine that an object was vibrating at 200 Hz, but we did not know this was its frequency of vibration. Further imagine a group of resonators with known resonance frequencies—for instance, 100, 200, and 300 Hz. The three resonators could then be driven by the driver with the unknown frequency. Whichever resonator vibrated with the greatest amplitude must have a resonance frequency close to the driving frequency. In the case just described the 200-Hz resonator would vibrate with the greatest amplitude since the driver has a 200-Hz driving frequency. A graph such as that shown in Figure 3.1 could be drawn to indicate the amplitudes of the three resonators as they are driven by the unknown (200-Hz)

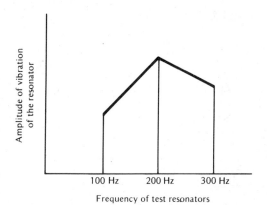

Amplitude of vibration
of the resonator

100 Hz   200 Hz   300 Hz

Frequency of test resonators

Figure 3.1 Relative amplitudes of three resonators driven by a 200-Hz driving frequency. The 200-Hz resonator is driven with the greatest amplitude.

object. The peak of the graph indicates the spectral area of the *driving frequency*. Thus a series of resonators may be used to determine the frequency of any vibrating object.

So far only such resonators as glass have been discussed; however, a closed tube in which there are standing waves can also act as a resonator. If a driving force creates standing waves within a closed tube, the standing wave will produce a vibration that will oscillate at the tube's resonance frequency. It is possible to drive a tube with a vibration of small amplitude and produce resonant vibration with a very large amplitude within the tube. This point will become significant when we consider sound waves entering the ear canal. Does the ear canal resonate and amplify the sound coming in? If so, what is the resonance frequency of the ear canal and other parts of the auditory system?

Resonators may be especially designed either to determine or modify the frequency of vibrating objects; such resonators are called *filters*. A filter is a resonator that vibrates in response to a very large range of frequencies. We refer to those frequencies to which the filter vibrates as the ones the filter will *pass*. That is, if a filter passes sinusoids with fre-

quencies between 200 and 400 Hz and if the filter is driven with these sinusoids, the amplitudes of these sinusoids at the output of the filter will be relatively unaffected by the filter. The amplitude of all other sinusoids will be attenuated (reduced) as a result of the filter. Thus if the filter passes sinusoids with frequencies between 200 and 400 Hz and if the driving force has a frequency of 200 to 400 Hz, these sinusoids will have amplitudes at the output of the filter that equal their driving force amplitudes. If an object with a driving frequency of 100 Hz and an intensity of 80 dB SPL drives a 200- to 400-Hz filter, then at the output of the filter the 100-Hz vibration *might* have an intensity of only 20 dB SPL. Thus a filter produces sinusoids either with no reduction in amplitude or with attenuated amplitudes.

There are three general types of filters: *low-pass, high-pass,* and *band-pass.* A low-pass filter will pass all sinusoids with frequencies below a particular value; sinusoids with frequencies above that value will have their amplitudes attenuated. A high-pass filter passes sinusoids with frequencies above a particular value. A band-pass filter will pass all sinusoids with frequencies between two particular values. The frequency values above, below, or between which the filter passes the sinusoids without reducing their amplitudes are called the *cutoff frequencies* of the filter. Thus, a low-pass filter with a cutoff of 1000 Hz will pass all sinusoids with frequencies below 1000 Hz and will attenuate the amplitudes of all sinusoids with frequencies above 1000 Hz. A 1000-Hz cutoff high-pass filter will do just the opposite. A band-pass filter with cutoffs at 500 Hz and 1000 Hz will pass only sinusoids with frequencies between 500 and 1000 Hz. Figure 3.2 shows the three types of filters (notice the similarity to the resonance curve shown in Fig. 3.1). The amount of attenuation given to the amplitude of sinusoids beyond the cutoff frequency is expressed in decibels of attenuation per *octave*

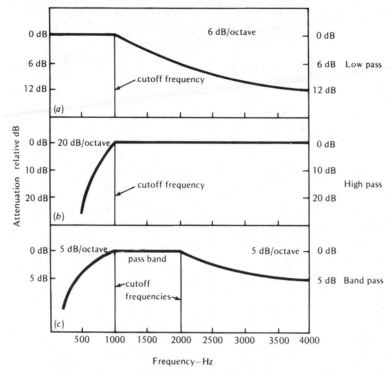

Figure 3.2 Three filters. **3.2a:** low-pass filter with 1000-Hz cutoff and 6 dB/octave roll-off; **3.2b:** high-pass filter with 1000-Hz cutoff and 20 dB/octave roll-off; **3.2c** band-pass filter with 1000-Hz and 2000-Hz cutoffs and 5 dB/octave roll-off. The amount the filter attenuates the sound is shown as a function of frequency.

of frequency. The octave is expressed relative to the cutoff frequency of the filter. An octave indicates a doubling of frequency. The first octave of 200 Hz is 400 Hz, the second octave is another doubling, or 800 Hz, the third octave is 1600 Hz, and so on. Table 3.1 shows the harmonics and octaves of a 1000-Hz sinusoid. Octaves should not be confused with harmonics; octaves express a ratio scale, with the ratio being 2 to 1.

If a low-pass filter has a 1000-Hz cutoff and an attenuation rate of 6 dB per octave, then the filter passes all sinusoids with frequencies below 1000 Hz, and the amplitudes of sinusoids with frequencies above 1000 Hz are attenuated at the rate of 6 dB for each doubling

Table 3.1 Harmonic and Octave Relations of a 1000-Hz Tone

Tone	Harmonics	Octaves
Fundamental frequency	1000 Hz	1000 Hz
2nd harmonic and 1st octave	2000 Hz	2000 Hz
3rd harmonic	3000 Hz	
4th harmonic and 2nd octave	4000 Hz	4000 Hz
5th harmonic	5000 Hz	
6th harmonic	'6000 Hz	
7th harmonic	7000 Hz	
8th harmonic and 3rd octave	8000 Hz	8000 Hz

of the cutoff frequency, 1000 Hz. Thus the amplitude of a 2000-Hz sinusoid would be attenuated 6 dB below its amplitude at the input. For a 4000-Hz sinusoid the attenuation is 12 dB, for an 8000-Hz sinusoid the attenuation is 18 dB, and so forth. In Figure 3.2a the "roll-off," or rate of attenuation, for the various filters is 6 dB per octave, in Figure 3.2b it is 20 dB per octave, and in Figure 3.2c it is 5 dB per octave.

Filters are used in the same way as resonators to determine the frequency spectra of unknown signals. That is, filters can be used to perform a type of Fourier analysis of a complex waveform. Chapter 1 described how to compute the time-domain waveform from the amplitude and phase spectra but not how to determine the spectra from the time-domain waveform (Fourier analysis). To determine the spectral components of a waveform we can establish a series of band-pass filters with, for instance, the following cutoff frequencies: 95–105 Hz, 195–205 Hz, 295–305 Hz, and 395–405 Hz. If we found after analyzing an input waveform with these filters that the second filter (195–205 Hz) and the fourth filter (395–405 Hz) passed much more intensity than did the other two filters, then the input waveform must have more intensity in the 200-Hz and 400-Hz regions of the spectrum than in the 100-Hz and 300-Hz regions. The actual amount of intensity coming through each filter can be used to determine an amplitude spectrum for the unknown input waveform. In this case we plot the intensity at the output of each filter as a function of the center frequency of each band-pass filter. This is a very simple, practical, and economical way to obtain the amplitude spectrum of a waveform given in the time domain.

Another use of filters involves "shaping" the spectra of signals. Imagine that a complex waveform with the amplitude spectrum shown in Figure 3.3a is passed through the filter shown in Figure 3.3b. The complex wave will have at the output of the filter the amplitude spectrum shown in Figure 3.3c. Since the filter is a band-pass filter, the amplitudes of the sinus-oids within the band of frequencies passed (the *passband*) have not been attenuated, whereas those outside the passband have been attenuated from their input values by 20 dB per octave. If the amplitude spectrum and attenuation of the filter are expressed in decibels, then the amplitudes in the output spectrum in decibels are obtained by subtracting the attenuation values introduced by the filter from the amplitudes in the input spectrum. Thus a filter has been used to alter the amplitude spectrum of a complex waveform.

Filters also introduce a phase delay to signals that pass through them. Thus to describe a filter fully, we must indicate not only the type of filter, the cutoff frequencies, and the roll-off rate, but also how the phase of each sinusoid is altered. Although the phase shift a filter may introduce is not as easy to describe as the attenuation rate, *all* of these values must be known if the waveform at the output of the filter is to be determined exactly (given an exact description of the input waveform). If any of the information concerning the filter is missing, the picture of the output waveform will be incomplete.

As described in Chapter 1, if the amplitude or the phase spectrum of a complex wave is modified, then generally the time waveform representing the complex wave will also be altered. Since filters modify spectra, they will also alter time waveforms. Thus a filter may change the time-domain representation as well as the spectrum of a signal.

Many objects act as filters when they are driven by waveforms. One type of object, the resonator, has already been described. *Any* object that has mass and is moved by a driving force can act as a filter. The cone of a speaker, fluids, and the eardrum all act as filters; when these objects are driven by some vibratory force, they follow this vibration. When the driving force pushes on the speaker cone, the cone moves outward; and when the driving force draws in, the speaker cone does likewise.

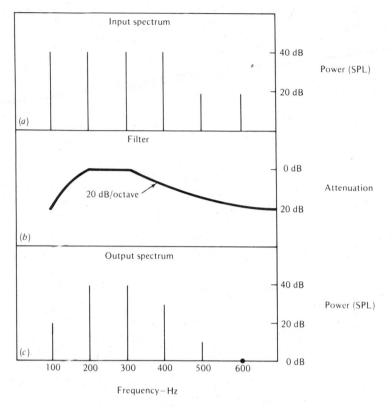

Figure 3.3   An input stimulus with the amplitude spectrum shown in **3.3a** is passed through the filter described in **3.3b**; the output stimulus has the amplitude spectrum shown in **3.3c**. The output spectrum is obtained by subtracting the attenuations (dB) shown in **3.3b** from the input amplitudes (dB) (3.3a).

When the frequency of the driving force is low, the speaker cone can follow the driving vibration with no loss in amplitude. However, as the driving frequency increases, the speaker cone cannot easily follow the driving force, and hence the amplitude of the speaker cone movement will be reduced. This happens because the cone has mass, and mass requires time to move. When the driving force has a high frequency, the speaker cone responds to the outward push after a small time delay due to the force attempting to move some mass. Thus, by the time the speaker cone begins to move outward, the driving force is moving inward, so the speaker cone also tries to move inward. The result is that the cone does not move as far outward as it did at lower frequencies, creating a lower amplitude at this high frequency. The speaker cone thus acts as a low-pass filter. The eardrum and other structures within the ear have mass and are driven by vibrations; they can react like a speaker cone. It is reasonable to assume that they would act as low-pass filters for the waveforms arriving at the ear. This will be discussed in greater detail in the next few chapters.

NONLINEARITIES

Thus far the discussion has concerned situations in which the *input* to *some object,* such as a filter, has been modified by an increase or decrease in the magnitude of the input value. If a waveform consisting of 100, 200, and 300 Hz is the input to a filter, the filter will alter only the amplitudes and phases of these sinusoids. There are, however, objects and systems that not only *modify* the values of the input but also *add* other frequencies. For instance, a complex waveform with values of 100, 200, and 300 Hz might be the input to such a system, but at the output of the system the values measured would consist of 100, 200, 300 Hz and perhaps the additional frequencies of 400, 500, and 600 Hz. That is, sinusoids are present in the output of this system in addition to those present in the input. A system that adds additional sinusoids to the input waveform is called a *nonlinear system,* whereas a system that only changes the amplitudes and phases of the input sinusoids is referred to as a *linear system.*

The interaction of a nonlinear system and waveforms will be discussed in terms of two waveforms: one, a simple waveform consisting of only one frequency, f_1; the other, a complex waveform consisting of two frequencies, f_1 and f_2. If one frequency f_1 is an input to a nonlinear device, then the output contains f_1 and its higher *harmonics:* $2f_1$, $3f_1$, $4f_1$, and so on. Thus if f_1 is 1000 Hz, the nonlinear device would yield at the output the following nonlinear frequency components: 2000 Hz, 3000 Hz, 4000 Hz, and so on.

If the two frequencies f_1 and f_2 are inputs, then the nonlinear outputs consist of the harmonics of each frequency: $2f_1$, $2f_2$, $3f_1$, $3f_2$, and so on, as well as frequencies consisting of the combination of f_1 and f_2. These frequencies, called *combination tones,* consist of two types: *summation tones* and *difference tones.* Typical summation tones are $f_1 + f_2$, $2f_1 + f_2$, $f_1 + 2f_2$, and typical difference tones are $f_1 - f_2$, $2f_1 - f_2$, $2f_2 - f_1$. If the input frequencies were 100 and 250 Hz, the nonlinear combination tones could be 350 Hz, 450 Hz, and 600 Hz (summation tones), and 150, 50, and 400 Hz (differ-

ence tones). Thus the total nonlinear output contains such harmonics and combination tones as 350, 200, 150, 50, 450, and so on. In general, a nonlinear device produces harmonics and combination tones according to this equation:

$$mf_1 \pm nf_2 \qquad (3.1)$$

where $m = 0, 1, 2, 3, \ldots$ and $n = 0, 1, 2, 3, \ldots.$

Table 3.2 Some Combination (Summation and Difference) Tones and Harmonics Resulting from Two Input Frequencies, 100 Hz (f_1) and 250 Hz (f_2)

Symbol	Harmonic Tones	Combination Tones Summation Tones	Combination Tones Difference Tones
f_1	100 Hz		
f_2	250 Hz		
$2f_1$	200 Hz		
$3f_1$	300 Hz		
$2f_2$	500 Hz		
$3f_2$	750 Hz		
$f_1 + f_2$		350 Hz	
$f_1 + 2f_2$		600 Hz	
$f_1 + 3f_2$		850 Hz	
$2f_1 + f_2$		450 Hz	
$3f_1 + f_2$		550 Hz	
$2f_1 + 2f_2$		700 Hz	
$2f_1 + 3f_2$		950 Hz	
$3f_1 + 2f_2$		800 Hz	
$f_1 - f_2$			150 Hz
$f_1 - 2f_2$			400 Hz
$f_1 - 3f_2$			650 Hz
$2f_1 - f_2$			50 Hz
$3f_1 - f_2$			50 Hz
$2f_1 - 2f_2$			300 Hz
$2f_1 - 3f_2$			550 Hz
$3f_1 - 2f_2$			200 Hz

Table 3.2 displays combination tones for input frequencies of 100 and 250 Hz. The amplitudes and phases of the nonlinear components present in the output depend on the frequencies, amplitudes, and phases of the input and on the nature or type of nonlinearity.

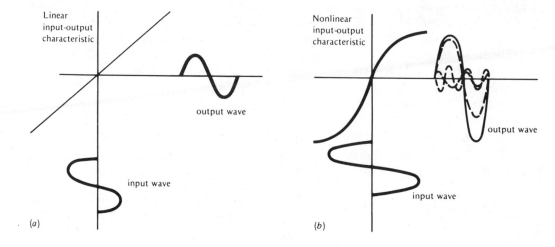

Figure 3.4 **3.4a:** A linear system is viewed as multiplying the values of an input stimulus by a straight-line function. The result is a sinusoid (if the input is a sinusoid) that will change only in phase and amplitude. **3.4b:** A nonlinear system is viewed as multiplication by a curved (nonlinear) function. The result for a sinusoidal input is a complex wave consisting of the input sinusoid (shown as the solid line) plus its higher harmonics (shown as dashed lines in 3.4b).

So far a nonlinear device has been discussed in terms of changes in the frequency domain; waveforms are also changed in the *time domain* by nonlinear devices. The difference between simple linear and nonlinear devices can be illustrated as in Figure 3.4. A simple linear device is one that changes only the amplitude or the phase of the input. This is like taking the input and multiplying it by a straight line (a linear device is, therefore, represented by a straight line). A nonlinear device modifies the input by changing it from a simple to a complex waveform, which is like multiplying the input by a line that is not straight (thus, a curved line represents a nonlinear device). The change in the time-domain representation resulting from a nonlinear device is sometimes called *distortion*. Thus, the output time wave-

form of a nonlinear device differs from the input time waveform. This, of course, is also true for a linear filter (a complex linear system), which will modify the input time waveform. Therefore we cannot investigate simply the difference between the input time waveform and the output time waveform to decide whether a system is nonlinear; we must also investigate changes in the frequency domain. If there are frequencies present in the output spectrum that are not present in the input spectrum, then the system is nonlinear. One question of great interest to the hearing scientist is whether the auditory system is linear or nonlinear. If it is a nonlinear system, what types of nonlinearities are produced? This question will be discussed in the later chapters of this book.

Summary Resonators and filters can be used to determine the amplitude spectrum of an unknown waveform. There are three general types of filters (low-pass, high-pass, and band-pass), and each is characterized by its cutoff frequency and the attenuation roll-off in decibels per octave. Filters also modify the spectrum of a waveform. A linear system changes only the phase and amplitude of an input waveform, whereas a nonlinear system adds additional sinusoids to the input. These nonlinear additional sinusoids are harmonics and combination tones (summation and difference tones) of the input sinusoids. Although filters and nonlinear devices are usually described in terms of altering the frequency domain of waveforms, both types of systems also alter the time domain of the waveform.

Supplement

Filter theory and the theory of nonlinear systems are complex matters dealing with acoustics and electrical engineering. The purpose of this chapter is to acquaint you with some of the terms used to describe filters and nonlinear systems. Further discussions of these effects are given in the remaining chapters of the book and in Appendix A. Licklider's chapter in Stevens' (1951) *Handbook of Experimental Psychology,* the book by Scott (1964) on *Linear Circuits,* and most of the reference books mentioned in Chapter 14 cover the topics of filtering and nonlinearity. It should be emphasized that filtering and nonlinearity are two *independent* aspects of any object that vibrates or any system that analyzes vibration.

The cutoff frequency of a filter is usually defined as that frequency at which the power of the signal has been attenuated by half of its maximum value. In decibels this means that the cutoff frequency is determined at the frequency at which the intensity is 3 dB below the maximum value obtained in the passband of the filter.

Appendix A should now be consulted for further information on how to obtain the nonlinear combination tones from a nonlinear system.

CHAPTER 4
The Outer and Middle Ears

Structure of the Outer Ear
Structure of the Middle Ear
Functions of the Outer and Middle Ears

The previous chapters have discussed the nature, transmission, and analysis of sound. The next four chapters will investigate how acoustic energy is collected by the outer ear and transmitted to the fluids of the inner ear, how the inner ear transforms this energy into neural impulses, and how these neural impulses may code or analyze acoustical information.

Figure 4.1 summarizes the structure, mode of operation, and function of four gross divisions of the auditory system: *outer ear, middle ear, inner ear,* and *central auditory nervous system.* The central auditory nervous system includes all of the complex interconnections in the auditory system from the auditory branch of the eighth cranial nerve to and including the auditory cortex. (The central auditory nervous system is therefore not diagramed in Fig. 4.1.) Chapter 7 discusses the central auditory nervous system, Chapter 6 the function of the inner ear, and Chapter 5 the structure of the inner ear. The present chapter deals with the outer and middle ears. First, we shall describe in detail the structures of the outer

and middle ears. This process will necessarily involve learning a new vocabulary. Second, we shall discuss the function of each of these structures.

Acoustic pressure is transmitted to the fluids of the inner ear via the outer and middle ears in a variety of ways. The outer and middle ears help to overcome middle and inner ear impedances (Chapter 2) and thus allow for a very efficient transmission of the acoustic stimulus to the inner ear. The outer and middle ears also provide protection to the inner ear against excessive changes in the environment.

Appendixes C and D will assist the reader in understanding the general areas of anatomy (the structure of an animal body and the relation of its parts) and physiology (the function of an anatomical system).

STRUCTURE OF THE OUTER EAR

The changing acoustic pressures that constantly impinge upon us are collected by the *outer ear.* The outer ear consists of the visible

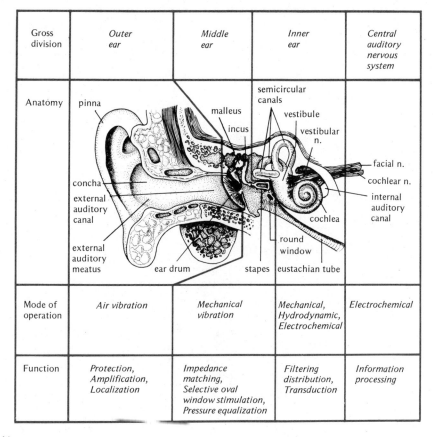

Gross division	Outer ear	Middle ear	Inner ear	Central auditory nervous system
Anatomy				
Mode of operation	Air vibration	Mechanical vibration	Mechanical, Hydrodynamic, Electrochemical	Electrochemical
Function	Protection, Amplification, Localization	Impedance matching, Selective oval window stimulation, Pressure equalization	Filtering distribution, Transduction	Information processing

Anatomy labels: pinna, concha, external auditory canal, external auditory meatus, ear drum, malleus, incus, stapes, eustachian tube, semicircular canals, vestibule, vestibular n., cochlea, round window, facial n., cochlear n., internal auditory canal

✳ Figure 4.1 Cross section of human ear, showing divisions into outer, middle, and inner ears. Below are listed the predominant mode of operation of each division and its suggested function. *(Adapted from Ades and Engstrom, 1974; Dallos, 1973, by permission)*

part of the ear (*pinna*) and the canal leading to the eardrum. The human pinna (illustrated in Figure 4.1) is formed primarily of cartilage without useful muscles. The deep center portion of the pinna is called the bowl, or *concha* (cave). The concha has a diameter of 1 to 2 cm (1 inch = 2.54 cm = 25.4 mm) and leads to an opening with a diameter of about 5 to 7 mm. This opening (or meatus) is called the *external auditory meatus;* it opens into a canal 2 to 3 cm in length called the *external auditory canal.* The lateral (toward pinna) third of the canal consists of cartilage containing glands and lined with hairs; the rest of the canal is bony, with a tight skin lining close to the eardrum or *tympanic membrane.*

STRUCTURE OF THE MIDDLE EAR

The tympanic membrane is held in place by fibers and cartilage situated in a bony groove. The tympanic membrane denotes anatomically one boundary of the large cavity known as the *middle ear cavity* or tympanum. The main portion of the middle ear cavity lies between the tympanic membrane and a bony wall, which contains the cochlea of the inner ear.

The middle ear cavity is about 2 cubic centimeters (cm³) in volume and includes a smaller upper cavity called the *epitympanum* or *epitympanic recess*. The middle ear cavity is connected to the nasopharynx (nose cavity) by a long (35 to 38 mm) tube known as the *eustachian* or *auditory tube*.

The tympanic membrane is a cone-shaped, relatively transparent membrane, 55 to 90 mm² in area. It is constructed of layers of tissue, of which the central fibrous layers are structurally the most important. The tympanic membrane consists of two sets of fibers: one set radiates from the center to the outside of the membrane, and the other set is composed of rings of fibers. The fibers are very sparse in the upper (superior) portion (toward the epitympanum) of the tympanic membrane called the *pars flaccida* (Fig. 4.2). The region of maximum concavity of the tympanic membrane is

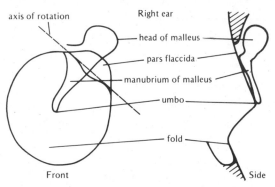

Figure 4.2 Front and side views of a right tympanic membrane and its connection to the malleus.

the *umbo* (the Latin word for the knob on a warrior's shield). The tympanic membrane is attached to the *manubrium* (handle) of the *malleus*, the outermost (lateral) of the three middle ear bones or *ossicles*. The head (upper portion) of the malleus is the rounded part that occupies half of the *epitympanic recess*. The head of the malleus connects with the

next ossicle, the *incus*. The ossicles and their relation to one another can be seen in **Figure 4.3.**

The incus lies medial (toward the center of the head) to the malleus, and the head of the malleus and the body of the incus are connected at a double saddle joint occupying most of the epitympanic recess. The *inferior process* (also called the long process) of the incus projects downward and then bends toward the inner ear to form the *lenticular process*, which joins with the third ossicle, the *stapes*.

The *stapes,* which is the smallest bone in the body, consists of the *head* (or capitulum), two bony struts called *crura* (singular *crus*), and a flat oval bone called the *footplate*. The footplate is implanted in the oval window (part of the inner ear) and is attached to its head by the crura. The stapes' footplate is surrounded at its rim by a ring-shaped ligament situated along the edge of the oval window. This ligament, called an *annular ligament,* assists in supporting the footplate in the oval window. Thus, the tympanic membrane is directly joined or "coupled" to the inner ear by the three ossicles. The three ossicles are suspended in the tympanic cavity by means of ligaments. Those ligaments most important for suspension are the *axial ligaments*. The axial ligaments consist of the *posterior ligament of the incus* and the *anterior ligament of the malleus,* as shown in Figure 4.4. Also shown in Figure 4.4 are the middle ear muscles. One of the middle ear muscles is the *tensor tympani muscle,* which is about 25 mm in length. Most of this muscle is enclosed within a bony canal which runs parallel to and above the eustachian tube. A tendon emerges from the bony canal to connect the muscle to the upper part of the manubrium of the malleus. The other middle ear muscle, the *stapedial muscle,* also originates within a bony canal. Only about 6 mm in total length, it is the smallest muscle in the body. The tendon of

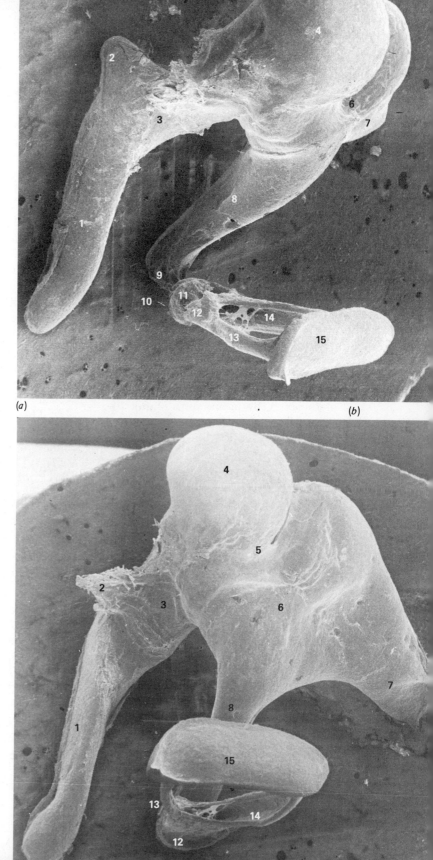

Figure 4.3 Middle ear ossicles. **4.3a:** From the front (anterior aspect); **4.3b:** from within the inner ear (medial aspect). Parts of the *malleus:* 1: manubrium; 2: anterior process; 3: neck; 4: head. Parts of the *incus:* 6: body; 7: short process; 8: long process; 9: lenticular process. Parts of the *stapes:* 11: head; 12: neck; 13: anterior crus; 14: posterior crus; 15: footplate. Also: 5: incudomalleal articulation; 10: incudostapedial articulation. *(Photographs courtesy of Dr. Ivan Hunter-Duvar, Hospital for Sick Children, Toronto)*

(a)

(b)

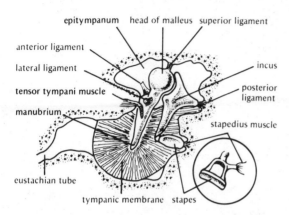

Figure 4.4 Schematic drawing of human middle ear (right side) seen from within: medial view. *(Adapted from Moller, 1970, by permission)*

the stapedial muscle completes the attachment to the head of the stapes.

Thus we can see that the inner ear communicates with the acoustic environment outside of the body by means of a funnel (the pinna), a short tube (the external auditory canal), a thin membrane (the tympanic membrane), and three small bones.

We shall now consider the functions served by the pinna, external auditory canal of the outer ear, tympanic membrane, and the ossicles of the middle ear.

FUNCTIONS OF THE OUTER AND MIDDLE EARS

Only mammals have pinnae, but among mammals there is great diversity in their form. In general, only animals with relatively high-frequency hearing have mobile pinnae. Since the pinnae of man and other primates have no useful muscles, they are relatively immobile. Mobile, and to some extent immobile, pinnae seem to help in localizing high-frequency sounds by funneling them toward the external auditory canal and possibly in distinguishing noises originating in front from those in back of the head.

One way to determine the effect of the exter-

nal ear on the auditory system is to observe what changes in the stimulus occur as a result of its presence. By producing a constant sound pressure level at a variety of frequencies in an empty sound field and comparing those SPLs with measurements made at the eardrum of a person placed in the field, we can determine the effects of the outer ear on stimulus intensity. The effect of the outer ear is to cause an increase or amplification in intensity of about 10 to 15 dB in a frequency range from roughly 1.5 kHz to 7 kHz (see p. 13). Experiments have shown that this frequency-dependent increase in SPL between the free field measurement and the measurement at the tympanic membrane is due mainly to the effects of the concha and the external auditory canal, as shown in Figure 4.5. In Chapter 3 we discussed the concept of resonance. It is the resonances of the concha and external canal that complement each other to produce a gain in acoustic pressure in the frequency range from 1.5 to 7 kHz. The resonance frequency of the external auditory canal is about 2.5 kHz, and the resonance frequency of the concha is closer to 5 kHz. The resonance curves are shown in Figure 4.5b.

The only other known function of the external ear is that of protection of the tympanic membrane against foreign bodies and changes in humidity and temperature. Since it completely seals off the external auditory canal, the tympanic membrane provides some protection for the middle ear against foreign bodies. The tympanic membrane vibrates as a result of the sound waves traveling in the external auditory canal, and this vibration is passed along to the ossicular chain. The vibratory pattern of the tympanic membrane has been the subject of much research since Helmholtz published his first experiments in 1868. Figure 4.6 shows a composite of the vibratory patterns found by two different experimenters. One of the simplest forms of vibration was described by von Bekesy for stimuli below 2000 Hz. He suggested that the membrane

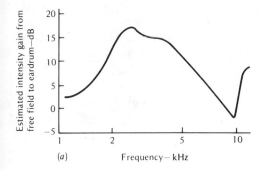

(a)

Frequency— kHz

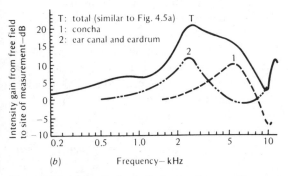

T: total (similar to Fig. 4.5a)
1: concha
2: ear canal and eardrum

(b)

Frequency— kHz

Figure 4.5 4.5a: Estimated change in sound pressure level from free field to the eardrum as a function of frequency. 4.5b: This average pressure (T curve) is divided among the various components that may contribute to the gain. Note that the concha and ear canal–eardrum, lines 1 and 2, are thought to contribute the most to the total gain. The concha has a resonant frequency near 5000 Hz and the ear canal–eardrum a resonant frequency near 2000 Hz. *(Adapted from Shaw, 1974, by permission)*

vibrates maximally at a point below the umbo and directly above the fold (see Fig. 4.6, point 15). Modern investigative methods show the complicated vibratory patterns illustrated on the bottom of Figure 4.6. It is generally agreed that the vibratory pattern of the tympanic membrane is the most complicated at higher frequencies and higher intensities. The complicated vibratory response illustrated by time-averaged holography show variations with the frequency of the stimulus. At the low frequency used in Figure 4.6b the point of maxi-

mum displacement is in the superior posterior (top rear) section of the membrane. These vibratory patterns found by Tonndorf and Khanna using holography fit the concepts first suggested by Helmholtz 100 years previously. This vibratory pattern of the tympanic membrane, though complicated and not completely understood, allows for a fairly efficient transfer of the acoustic stimulus from the outer ear to the middle ear and the middle ear structures. The vibratory pattern of the tympanic membrane provides resonance and filtering in addition to that performed by the outer ear.

Once the acoustic stimulus reaches the tympanic membrane, there are three methods by

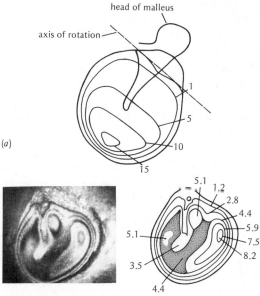

Figure 4.6 4.6a: The vibratory pattern of the right tympanic membrane to a 2 kHz tone. The closed curves represent contours of equal displacement amplitude on a relative scale; 15 is the maximum amplitude. This is von Bekesy's 1941 stiff-plate model. 4.6b: Tonndorf and Khanna's 1972 time-averaged holograph of the left tympanic membrane vibration. The stimulus was a 525 Hz, 121 dB SPL pure tone. In the explanatory drawing, each isoamplitude contour must be multiplied by 10^{-5} cm to obtain the actual displacement value. The point of maximum displacement was found in the upper rear portion of the membrane (8.2). *(Adapted from Tonndorf and Khanna, 1972, by permission)*

which it can be transmitted through the middle ear to the inner ear: (1) via bone conduction (that is, the sound could travel via the bones of the skull, bypassing the middle ear and going directly to the inner ear), (2) via the air in the middle ear cavity, and (3) across the middle ear cavity by means of the ossicular chain (the malleus, incus, and stapes) to the inner ear. As will be discussed, the ossicular chain is the most effective method of transmitting sound to the inner ear.

In order for the ossicular chain to operate efficiently, the middle ear must not be a closed cavity. If the middle ear cavity were completely closed, then changes in atmospheric pressure that occur frequently in elevators, airplanes, or under water would cause the tympanic membrane to move more in one direction than in the other because of the pressure differences. The eustachian tube allows for equalization of this type of pressure difference across the tympanic membrane, by providing another path (via the nasal passages) for the pressure. That is, the eustachian tube allows the tympanic membrane to operate efficiently in a variety of atmospheric pressures.

The inner ear is filled with a fluid that must be moved by the pressure exerted on the membrane (oval window membrane) leading into it. If this oval window membrane were pushed or driven by air, then air pressure would be the driving force. Since the fluid is denser than air, however, air would not be very efficient in moving the fluid. Thus, the auditory system would lose some of its sensitivity due to the impedance (Chapter 2) that the fluids of the inner ear provide for the propagation of the air-conducted sound. The difference between the impedance of air and water can be illustrated by the ease with which one can move a cupped hand through the air versus through water. The difference is referred to as an impedance mismatch. This impedance difference means that more pressure is required for a stimulus to be propagated in the cochlear

fluids than in the air. Nature has compensated for this mismatch, principally by the size difference between the areas of the tympanic membrane and the stapes footplate and, to a more limited extent, by the lever action of the ossicular chain.

When stimulated by high levels of pressure the tympanic membrane operates as a stretched membrane, and only part of the pressures acting on it are transferred to the manubrium of the malleus. Measurements show that only two-thirds of a total area of 85 mm^2 of the tympanic membrane is stiffly connected to the manubrium and thus vibrates at high intensities. Therefore, the effective surface area of the tympanic membrane is 55 mm^2. The stapes, which is the last part of the middle ear chain, makes contact with the oval window and the fluids of the inner ear. The area of the stapes footplate is about 3.2 mm^2, which is considerably less than the effective area of the tympanic membrane. This difference in surface area acts as an amplifier of the pressure exerted on the tympanic membrane. Consider that if all of the force that impinges on the tympanic membrane is transferred to the stapes footplate, then more force per unit of area ($p = F/A$) must be at the footplate since it is smaller than the tympanic membrane. Mathematically, the increase in pressure can be expressed as the ratio of the effective area of the tympanic membrane to that of the stapes footplate; that is, $55/3.2 = 17$. Thus, the pressure at the footplate is 17 times greater than at the tympanic membrane, and therefore it is more capable of stimulating the fluid-filled inner ear.

The transfer of the force from the tympanic membrane to the stapes footplate is dependent on the action of the ossicles. The ossicles work as a lever system because the length of the manubrium and neck of the malleus is longer than the long process of the incus (see Fig. 4.3). The lever action of this system is 1.3 to 1; that is, the force at the tympanic membrane is increased by a factor of 1.3 at the stapes. Thus the pressure increase of a factor of 17 due to the area difference of the tympanic membrane and stapes footplate is further amplified by 1.3, resulting in a theoretical maximum total pressure increase of 17×1.3, or 22 (a pressure increase of 22 to 1 corresponds to 27 dB, see Appendix B) at the stapes footplate. The actual pressure transformation is dependent on the frequency of the acoustic stimulus. Figure 4.7 shows the increase of the pressure between the eardrum and stapes as a function of frequency. This figure indicates that the increase between the eardrum and stapes is 20 dB or more, up to about 2500 Hz. Above this frequency, the ratio decreases. In addition, as we showed earlier, the resonances of the concha and external canal are in the 2-kHz to 5-kHz range, thus causing a significant amount of amplification across a wide frequency range that is important for the perception of speech. Therefore the outer and middle ear provide the amplification necessary for air pressure to move the dense fluids of the inner ear. Nature has designed an ingenious system.

Previously we described the suspension sys-tem of the ossicles and stated that there were several ligaments that performed this function. Interestingly, this suspension does not alter the vibratory pattern of the middle ear. Von Bekesy's experiments on the axial ligaments are a case in point. He cut the axial ligaments and found no effect upon the vibratory amplitude of the stapes when driven by acoustic stimulation (above 200 Hz) introduced into the meatus.

Two important components of the ossicular suspension system are the middle ear muscles. These muscles are normally in a state of tension, but when the ear is excited by sound, they exert an increased pull, which is a reflex action. The sound which elicits the reflex must be about 80 dB above the quietest sound a person can hear (80 dB SL). Contraction of the middle ear muscles reduces the transmission of pressure through the ossicular chain. The reduction in transmission has a maximum value of about 0.6 to 0.7 dB per decibel increase in stimulus intensity above the threshold of the reflex. The reduction amounts to approximately 10 dB to 30 dB for loud sounds and is frequency-dependent, having

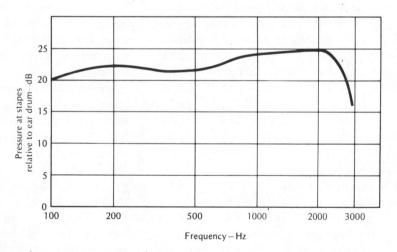

* **Figure 4.7** Pressure at the stapes is increased over pressure at the tympanic membrane by the dB value shown as a function of the frequency of the stimulus. *(Adapted from von Bekesy, 1960, by permission)*

more effect for low frequencies than for high, and probably having no effect for frequencies above 2 kHz. The time for the reflex action to occur is a minimum of 10 ms for very loud sounds and can be as long as 150 ms for stimuli at very low intensities. Therefore, short-duration sounds of sudden onset are not greatly attenuated or reduced by the middle ear reflex. The muscles can thus provide a type of protection since they can reduce the amount of fatigue and damage from exposure to high-intensity, low-frequency steady sound.

Another possible function of the middle ear muscles is to limit *distortion* (nonlinearities). If the contact pressure between two vibrating bodies is smaller than the driving pressure acting during the vibration, the two bodies (such as the ossicular bones) will separate, and as a result of the separation a distortion of the transmitted signal could easily occur at the joint. In the middle ear when the vibrations are small, the elastic ligaments are able to exert a pressure sufficiently great that the bones do not separate. For larger vibrations, however, the pressure of the ligaments may not be sufficient, and the muscles work in opposition to one another to press the stapes against the incus, thus limiting the separation. Anatomically it is also interesting that each of the middle ear muscles is enclosed throughout its length in a long narrow canal. This permits the muscles to produce only a pull and not to be set into vibration themselves. If the muscles did vibrate due to acoustic stimulation, they would produce harmonics (nonlinearities) that could be translated to the fluids of the inner ear and could become audible.

The ossicular chain does not move in a simple manner for all frequencies and intensities. Due to the size of the heads of the malleus and incus, the mass of the ossicles is distributed evenly around an axis through the two large ligaments of the malleus and the short process of the incus. At moderate intensities the ossicular chain moves in such a way that the footplate of the stapes swings about an imaginary axis drawn vertically through the posterior crus much like a swinging door pivoting about its hinges. The anterior portion of the footplate therefore pushes into and out of the cochlea like a piston. This pivotal action is possible because of the asymmetric fiber length of the annular ligament. At very low frequencies (below 150 Hz) and at extremely high intensities this rotation of the footplate is thought to change dramatically. Under these conditions the axis of rotation is through the crura, becoming perpendicular to the previous vertical axis. The motion of the stapes becomes a rocking motion around the axis much like that of a seesaw, as seen in Figure 4.8. The motion can be illustrated by putting your pencil on the table and centering the back cover of your book on top of it. Rocking the book back and forth on the pencil illustrates how half of the stapes footplate is going into the cochlea while the other half is coming out. The resultant displacement of the cochlear fluids is zero. At very high intensities as the frequency increases above 150 Hz, the motion of the footplate consists of both types of rotations simultaneously. Because of this complex form of rotation, further increases in intensity result in very little motion of the fluids of the inner ear. This complex motion is thought to help protect the inner ear from being overstimulated. Recent experiments with cats, however, have shown that the stapes has an effective pistonlike motion for low frequencies even at sound pressures as high as 130 dB SPL. It was not until 150 dB SPL was reached that a rocking motion was added to the pistonlike motion. Thus, the protection provided by the rocking motion occurs only at very high intensities not often encountered in nature. Some man-made noises, however, especially ones of short duration, may reach this extremely high level.

Despite the claims that the middle ear reflexes and stapes footplate motion may provide protection, deafness caused by exposure

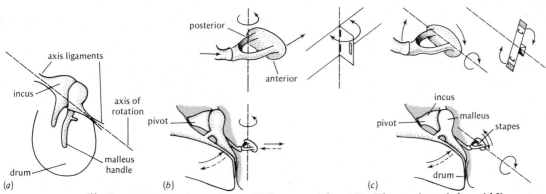

✳ Figure 4.8 Motions of the middle ear ossicles. 4.8a: The motion of the middle ear ossicles is a rocking motion about an axis drawn through the axial ligaments and the short process of the incus. Since the large heads of the malleus and incus offset the rest of the mass of the ossicular chain, this axis is also the center of gravity. **4.8b:** The normal stapes motion is like that of a swinging door with the posterior section as the hinge and the anterior section pushing in and out of the oval window like a plunger. **4.8c:** At very high intensities the stapes is thought to rock around an axis drawn through the crura. This seesaw motion affects the inner ear fluid only slightly. *(Adapted from von Bekesy, 1936a, by permission)*

⌐ ┌Rocks like a door that is hindged on one side - otoschlerosis hindges both
└sides

to man-made environmental noises such as some industrial noises does seem to be positive evidence of the fact that the ear does not really have an adequate protective mechanism against our present levels of acoustic stimulation.

From a developmental point of view it is not surprising that as animals developed from living in water to living on land, a middle ear system evolved that matched the high impedance of the fluid-filled cochlea with the airborne stimulation. But what about the pathways to the inner ear other than the middle ear ossicles—that is, direct air conduction and bone conduction? If the middle ear ossicles were missing, the inner ear could be stimulated directly by air pressure variations in the middle ear cavity. This would provide an additional loss due to the fact that both the entries to the inner ear would be stimulated simultaneously and in phase at some frequencies of stimulation. We shall see in the next chapter that the *round* and *oval windows* lead to the inner ear on opposite sides of the basilar membrane. Positive pressure on the round window will cause the basilar membrane to move in one direction, and positive pressure

on the oval window will cause basilar membrane motion in the opposite direction. Having the same pressure applied to both windows simultaneously results in a very inefficient system since the basilar membrane would not move. A hearing loss of 60 dB is often found in patients who have no middle ear system unless the round window is shielded from the air pressure variations. Thus another function of the middle ear system is to direct the stimulation to the oval window, allowing the round window to move according to pressure variation within the inner ear.

Stimulation of the inner ear by bone conduction does not occur as an important part of normal auditory function. If, however, a vibrator is applied to the skull, the inner ear can be stimulated (vibrated) via conduction of the sound through the bones of the skull. This may be employed to a practical advantage in the event of damage to the middle ear. That is, stimulation of the skull by a vibrator can be used during diagnosis to test the viability of the inner ear, thus bypassing the damaged middle ear.

Summary The outer ear consists of the pinna and the external auditory canal and ends at the lateral border of the tympanic membrane. The three ossicles (malleus, incus, stapes) in the middle ear couple the tympanic membrane to the inner ear. Two muscles and several ligaments help support these ossicles. The resonance of the external auditory canal and the tympanic membrane, along with the lever action of the ossicular chain and the area difference between the tympanic membrane and oval window membrane, help amplify the air pressure at the external auditory meatus so that the air pressure can drive the dense fluids of the inner ear. In some limited fashion the muscles may help protect the auditory system. For higher intensities, motion of the ossicular chain varies as the frequency and intensity of the input stimulus change.

Supplement

The early research on the function of the external ear was conducted by von Bekesy (1941, 1960), Wiener (1947), and Wiener and Ross (1946). The recent research that illuminated the role of the concha determining the resonances of the external ear was performed by Shaw (1974).

The vibratory pattern of the tympanic membrane and the middle ear ossicles has been the subject of research since Helmholtz published his work in the first issue of *Pfluegers Archiv fur die Gesamte Physiologie des Menschen und der Tiere* in 1868. Von Bekesy's (1941) description of the tympanic membrane was widely accepted for many years. In the late 1950s and early 1960s two classic works on the middle ear were published (Kobrak, 1959; Kirikae, 1960). Kirikae suggested an alternative vibratory pattern for the tympanic membrane. Recently, Tonndorf and Khanna (1972) have suggested the complicated vibratory pattern shown in Figure 4.6. Their results are consistent with those of Helmholtz and Kirikae.

Recent advances in investigative techniques have allowed scientists to study, in detail, the middle ear ossicles (Moller, 1973a, 1974). Basically the function of the middle ear is to act as an impedance matching system and to direct the acoustic stimulation to the oval window, leaving the round window free to vibrate. Although we have discussed only the resistance of the fluid-filled cochlea, the ossicles and tympanic membrane also have a form of impedance known as reactance. The ossicles have mass, which offers impedance to the tympanic membrane motion; the tympanic membrane, although it has little mass, acts much like a spring, thus offering its own impedance to acoustic stimulation. The total impedance of the middle and inner ear is the subject of many current investigators (Moller, 1974; Dallos, 1970). The impedance of the middle ear can be easily measured with an instrument called an electroacoustic impedance bridge. This type of measurement is currently used as a method of assessing the condition of the middle ear. That is, changes in abnormal middle ear structures can be detected as abnormal impedances. For a detailed discussion of the measurement of middle ear impedance and its value as a diagnostic tool, read Jerger's (1975) book.

It is often stated about the middle ear muscles that they serve as a protector against high-intensity stimulation. The middle ear reflex has a threshold of 80 dB SL and a minimum latency of 10 ms. Its attenuation is primarily to stimulation below 2 kHz (Moller, 1974), and it probably does not attenuate by more than about 10 dB. Thus it is protective only for gradual-onset low-frequency sounds. Von Bekesy (1960) suggested that the middle ear muscle may serve to reduce distortion by tightening the joint between the malleus and stapes at high intensities. Von Bekesy (1936, 1960) has also suggested that the rocking motion of the stapes at high intensities offered a protective device against overstimulation. Guinan and Peake's (1967) work suggests, however, that a stimulus of 150 dB SPL is needed before a rocking motion occurs. Therefore we can conclude that while the external and middle ears are efficient in collecting, amplifying, and transmitting acoustic information to the inner ear, the high incidence of deafness due to overstimulating the inner ear makes explicit the inability of any of the suggested protective mechanisms to deal completely with present levels of stimulation.

SUMMARY OF HUMAN OUTER AND MIDDLE EAR MEASUREMENTS

Most of the data listed here come from Wever and Lawrence's *Physiological Acoustics* (1954). Their Appendix D is a compilation of many authors' work, from which we have chosen the data to illustrate the range of measures. When available, a mean value is given. Additional data from recent investigations have also been added.

Pinna (Male)

length: 60–75 mm, mean = 67 mm
breadth: 30–39 mm, mean = 34.5 mm
angle that length axis is inclined to head: 15°
concha volume: 2.5 cm³
concha resonance frequency: 4.5 kHz

External Auditory Meatus

cross section: 0.3–0.5 cm²

External Auditory Canal

cross section: 0.3–0.5 cm²
length: 2.3–2.97 cm
diameter: 0.7 cm
volume: 1.0 cm³
resonance frequency: 2.6 kHz

Tympanic Membrane

diameter along the manubrium: 7.5–9 mm
diameter perpendicular to the manubrium: 7.5–9 mm
area: 0.5–0.9 cm²
effective area: 42.9–55 mm²
inward displacement of umbo: 2 mm
thickness: 0.1 mm
weight: 14 mg
breaking strength: 0.4–3.0×10^6 dynes/cm², mean = 1.61×10^6 dynes/cm²
displacement amplitude for low-frequency tones at threshold of feeling: 10^{-2} cm
displacement amplitude for a 250-Hz tone: 12.5 Å at 75 dB SPL, 7.5 Å at 70 dB SPL, 5 Å at 65 dB SPL

Middle Ear Cavity

total volume: 2.0 cm³
volume of ossicles: 0.50–0.8 cm³

Malleus

weight: 23–27 mg
length from end of manubrium to end of lateral process: 5.8 mm
total length: 7.6–9.1 mm

Incus

weight: 25–32 mg
length of long process: 7.0 mm
length of short process: 5.0 mm

Stapes

weight: 2.05–4.34 mg, mean = 2.86 mg
height: 2.50–3.78 mm, mean = 3.26 mm
length of footplate: 2.64–3.36 mm, mean = 2.99 mm
width of footplate: 1.08–1.66 mm, mean = 1.41 mm
area of footplate: 2.65–3.75 mm², mean = 3.2 mm²
width of elastic ligament: 0.015–0.1 mm
amplitude of displacement for a constant eardrum pressure of 1 dyne/cm²:

125 Hz	75×10^{-8} cm
200 Hz	28×10^{-8} cm
400 Hz	20×10^{-8} cm
750 Hz	18×10^{-8} cm
1500 Hz	10×10^{-8} cm
2000 Hz	6×10^{-8} cm
2500 Hz	2×10^{-8} cm

maximum displacement: 0.1 mm

CHAPTER 5

Structure of the Inner Ear and Its Mechanical Response

Structure of the Inner Ear
Mechanical Response of the Inner Ear
How the Traveling Wave Excites the Hair Cells

In Chapter 4 we considered the course of the acoustic stimulus as it traveled from the environment toward the inner ear. Reference has already been made to the fluids of the inner ear; this chapter will describe the remaining anatomy of the inner ear and how this anatomy relates to the vibratory stimulation it receives from the stapes.

In general, the motion of the stapes moves the fluid and other structures of the inner ear. This motion causes the hair cells of the inner ear to be stimulated and to elicit neural discharges in the auditory nerve. Thus the mechanical energy of sound vibration is changed into neural information within the inner ear. The inner ear provides the nervous system with information about the frequency, intensity, and temporal content of acoustic stimulation. Part of the spectral analysis of sound is provided by the mechanics of the inner ear in a way that can be described as filtering.

STRUCTURE OF THE INNER EAR

The inner ear can be divided into three parts: the semicircular canals, the vestibule, and the cochlea, all of which are located in the temporal bone. There are three semicircular canals that open into the vestibule: superior, posterior, and lateral. Under normal circumstances these structures affect balance (the *vestibular system*) rather than hearing. They are, however, part of the total system to which acoustic disturbances are delivered. The sensory receptor cells of the vestibular system, as in the auditory system, are hair cells, and the two systems are often discussed together. Since our main interest is in presenting the fundamentals of hearing, we shall not cover the structure and function of the vestibular system.

The vestibule is the central inner ear cavity

(see Fig. 5.1). It is about 5 mm front to back and top to bottom and about 3 mm in width. The vestibule is bounded on its lateral side by the *oval window*, which is located in its wall facing the middle ear cavity (tympanic wall). The footplate of the stapes connects to the oval window. The vestibule contains the *utricle* and the *saccule,* which are sense organs of the vestibular system.

The cochlea, the small shell-shaped part of the bony labyrinth shown in Figure 5.2 and

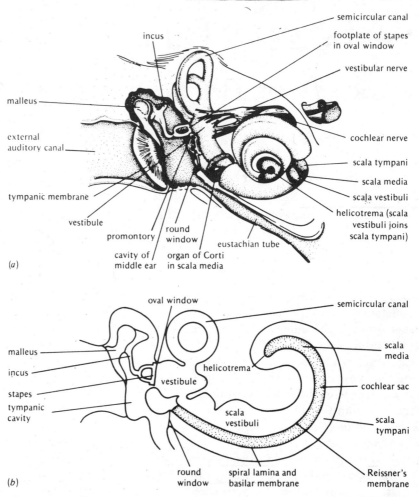

(a)

(b)

Figure 5.1 **5.1a:** Main components of the inner ear in relation to the other structures of the ear. *(Adapted from Dorland, 1965)* **5.1b:** Schematic diagram of middle ear and partially uncoiled cochlea, showing the relationship of the various scalae. *(Adapted from Zemlin, 1968, by permission)*

illustrated schematically in Figure 5.1, contains the primary auditory organ of the inner ear. It resembles a tube of decreasing diameter, which is coiled increasingly sharply upon itself—2⅝ times in humans. The cochlea terminates blindly in its third turn at the *apex*. Its central axis is called the *modiolus*, which acts as an inner wall. The spiral canal of the cochlea is about 35 mm long and is partially divided throughout its length by a thin spiral shelf of bone projecting from the modiolus, known as the *osseous spiral lamina* (Figs. 5.2 and 5.3). Across this shelf the tough *basilar membrane* connects to the outer wall of the bony cochlea at the *spiral ligament* and completes the division of the canal into two passages the full extent of the canal, except for a small opening at the apex called the *helicotrema*. The lower passage of the canal (scala tympani) has an opening, known as the *round window*, which is covered with a thin membrane (round window membrane) separating the scala tympani from the tympanic cavity. A delicate membrane, *Reissner's membrane,* extends upward diagonally from the osseous spiral lamina to a region of the outer wall slightly above the basilar membrane; it extends the length of the cochlea to the apex, where it joins the basilar membrane at the helicotrema. Thus there is a completely sealed sac within the middle of the cochlea, called the *cochlear sac* (or cochlear duct), which runs the length of the cochlea except for a small portion at the apex. The cochlear sac is bounded "above" by Reissner's membrane, "below" by the basilar membrane, and on its one "side" by the stria vascularis; surrounded by a watery fluid called *perilymph*, it contains its own fluid called *endolymph*.

Cross sections of the cochlea, as in Figure 5.3, show the canal divided into three parts or ducts. These three ducts are *scala vestibuli, scala tympani*, and *scala media*. Scala vestibuli extends from the oval window in the vestibule to the helicotrema. In cross sections (Figure 5.3) of the cochlea it is usually shown as the upper scala. Scala tympani extends from the round window to the helicotrema. In cross section it is often shown at the bottom. The scala media is the central duct, which is bounded by the basilar membrane, a portion of the outer wall of the cochlea, and Reissner's membrane. The outer wall of the scala media is covered by the *stria vascularis*, which has a dense layer of blood capillaries and specialized cells. Scala vestibuli and scala tympani contain perilymph, and scala media contains the endolymph. It is easy to remember the names of the different scalae, since scala vestibuli lies opposite the vestibule, scala tympani communicates with the tympanic cavity via the round window, and scala media lies in the middle. The two *peri*pheral scalae, scala tympani and scala vestibuli, contain *peri*lymph and the middle or *en*closed scala, scala media, contains *endo*lymph.

Whereas the bony cochlea becomes smaller and smaller in cross-sectional area as the apex is approached, the basilar membrane lying within the cochlea becomes progressively wider as it approaches the apex, as shown in Figure 5.4. The osseous spiral lamina is broadest at the vestibular (basal) end, where the basilar membrane is about 0.16 mm wide; near the helicotrema the basilar membrane has broadened to 0.52 mm. Measuring the various characteristics of the basilar membrane was of primary interest to von Bekesy, who later was able to build a model of the membrane and describe its complicated pattern of motion.

From von Bekesy's work it may be concluded that the human basilar membrane is a stout layer of closely attached fibers about 34 mm long from base to helicotrema. *It is wider, more flaccid, and under no tension at the apical end. The base end is narrower and stiffer than the apical end and may be under a small amount of tension.* These facts become important in considering the vibratory pattern of the membrane in response to acoustic stimulation.

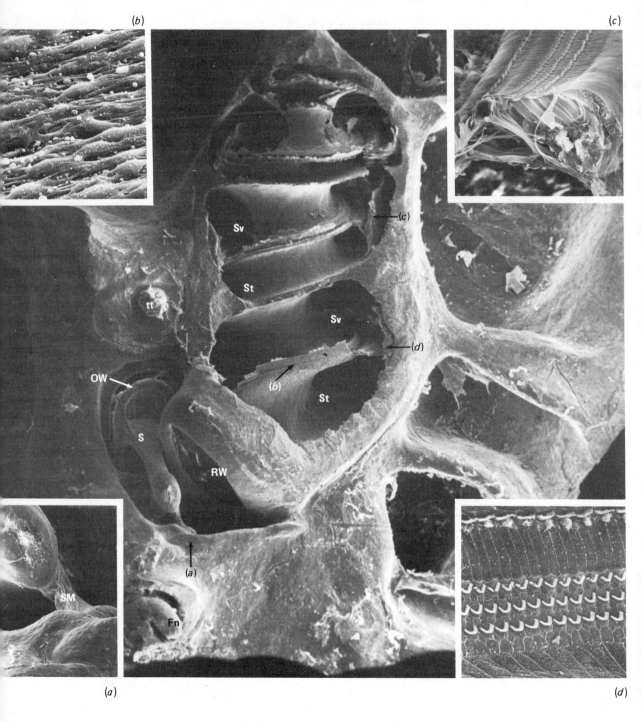

(b)

(c)

(a)

(d)

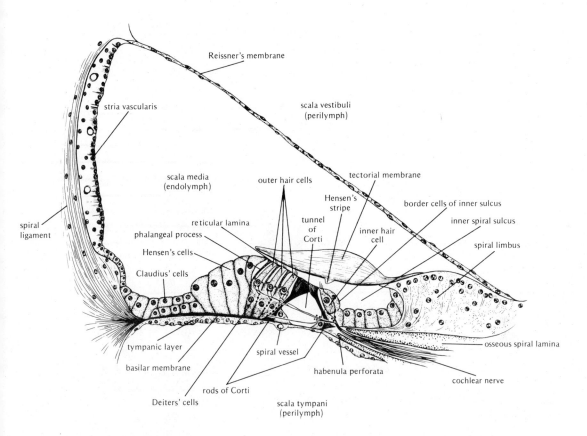

On the scala media surface of the basilar membrane lies the *organ of Corti* (see Figs. 5.3 and 5.5). The organ of Corti is divided into inner and outer portions by the *pillars* or *rods of Corti*. The rods of Corti form a tunnel that is almost triangular in cross section and

Figure 5.2 Scanning electron micrograph showing the coiling of the chinchilla cochlea (3¾ turns). Also shown: S: Stapes; OW: oval window; RW: round window. The inserts show details at the points indicated on the central photograph: **5.2a:** SM: stapedial muscle. **5.2b:** Tympanic layer below the basilar membrane. **5.2c:** Cross section of the organ of Corti. **5.2d:** Cilia of the inner and outer hair cells. Sv: scala vestibuli; St: scala tympani; tt: attachment of tensor tympani; Fn: facial nerve. *(Photograph courtesy of Dr. Ivan Hunter-Duvar, Hospital for Sick Children, Toronto)*

Figure 5.3 Drawing of a cross section of the cochlea showing the organ of Corti situated in the scala media on the basilar membrane. *(Drawing by Sarah Crenshaw McQueen, Henry Ford Hospital, Detroit)*

runs the length of the cochlear sac. The space between the rods is called the *inner tunnel of Corti*, which contains a fluid called *cortilymph*. The inner portion of the organ of Corti is on the modiolar side (inside) of the rods, and the outer portion lies toward the bony cochlear wall (toward stria vascularis).

On the inner side of the inner rods is a single row of hair cells, called the *inner hair cells*, and on the outer side of the outer rods are three or four rows of smaller hair cells, called the *external* or *outer hair cells*, with various supporting cells. The inner and outer

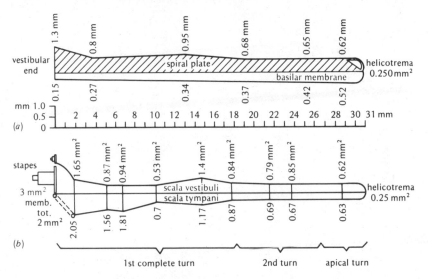

Figure 5.4 Schematic diagrams. **5.4a:** Dimensions of the basilar membrane. **5.4b:** Dimensions of the scalae of the human cochlea. The basilar membrane is wider at the apical end than at the basal end, but the scalae are smaller at the apex than at the base. *(Adapted from Fletcher, 1953; data are from Wrightson and Keith, 1918, by permission)* Additional inner-ear measurements are listed in the Supplement to this chapter.

hair cells slant toward each other and are held in place in three ways. First, cells of *Deiters* and *Hensen* serve as lateral buttresses for the outer hair cells, and the *border cells* of the *inner sulcus* serve the same purpose for the inner hair cells. Second, a *reticular membrane* (or lamina) holds the upper ends of the hair cells and assists in maintaining their alignment. Third, the *Deiters' cells* are found below the hair cells, with one Deiters' cell per hair cell. The upper end of the cylindrical Deiters' cell is a cup-shaped structure that encloses the base of the hair cell. From the cupped end of the cylindrically shaped Deiters' cell a slender process passes to the surface of the organ of Corti, forming a *phalangeal process* and a part of the reticular membrane (see Figs. 5.5 and 5.6). These Deiters' cells and phalangeal processes form the main vertical supportive mechanism for the hair cells.

Figure 5.7 shows the detailed structure of the inner and outer hair cells and the difference in their shape. The upper surface of each inner hair cell consists of a membrane with cuticle (below) into which the bases of the stereocilia (*cilia*, or tiny hairs) are rooted. On each inner hair cell are about 40 cilia, arranged in two or more parallel rows which form a very shallow U (Figs. 5.8 and 5.9a). One small area of the surface of the hair cell is cuticle-free, and in this area a basal body or modified kinocilium is usually found. A kinocilium is an extremely long cilium found in other hair cell receptor systems. During embryonic life, the human cochlea hair cells also have a long, coarse kinocilium. After birth the kinocilium generally disappears, and only a basal body remains, although a rudiment of the kinocilium may also remain. The basal body of the inner hair cell is located on the outer edge of the cell, that is, away from the modiolus, toward the inner rods of Corti.

The upper surface of the outer hair cell contains about 150 stereocilia arranged in three or more rows on each cell in the shape of a V or W (Figs. 5.8 and 5.9b). The basal

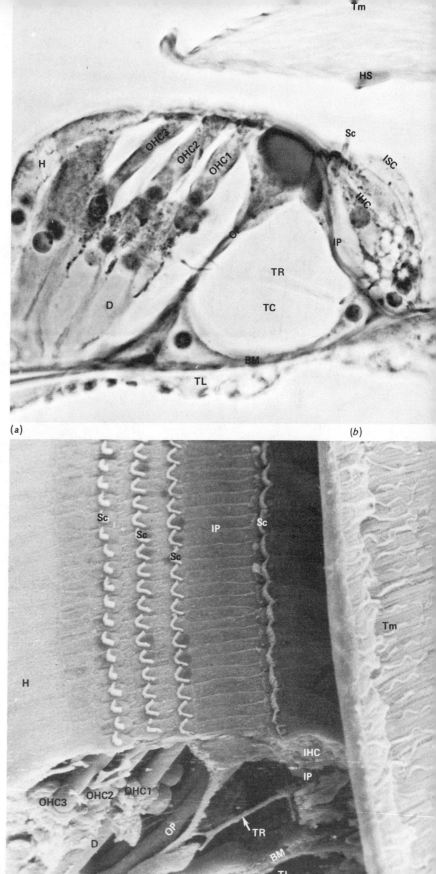

Figure 5.5 5.5a: Light micrograph of a cross section of a chinchilla organ of Corti. Clearly shown are: IHC: inner hair cell; OHC: the three rows of outer hair cells; OP, IP: outer and inner pillars of Corti; TC: tunnel of Corti; BM: basilar membrane; TL: tympanic layer of cells below BM; D, H: supporting cells of Deiters and Hensen; Tm: tectorial membrane; HS: Hensen's stripe; ISC: inner sulcus cells; TR: a tunnel radial nerve fiber. 5.5b: Scanning electron micrograph of a cross section of a chinchilla organ of Corti. Many of the same parts of the organ of Corti are shown, but with the advantage of added dimensionality. This view also shows the head of the IP cells between the stereocilia (Sc) of the inner and outer hair cells. Tm is pulled back to expose the stereocilia. *(Photographs courtesy of Dr. Ivan Hunter-Duvar, Hospital for Sick Children, Toronto)*

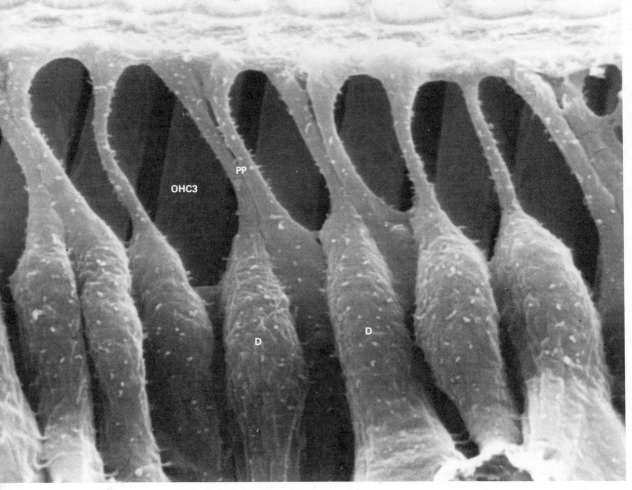

Figure 5.6 Scanning electron micrograph showing the supporting structure of the organ of Corti provided by Deiters' cells (D) and their phalangeal processes (PP) in relation to the outer row of outer hair cells (OHC3). The phalangeal processes arise from the top of the Deiters' cells and form part of the reticular lamina at the top of the hair cells. The stereocilia (Sc) are above the reticular lamina; the body of each hair cell sits in the cup-shaped top of a Deiters' cell. (*Chinchilla photograph courtesy of Dr. Ivan Hunter-Duvar, Hospital for Sick Children, Toronto*)

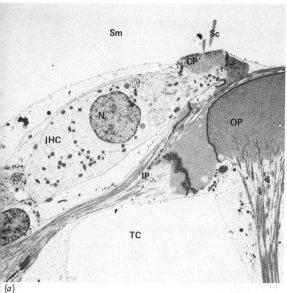

(a)

Figure 5.7 5.7a: Transmission electron micrograph showing the detailed structure of an inner hair cell (IHC). The stereocilia (Sc) of the hair cell project into the scala media (Sm) and are rooted in the cuticular plate (CP). The nucleus (N) of the inner hair cell is clearly seen. At the base of the hair cell, nerve fibers of the inner spiral bundle (IS) are visible. Also shown: inner and outer pillars (IP, OP) of the tunnel of Corti (TC). 5.7b: Transmission electron micrograph of the outer hair cells (OHC). Note the difference in shape between IHC and OHC. The OHC is seen sitting in the cup-shaped Deiters' cell (D). At the base of OHC, an efferent nerve fiber (E) is also seen. The space between OHCs is the space of Nuel (SN); within SN parts of the phalangeal processes (PP) are seen. The tops of PP form part of the reticular lamina and separate and hold in place the hair cells. *(Chinchilla photographs courtesy of Dr. Ivan Hunter-Duvar, Hospital for Sick Children, Toronto)*

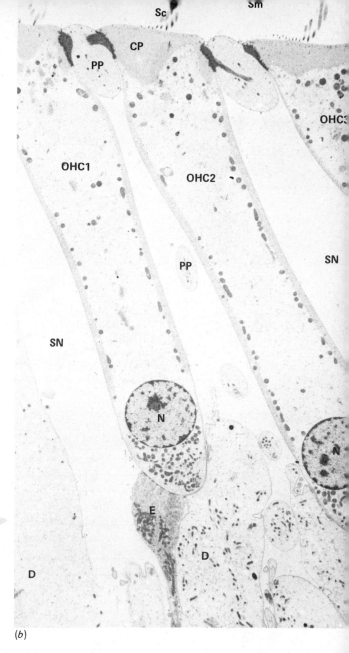

(b)

body lies at the bottom of the W, toward the stria vascularis. The tips of the tallest row of cilia of each outer hair cell are in contact with a structure of colorless fibers, known as the *tectorial membrane* (Fig. 5.10). The tectorial membrane is a soft, ribbonlike structure, attached along one edge to the spiral limbus and perhaps attached along the other edge to the outer border of the organ of Corti (near the supporting cells).

The photographs of the inner ear anatomy used in this chapter were taken by means of various photomicroscopic techniques. The reader will find Appendix C helpful in understanding how these photographs were made with different types of microscopes.

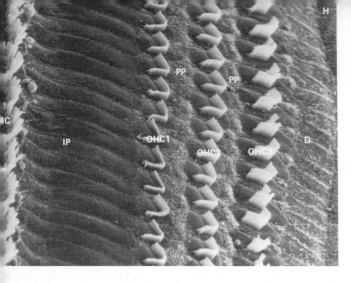

Figure 5.8 Scanning electron micrograph of the top of the organ of Corti, with the tectorial membrane removed to expose the stereocilia of the inner and outer hair cells. One row of inner hair cells and three rows of outer hair cells are clearly seen. Between the inner and outer hair cells, the heads of the inner pillar cells (IP) are seen. Between the tops of the rows of outer hair cells, the tops of the phalangeal processes (PP) are seen. The supporting cells of Deiters (D) and Hensen (H) are at the outer edge. Note that the W formation of the stereocilia of the outer hair cells is slanted in relation to the inner hair cells and is slightly different for each row. *(Chinchilla photograph courtesy of Dr. Ivan Hunter-Duvar, Hospital for Sick Children, Toronto)*

Figure 5.9 **5.9a:** Scanning electron micrograph showing the stereocilia (Sc) of an inner hair cell (IHC) in detail. Also shown: the head of an inner pillar cell (IP) and some small cilia called microcilia (m). **5.9b:** Scanning electron micrograph showing the stereocilia (Sc) of an outer hair cell (OHC) in detail. In both photographs, the graduation in size of the stereocilia is clearly seen. *(Chinchilla photographs courtesy of Dr. Ivan Hunter-Duvar, Hospital for Sick Children, Toronto)*

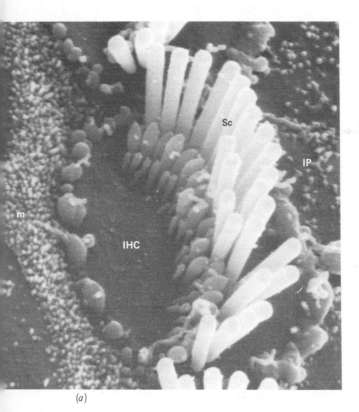

(a)

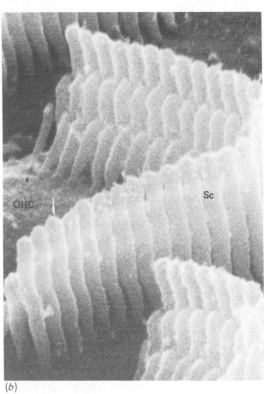

(b)

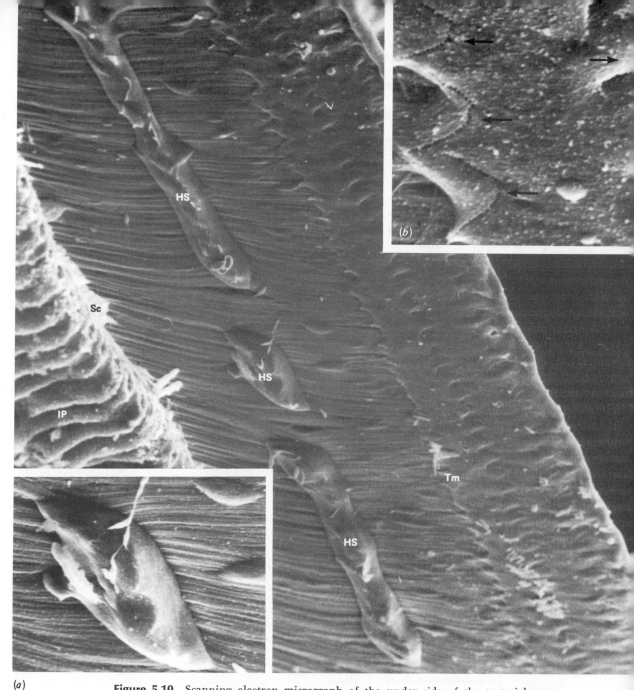

(a)

(b)

Figure 5.10 Scanning electron micrograph of the under side of the tectorial membrane (Tm). The inner pillar cells (IP) of the tunnel of Corti and the stereocilia (Sc) of the inner hair cells are shown at left for reference. The inserts, further magnified, show: **5.10a:** Hensen's stripe (HS); **5.10b:** the W imprint of the tallest row of stereocilia for each outer hair cell. These imprints are evidence that the stereocilia of the outer hair cells are in contact with the tectorial membrane. There are no imprints in the tectorial membrane corresponding to the stereocilia of the inner hair cells. (*Chinchilla photograph courtesy of Dr. Ivan Hunter-Duvar, Hospital for Sick Children, Toronto*)

MECHANICAL RESPONSE OF THE INNER EAR

The vibratory patterns representing the acoustic message reach the inner ear via the stapes. As we have seen, the stapes moves the oval window, which leads into a fluid-filled system (cochlea) that contains the cochlear sac. Within the cochlear sac at the organ of Corti these vibratory undulations contain the information that must be coded into neural information. One of the key factors in this process is the mechanical response of the basilar membrane and the organ of Corti. Here we shall refer to the basilar membrane instead of the whole cochlear sac; since its vibratory patterns are more easily illustrated, it is usually the structure discussed.

The general function of the cochlea, and hence of the basilar membrane, is to translate the mechanical vibrations of the stapes and the inner ear fluids into neural responses in the auditory branch of the eighth cranial nerve. The auditory nerve interacts with the hair cells by way of synaptic junctions, and the hair cells are attached to the basilar membrane by the supporting cells. Thus the vibration of the fluids causes the basilar membrane to move, which in turn causes the cilia of the hair cells to bend. The bending of the cilia somehow causes the nerve at the base of the hair cell to initiate a neural potential, which is sent along the auditory nerve. Thus the hair cells, in connection with the basilar membrane, translate mechanical information into neural information.

Most of the work that demonstrates the importance of the vibration of the basilar membrane was done by von Bekesy, using both direct observation of the cochlea and cochlear models. By very careful and tedious experimentation von Bekesy was able to determine which physical factors of the cochlea affect the vibratory pattern of the basilar membrane. Changing the elasticity of the round window or the length of the cochlear canals did not affect the vibratory pattern of the basilar membrane. Even altering the position of the stapes and changing the fluid did not produce any variation from the vibratory pattern of the normal model. Thus the vibratory pattern of the basilar membrane remains very stable under a number of conditions. This implies that the vibratory pattern must depend heavily on the characteristics of the basilar membrane itself—that is, the changes in elasticity and width discussed previously.

We shall now discuss in some detail the motion of the basilar membrane and how this motion bends the cilia of the hair cells. In particular, we shall determine how the frequency and intensity of an auditory stimulus affect this movement.

Each point along the basilar membrane that is set in motion vibrates at the same frequency as the stimulus. However, the amplitude of the membrane vibration is different at different locations, depending on frequency and intensity of the input stimulus. In a sense, a wave motion is set up along the membrane as the fluids in the inner ear are driven by the stapes.

Since the basilar membrane becomes wider as the distance from the stapes to the helicotrema increases and since its flaccidity also increases toward the helicotrema, the natural period of vibration of the basilar membrane decreases toward the helicotrema. Because of the variation in stiffness, *different frequencies will cause maximum vibration amplitude at different points along the membrane.* If two different frequencies are received by the cochlea simultaneously, they will each create maximum displacement at different points along the basilar membrane. This separation of a complex signal into different maximal points of displacement along the basilar membrane, corresponding to the sinusoids of which the complex signal is composed, means that the basilar membrane is performing like a series of bandpass filters (Chap. 3).

The response of the membrane is a *traveling wave*. The wave motion of the membrane appears to travel toward the helicotrema. The pressure of the sound is distributed immediately throughout the cochlea because the stapes is transmitting the pressure variations to a relatively incompressible fluid environment. An example of the vibratory pattern along the membrane that is "frozen" or stopped at an instant in time is called an *instantaneous waveform*. Figure 5.11 shows a representation of two instantaneous waveforms of the traveling wave along the basilar membrane. This figure presents a more realistic representation than usual because the basilar membrane is shown attached at its two edges and is displaced or bent in response to sound in a transverse (medial or crosswise) direction as well as in the longitudinal direction. Most instantaneous waveforms of basilar membrane displacement are shown as if Figure 5.11a were viewed from the side, the basilar membrane

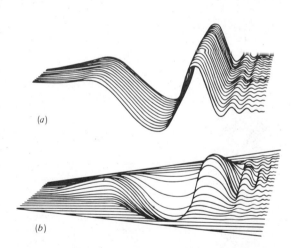

(a)

(b)

Figure 5.11 Instantaneous waveform of a traveling wave along the basilar membrane. 5.11a: The waveform that would result if the membrane were ribbon-like. 5.11b: The membrane vibration illustrated more realistically; since the basilar membrane is attached along both edges, it must vibrate in a radial or transverse direction, as in 5.11b. *(Adapted from Tonndorf, 1960, by permission)*

being represented as a single line (see Fig. 5.12). One should always keep in mind that the condition shown in Figure 5.11b is more accurate. Figure 5.12 shows a number of instantaneous waveforms in successive temporal order (1–4) for a sinusoidal input. That is, curve 1 shows the basilar membrane displacement for the first instant in time, curve 2 shows the next instant in time, and so on. These instantaneous waveforms indicate that one part of the basilar membrane may be displaced toward scala tympani, while at the same time an adjacent part may be deflected in the opposite direction. This is also obvious in Figure 5.11. This difference in direction of displacement can be viewed as a phase difference between the vibratory pattern of two adjacent portions of the membrane. This phase difference is greater in the apical portion of the wave than in the basal portion.

If a line is drawn through the points of maximum displacement for each point along the membrane for a specific traveling wave, the resulting curve is the *envelope* of the traveling wave. The envelope of the maximum points of positive and negative displacement of the traveling wave of Figure 5.12 are illustrated as the solid line; however many illustrations of the envelope of the traveling wave show only the positive envelope. Figure 5.13 is a schematic representation of the cochlea and the envelope of the traveling wave that would occur for stimuli of three different frequencies. An instantaneous waveform is also shown for each frequency. Notice that the maximum point of displacement, as indicated by the maximum of the envelope, is different for each frequency. For the lowest frequency (60 Hz) the maximum displacement is near the apical end, for the highest frequency (2 kHz) the maximum displacement is near the base, and the intermediate frequency has its maximum between the other two. This relationship between point of maximum displacement and frequency is further depicted in

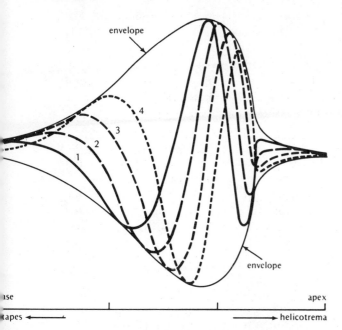

base   apex

stapes ←   → helicotrema

Figure 5.12 Four successive instantaneous wave-forms (1–4) of a traveling wave. The envelope (solid line) of the traveling wave formed by connecting all the points of maximum amplitude along the membrane is also shown. *(Adapted from Ranke, 1942, by permission)*

Figure 5.14. Figures 5.13 and 5.14 also illustrate another important point—that lower frequency stimulation will stimulate not only the basal end of the membrane but also the apical end, where the point of maximum displacement occurs. Higher frequencies, however, stimulate only the basal end of the cochlea. As shown by the envelopes of the traveling waves created by high-frequency stimulation, the amount of displacement apical to the point of maximum displacement is reduced rapidly. In contrast, the amount of displacement basal to the point of maximum displacement is reduced slowly in a basal direction for all frequencies and extends completely to the base. An unusual feature of the traveling-wave motion of the basilar membrane is that it *always* starts in the base and travels toward the apex. In most natural situations where traveling waves

are found, the wave motion is in a direction away from the driving force. If the placement of the driving force is changed, the direction of the wave motion is similarly altered. The driving force in the cochlea is the stapes motion, and the wave motion does travel away from the stapes as expected. The unusual feature is that if the stapes is placed at the apical end, the motion of the traveling wave would still start in the base end and travel toward the apex. The fact that the direction of

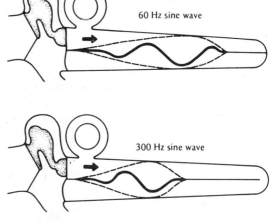

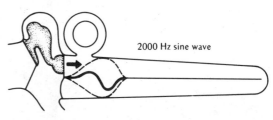

Figure 5.13 Instantaneous waveforms and envelopes of traveling waves of three different frequencies shown on a schematic diagram of the cochlea. Note that the point of maximum displacement, as shown by the high point of the envelope, is near the apex for low frequencies and near the base for higher frequencies. Also, note that low frequencies stimulate the apical end as well as the basal end, but that displacement from higher frequencies is confined to the base. *(Adapted from Zemlin, 1968, by permission)*

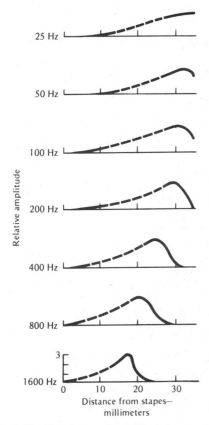

Figure 5.14 Envelopes of traveling waves of seven different frequencies, showing that the point of maximum displacement shifts toward the stapes as frequency increases. Solid lines represent von Bekesy's measurements, and the dotted lines are estimates of the envelopes. *(Von Bekesy, 1943, by permission)*

the wave motion would not change with the change in driver placement is called the *traveling-wave paradox*. We may conclude then that the traveling wave always travels from the base toward the apex. How far toward the apex it travels depends on the frequency of stimulation; lower frequencies travel farther.

If we measure the phase relationship between the stapes and the various locations along the basilar membrane for various frequencies of stimulation, we can calculate the time it takes for the traveling wave to "travel"

to a particular location on the membrane. Figure 5.15 shows the phase shift between a point on the membrane (horizontal axis) and the motion of the stapes. For instance, a 200-Hz tone will set up a vibration that moves in phase with the stapedial motion at 20 mm from the stapes. At about 27 mm from the stapes the vibration from the 200-Hz tone is 180° out of phase with the stapes. Since a 200-Hz tone has a 5-ms period, the 180° phase shift indicates that the vibration at 27 mm from the stapes occurs 2.5 ms (that is, one-half period) after the stapes moves. That is, the time delay between displacement at the apex and that at the base (or stapes) results in a phase shift along the cochlear partition for various frequencies. The amount of phase shift depends on the frequency of the stimulus since the time delay from base to apex is constant. In addition, the membrane displacement increases as the intensity of the sound is increased.

 In trying to visualize these traveling-wave patterns we should keep in mind some of the basic characteristics of the basilar membrane. *First, the basal end of the basilar membrane responds best to high-frequency stimulation, but it can also respond to low-frequency stimulation. The apical end of the basilar membrane vibrates only to low-frequency stimulation. Furthermore, there is a time lag between the stapes movement and the movement of the apical end of the basilar membrane.* Thus high-frequency stimulation causes maximum displacement in the basal end of the membrane. Low-frequency stimulation causes the basal end to vibrate first, with a small displacement.

With a constant, moderately intense input a particular location along the basilar membrane will be displaced maximally by only one frequency. It is also true that for that particular location the basilar membrane will be displaced by frequencies lower than the one that displaces it maximally. In contrast, higher

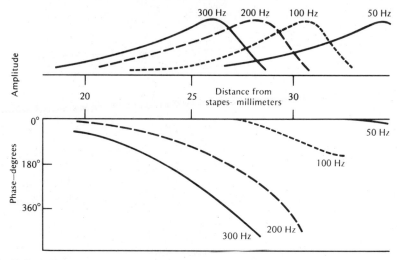

Figure 5.15 Above: envelopes of traveling waves of four different frequencies. Below: the phase shift in degrees between the motion of the stapes and a point on the basilar membrane. By calculating the period of the sinusoid and the amount of phase shift, one can calculate the time for the traveling wave to "travel" to a particular point on the membrane. See text for an example. *(Adapted from von Bekesy, 1947b, by permission)*

frequencies will displace that location on the membrane only a little, if at all, even at high intensities. From our discussion of filters in Chapter 3 it can be seen that a given location along the basilar membrane acts as a filter with a sharp high-frequency roll-off. That is, a location along the basilar membrane will pass (or vibrate to) only frequencies below a given value. Since lower frequencies progressively displace the membrane less and less at that location, that location also has a gradual low-frequency roll-off. Thus a particular location along the basilar membrane acts as a band-pass filter of the vibrating motion. This filter has a sharp high-frequency roll-off and a very gradual low-frequency roll-off for a constant, moderately intense input. We might expect that the neural output of the cochlea would reflect this filtering characteristic of the basilar membrane. In Chapter 6, we examine this neural output, and the band-pass filtering characteristics described above will be seen in the discharges of the individual nerves that leave the cochlea (see Fig. 6.17).

HOW THE TRAVELING WAVE EXCITES THE HAIR CELLS

Situated at the top of the organ of Corti is the tectorial membrane, which runs parallel to the basilar membrane. When the basilar membrane vibrates, the tectorial membrane must also move, but there is an important difference in the motion of the two membranes due to differences in their support. As shown in Figure 5.16, the tectorial membrane is hinged on one end at the spiral limbus, whereas the modiolar edge of the basilar membrane is thought to be hinged on the osseous spiral lamina. As the basilar and tectorial membranes are displaced, they pivot about the two different hinging points, and the indicated shearing forces are created. To get a "feel" for this shearing force, try to model the two membranes with your hands. Put your right hand palm up, and place your left hand on it palm down. Slide your right hand forward so that the fingers of the right hand extend about ½ inch further than those of the left. Now, keep-

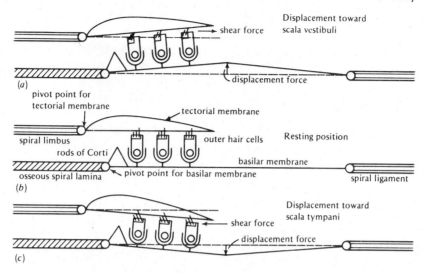

Figure 5.16 Schematic diagrams of shearing forces created between the hair cells and the tectorial membrane as a result of basilar membrane displacement. **5.16a:** Shearing force that results from displacement of the basilar membrane toward the scala vestibuli. **5.16b:** Relationship between hair cells and tectorial membrane with no stimulation. **5.16c:** Shearing forces in the direction opposite to that in 5.16a for displacement in the opposite direction. The shearing of the cilia is thought to activate the neurons at the base of the hair cells. *(Adapted from Zemlin, 1968, by permission)*

ing your palms still and your fingers stiff, move the fingers of both hands up and down simultaneously, and you can feel the shearing forces in your fingers. The effect of these shearing forces on the cilia is thought to be the stimulation of the nerve fibers at the base of the outer hair cells. Thus mechanical energy is transduced into electrochemical activity by the hair cells. At present we do not fully understand how the mechanical shearing of the cilia triggers the nerve impulse. In the next chapter we shall discuss the anatomical relationship between the hair cells and the nerve fibers. Then we shall describe the response of the nerve fibers to variations in frequency and intensity of sound. By comparing these neural responses to the mechanical motion of the basilar membrane we can obtain some insight into how the cochlea transforms the hydromechanical events described in this chapter into neural impulses.

Summary The main part of the three inner ear structures is the cochlea, which is divided into three sections: scala vestibuli, scala media, scala tympani (by the basilar membrane and Reissner's membrane). The scala vestibuli and scala tympani contain the fluid perilymph, and the scala media contains endolymph. The basilar membrane is supported on the modiolar side by the osseous spiral lamina and on the stria vascularis side by the spiral ligament. The basilar membrane is wider, more flaccid, and under no tension at the apical end. The base end is narrower and stiffer than the apical end and may be under a small amount of tension. In the scala media is the organ of Corti. On the inner (modiolar) side of the tunnel of Corti are the inner hair cells. On the outer side of the tunnel of Corti are the three rows of outer hair cells; their cilia are in contact with the tectorial membrane. The hair cells and nerve fibers are held in place by supporting cells. The basilar membrane has a traveling-wave motion when excited by the stapes. The traveling wave yields maximal displacement only at the base for high-frequency stimuli and maximal displacement, after a time delay, at the apex for low-frequency stimulation. Intensity variations cause variations in amount of displacement of the basilar membrane. The differential motion of the basilar and tectorial membranes results in a shearing motion of the cilia of the hair cells, which in turn triggers the nerve fibers.

Supplement

There are several summaries of the anatomy of the inner ear. Some of the more recent take advantage of the scanning electron photomicrographs and therefore offer a pictorial presentation that cannot be equaled by the earlier methods (Ades and Engstrom, 1972, 1974; Angelborg and Engstrom, 1973; Bredberg, 1968; Engstrom and Ades, 1975; and Lim, 1969). In addition to these more recent works, one should read some of the older classical investigations referred to in the newer works to get a full appreciation of the anatomy of the inner ear. In addition, Iurato's (1967) book, *Submicroscopic Structure of the Inner Ear,* and Vinnikov and Titova's (1964) book *The Organ of Corti: Its Histophysiology and Histochemistry* are highly recommended.

Von Bekesy is the person most responsible for our understanding of the vibratory characteristics of the basilar membrane. Much of his work is summarized in his book *Experiments in Hearing* (1960). This book is an invaluable source of information for the serious student of audition. A good discussion of cochlear mechanics and hydrodynamics is given by Tonndorf (1970). An excellent summary of the traveling wave and its measurement by modern methods of laser light and Mössbauer methods is given by Eldredge (1974). For the reader who has some math and/or engineering background, a thorough discussion of cochlear mechanics can be found in Dallos (1973). In addition to von Bekesy's work, investigations of the traveling wave have been performed by Fletcher (1953), Kohlloffel (1972a–c), Johnstone et al. (1970), Johnstone and Boyle (1967), Peterson and Bogert (1950), Rhode (1971), Tonndorf (1959), Wever et al. (1954), and Zwislocki (1965). There are a number of films that show the traveling wave in a manner that a textbook cannot hope to replicate. The most readily available is an excellent film by the Bell Telephone Company, "Simulated Basilar Membrane Motion." For historical reasons, another excellent film is "Pendulums, Traveling Waves and the Cochlea," which was produced by von Bekesy and R. L. Grason while they were at the psychoacoustics laboratory of Harvard University.

The basilar membrane performs a filtering and distribution function by acting as a filter and by distributing maximal displacements at various places along the membrane according to the frequency of stimuli. Sitting on the basilar membrane is the complicated organ of Corti. Its function is to transduce the mechanical hydrodynamic undulations into neural impulses in some manner that is meaningful to the central nervous system. Because of its smallness, inaccessibility, and fragility, the organ of Corti is extremely hard to investigate in a systematic fashion. For instance, although it is well agreed that the tallest row of cilia of the outer hair cells are in contact with the tectorial membrane, it is still controversial as to whether the cilia of the inner hair cells touch the tectorial membrane. It is also controversial as to whether the tectorial membrane is attached to the organ of Corti at its outer edge (toward stria vascularis). Recent investigations have suggested that in newborn kittens the tectorial membrane is firmly attached to the Deiters' cells, but in adult cats it is less firmly attached, if at all (Lindeman and Bredberg, 1972). The following articles deal with these important questions of the microanatomy of the organ of Corti (Engstrom et al., 1962, 1966, 1970; Hilding, 1952; Iurato, 1962; Kimura, 1966; Lim, 1972; Lindeman and Bredberg, 1972; Naftalin et al., 1964; Tonndorf et al., 1962). These missing facts are crucial to explanations about how the organ of Corti performs its task. The careful reader will notice that in this chapter we have discussed the shearing motion of the tectorial membrane only on the outer hair cells and that the discussion is intentionally vague. The problem is that no one knows exactly how the hair cells are stimulated. Especially controversial are the inner hair cells. Some have proposed that the inner hair cells are stimulated by the subtectorial fluids; others have postulated tectorial membrane shearing forces. Lack of this fundamental knowledge makes for a fertile area of research at this time. The literature in this area (Billone and Raynor, 1973; Dallos et al., 1972; Davis et al., 1950; Helle, 1974; Steele, 1973; Wever, 1971; and Zwislocki and Sokolich, 1973) should be read critically. However, a thorough understanding of Chapters 5 and 6 is suggested before attempting it.

SUMMARY OF INNER EAR MEASUREMENTS

Since most of the experimental work on the inner ear has been performed with animals, both animal and human data are listed. The principal sources for these data are Angelborg and Engstrom (1973), Rauch and Rauch (1974), Spoendlin (1966), and Wever and Lawrence (1954). These sources are often secondary, so the data given here actually represent the results of measurements by many authors.

Oval Window

dimensions: 1.2×3 mm to 2.0×3.7 mm   *human*
area: 1.12–1.27 mm², mean = 1.20 mm²   *cat*
mean: 1.4 mm²   *guinea pig*

Round Window

dimensions: 2.25×1.0 mm   *human*
area: 2 mm²   *human*
    3 mm²   *cat*
    1 mm²   *guinea pig*

Cochlea

number of turns: 2⅝ *human*
volume: 98.1 mm³ (including the vestibule proper) *human*
length of cochlear channels: 35 mm *human*

Helicotrema

area: 0.08–0.04 mm² *human*

Basilar Membrane

length: 25.3–35.5 mm, mean = 34 mm *human*
　　　19.4–25.4 mm, mean = 22.5 *cat*
　　　mean = 18.8 mm *guinea pig*
width, basal end: 0.04–0.08 mm *human*
　　　　　　0.062 mm *guinea pig*
width, apical end: 0.423–0.651 mm, mean = 0.05 *human*
　　　　　　　0.194–0.240 mm, mean = 0.209 mm *guinea pig*

Organ of Corti

cross-sectional area, basal end: 0.00053 mm² *human*
　　　　　　　　　　　0.0055 mm² *cat*
cross-sectional area, apical end: 0.0223 mm² *human*
　　　　　　　　　　　0.0201 mm² *cat*

Outer Hair Cells

number: 12,000 *human*
cell body length: 20 Å (basal end), 50 Å (apical end) *human*
cell body width: 5 Å *human*
cilium width: 0.05 Å at its base to 0.2 Å at tip *human*
cilium length: 2 Å in basal turn, 6 Å in apical turn *human*
arrangement: 100–150 sterocilia per outer hair cell *human*
　　　cilia 6–7 rows in W or V pattern per outer hair cell *human*
　　　cilia 3 rows in W or V pattern per outer hair cell *cat and guinea pig*
　　　cilia of outermost row have tips embedded in the tectorial membrane;
　　　　angle in V shape 120° in the basal turn and 60° in the apical turn

Inner Hair Cells

number: 3500 *human*
　　　2600 *cat*
arrangement: 40–60 cilia per cell arranged in a shallow U shape, 2–4 rows of
　　　cilia per cell, length of cilia longer in apical turn than in basal turn,
　　　lengths and diameters vary among individual coils of the cochlea, and
　　　within a single cell

Spiral Ligament

　cross-sectional area: 0.543 mm² near basal end, 0.042 mm² at the apex *human*

Scala Vestibuli

volume: 54 mm³ including vestibule proper   *human*

Scala Tympani

volume: 37.4 mm³   *human*

Cochlear Duct

volume: 6.7 mm³   *human*
length: 35 mm   *human*

Perilymph

volume: scala vestibuli, 10–15 μl   *human*
        scala tympani, 6–8 μl   *human*
        total, 16–23 μl   *human*
volume: scala vestibuli, 15.6 μl   *cat*
        scala tympani, 9.3 μl   *cat*
        total, 24.9 μl   *cat*
K+ concentration: 4 meq/liter* (scala vestibuli)   *human*
Na+ concentration: 139 meq/liter (scala vestibuli)   *human*
pH: 7.4–7.8   *human;* 7.9   *guinea pig;* 7.3–7.87   *cat*
viscosity: 1.030–1.050, in relation to H_2O at 27°C = 1   *human* (at 27°C)
surface tension: 49.6 dynes/cm   *guinea pig* (at 23°C)
protein: 70–100 mg/100 ml   *human*
      142 mg/100 ml   *cat*
      70–107 mg/100 ml   *guinea pig*

Endolymph

volume: scala media, 2.7 μl   *human*
K+ concentration: 144 meq/liter   *human*
Na+ concentration: 13 meq/liter   *human*
pH: 7.5   *human* (postmortem); 7.4   *guinea pig;* 7.82   *cat*
viscosity: saccule, 1.030–1.050 in relation to H_2O at 27°C = 1   *human* (at 27°C)
surface tension: 52 dynes/cm   *guinea pig* (at 23°C)
protein: 20–30 mg/100 ml   *human*
      118 mg/100 ml   *cat*
      25 mg/100 ml   *guinea pig*

* Meq/liter: milliequivalents per liter.

CHAPTER 6

Electrophysiology of the Peripheral Auditory Nervous System

Cochlear Potentials
Structure of the Auditory Nerve
Function of the Afferent Auditory Nerve
Function of the Efferent System
Encoding of Frequency and Intensity

In Chapter 5 we emphasized the importance of the hair cell—the biological transducer for the auditory system. The mechanical shearing of the cilia results in neural discharges in the VIIIth (or auditory) nerve. Within the inner ear are many electric potential differences that may play a role in the transduction of mechanical energy into neural energy. Our purpose in this chapter is to describe these cochlear potentials and then to explain the function of the auditory nerve and its connections within the cochlea. We are particularly interested in determining how the frequency selectivity found along the basilar membrane is preserved or modified by the auditory nerve.

COCHLEAR POTENTIALS

The intricate motions and interactions of the various cochlear structures generate electric potentials which are relatively easy to study. Whether or not all of these potentials actually play an important role in the transduction process in an unanswered question. Even if they are nonfunctional by-products of the mechanics of the inner ear, they are of interest since they yield information about the cochlear transduction process. Four potentials can be recorded from the cochlea:

1. The resting potentials, which are dc (direct-current or nonalternating potentials), that exist without acoustic stimulation (see Appendix D).
2. The summating potential (SP), which is also dc, but appears only during acoustic stimulation.
3. The cochlear microphonic (CM), which is an ac (alternating-current) potential difference that appears only during acoustic stimulation.
4. The action potential (AP), which is also an ac potential difference, but is generated by the nerves rather than in the structures of the inner ear.

Each of these potentials is discussed in more detail below. In general, the potentials in the cochlea as well as those of the VIIIth nerve are measured with very small wire electrodes or glass micropipettes, as shown in Figure 6.1. The electrode measures the electric potential at the site of its penetration relative to some reference site. The reference site might be another part of the auditory system or, more often, a neutral location such as a neck muscle. Thus the potentials are the differences in electric charge between two points, for instance between points A and B in Figure 6.1.

Resting Potentials

Three dc potentials can be observed in the resting (as well as in the responding) cochlea. The one of greatest significance is the endocochlear or endolymphatic potential (EP). The

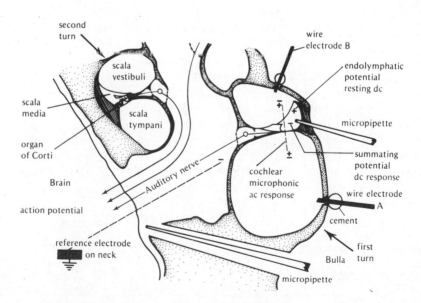

Figure 6.1 Drawing of a mid-modiolar section of the first and second turns of the guinea pig cochlea. The wire electrodes produce differential recordings of the CM, AP, and SP from the first turn. One glass micropipette records the EP, CM, and SP from the scala media of the first turn; the other records single neurons of the auditory nerve as they exit from the modiolus. (*Adapted from Davis, 1956, by permission*)

EP is located in the endolymph of the scala media (SM). The EP is about +80 millivolts (mV); that is, the electric charge in the scala media of a normal resting cochlea is 80 mV above 0 mV. This is the highest positive resting potential found in the body, and it is not found in the endolymph of the vestibular system despite the fact that the endolymph is continuous in both structures. This can be explained if the source of the EP is the stria vascularis, which is located on the wall of the cochlear duct but is not present in the other endolymphatic spaces of the inner ear. The exact function of the EP is not known. Since the hair cells have an intracellular resting potential of about –70 mV, the +80 mV of the endolymph makes the potential difference across the top of the hair cells about 150 mV, an extremely high potential difference to be found in the body. Because of this large potential difference it is thought that the EP could serve to increase the size of the electrical response of the hair cells. Damage to the stria vascularis will result in the loss, or decrease, of the EP, and without the EP the inner ear will not perform the mechanical to electrical transduction process.

In addition to the EP and the intracellular resting potentials of the organ of Corti, there is a third resting potential of unknown significance so far as its origin and function are concerned. A small dc potential difference is found between the scala vestibuli and the scala tympani, of about +2 to 5 mV, relative to the scala tympani. Figure 6.2 shows the resting potentials of the three scalae of the cochlea.

Summating Potential (SP)

The summating potential (SP) is a stimulus-related dc electrical response recorded from the cochlea. There is a baseline shift in the potentials recorded from the cochlea whenever a stimulus is present, as shown in Figure 6.3. Until recently the SP was considered a "high-

intensity, high-frequency" phenomenon. Recently experimenters who have attempted to quantify the SP have found it to be comprised of different potentials, which interact in a complicated manner. Thus we are not certain of the exact source of the SP, although six sources have been listed as possibilities.

Cochlear Microphonic (CM)

The CM is an ac potential that occurs only during the presentation of an acoustic stimulus. If the ear is stimulated with a 500-Hz pure tone of moderate intensity, the CM will appear as a 500-Hz electrical sine wave. In other words, the electric potential difference in the cochlea oscillates in the same manner as the driving stimulus. From observations of its growth and shape, it appears that over a fairly wide range of sound intensities the CM faithfully reflects the intensity and frequency components of the sound input. If the sound intensity becomes too high, however, the voltage increase of the CM stabilizes and then decreases in magnitude. The reason for this decrease in CM at high intensities is not known. Figure 6.4 is one example of the growth of the level of the CM output as a function of the level of the input sinusoid. Such intensity curves are sometimes called *input-output functions*. Repeated or lengthy stimulation at extreme intensity levels results in either temporary or permanent impairment of hair cell function, which is clearly manifest in a decline in CM output. Consequently, understanding the decline in the input-output function at high intensities may provide clues to preventing impairment of hair cell function due to overstimulation.

The source of the CM is thought to be the cilia-bearing end of the outer hair cells. The most convincing evidence for this notion is an experiment by Tasaki, who inserted a microelectrode up through the organ of Corti from the scala tympani. He found that as the elec-

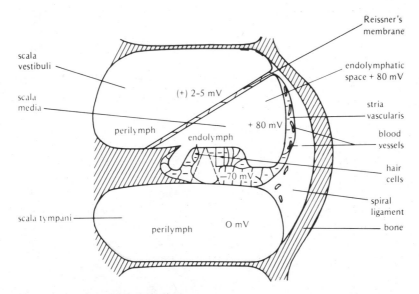

Figure 6.2 Schematic cross section of the cochlea showing resting potentials. The scala vestibuli is 2 to 5 mV more positive than the scala tympani. The scala media has a +80 mV potential called the endocochlear or endolymphatic potential (EP). In sharp contrast to the EP, the intracellular potentials of the organ of Corti are about –70 mV. Thus the potential difference across the top of the hair cells is about 150 mV. *(Adapted from Tasaki, Davis and Eldredge, 1954, by permission)*

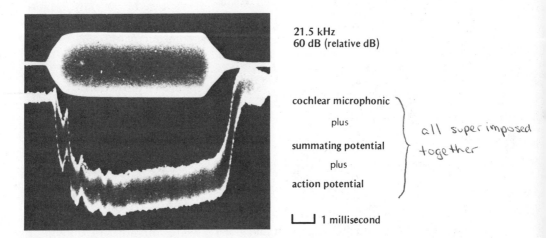

21.5 kHz
60 dB (relative dB)

cochlear microphonic

plus

summating potential

plus

action potential

all superimposed together

⌐_⌐ 1 millisecond

Figure 6.3 The trace above records the stimulus, a 21.5-kHz tone burst. The lower trace is a round-window electrode recording of the response to the stimulus. The downward dc shift of the trace during the presentation of the stimulus is the SP. The section of the recording that replicates the input signal is the CM. The wiggle at the beginning of the response as it begins its downward shift is the AP. The round-window recording technique, therefore, yields a composite response composed of SP, CM, and AP. *(Pestalozza and Davis, 1956, by permission)*

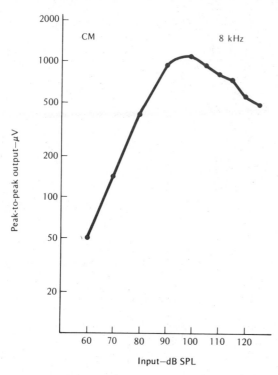

Figure 6.4 Input-output function (or intensity function) for the cochlear microphonic response recorded differentially from the first turn of the guinea pig cochlea (see Fig. 6.1 for electrode placements) to an 8-kHz tone burst. As the sound pressure level (SPL) increases to 90 dB, the CM increases linearly. From 90 to about 100 dB SPL, the CM increases at a slower rate. For this stimulus the CM is largest at about 100 dB SPL and then decreases as the input intensity increases beyond 100 dB SPL.

trode approached the top of the hair cell, the CM became larger and then reversed its electric signal (see Fig. 6.5). That is, if in the scala tympani the CM potential was positive, the CM became negative when the electrode entered the scala media. This growth and polarity reversal of the CM indicates that its generation is at the boundary of the hair cells and the scala media, near the level of the reticular lamina and the roots of the cilia of the hair cells.

The CM may be recorded from various posi-

tions close to the cochlea. The initial technique, which is still used, was to place an electrode on or near the round window. This technique has some characteristics that limit its usefulness. Since an electrode tends to record spatially near potentials better than spatially distant potentials, the *round window electrode* records potentials generated by the hair cells in the first turn (base) of the cochlea but gives little information about potentials generated in the apical end of the cochlea. Another characteristic of this technique is that a single electrode will record any potentials near it; thus even if studying the CM is of prime concern, the CM response will be contaminated by other potentials such as the action potential (AP). Figure 6.3 shows the CM, AP, and the summating potential, which were all recorded simultaneously with a round window electrode.

In order to record from small regions at either end of the cochlea *and* to separate the CM from the AP, the *differential recording* technique is utilized. This technique takes advantage of the shift in polarity of the CM observed by Tasaki (and other investigators) as the microelectrode was advanced up through the organ of Corti. This polarity shift indicates that if the CM is recorded from above the organ of Corti (from scala media or scala vestibuli), it will have an opposite polarity (charge) than when it is recorded from below the organ of Corti, that is, in the scala tympani. In contrast, the AP appears to have the same polarity when electrodes record it in any of the three scalae. The differential technique can take advantage of these differences in polarity to cancel the unwanted signal. If we are interested in studying the CM by the differential technique, we can place one intracochlear electrode in the scala tympani and the other in the scala vestibuli. These electrodes record the CM with opposite polarities but record the remote AP potential with the same polarity. The AP is then canceled by

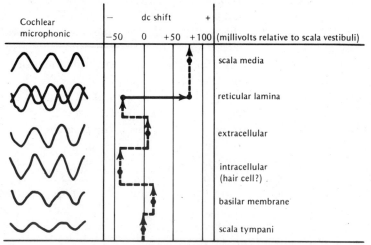

Cochlear microphonic	−	dc shift	+	
	−50	0 +50	+100	(millivolts relative to scala vestibuli)

scala media

reticular lamina

extracellular

intracellular
(hair cell?)

basilar membrane

scala tympani

Penetration of organ of Corti by a microelectrode
with phase reversal of CM at the reticular lamina

Figure 6.5 Microelectrode penetration of the organ of Corti. The electrode approaches the organ of Corti from the scala tympani, where the small sinusoid CM is first recorded as shown at bottom; here there is no added dc shift (0 dc). As the electrode penetrates the basilar membrane, there is a small dc shift and the CM begins to grow. Next, cells in the organ of Corti are penetrated, as indicated by the negative dc shift indicative of intracellular resting potentials. The CM continues to grow and maintains its original phase. Penetrating further, the electrode is thought to be between cells, because the dc shift returns to zero. The electrode then reaches the reticular lamina at the top of the hair cells; at this point the CM abruptly changes phase, as shown by the two CM recordings superimposed, and the dc potential shifts to positive, indicating that the tip has reached the scala media. In the scala media it records the EP and the CM, which has now shifted 180° in phase. (*Adapted from Tasaki, 1954, by permission*)

subtracting the outputs of the two electrodes. This subtraction not only cancels the AP but makes the resultant CM twice its original size. On the other hand, if we want to study the AP, we can simply add the outputs of the two electrodes: the CM will cancel and the AP will remain twice its size.

Another advantage of the differential recording technique is its use in measuring from small areas along the cochlear partition. The same technique of subtraction that cancels the AP also cancels CMs generated at a remote location. The differential electrodes record the nearer potentials better than the distant potentials simply on the basis of proximity. In addition, the differential electrodes can cancel the

remotely generated CM by subtraction, thereby limiting the area being recorded along the cochlear duct. Thus the differential electrode technique permits the measurement of cochlear activity at relatively discrete locations along the cochlear partition.

Von Bekesy has demonstrated that the *intensity of the CM is proportional to the displacement of the basilar membrane*. This fact, together with the ability to record from small areas along the cochlear partition by the differential electrode technique, has led to the electrophysiological investigation of the motion of the basilar membrane by means of the CM. That is, the CM can be used to measure the displacement action of the basilar membrane. Tasaki and his colleagues in 1952 first took advantage of these techniques by using guinea pigs, which have a cochlea that will allow placement of differential electrodes in each of their four turns. The first turn of the spiral cochlea is the base and the fourth, the apex. The outputs of the second, third, and fourth turns were compared with that of the first turn with respect to both amplitude and phase of the CM as a function of frequency. The resultant space-time pattern of the CM revealed a traveling wave that moved toward the apex to a location dependent on the frequency of the stimulus. The pattern agreed well with the mechanical movement observed by von Bekesy in his models. That is, the apical end of the cochlea responded to only low frequencies, but the basal end responded to all frequencies. Figure 6.6 shows that a low-frequency (500-Hz) tone generates a CM in all turns of the cochlea, along the entire basilar membrane. However, the amplitude of the CM is greatest at the apex (third turn), and a phase shift occurs (180° at 500 Hz) between the first-turn (base) recording and the third-turn recording. A high-frequency tone (8000 Hz), however, generates a CM only in the first turn (base) of the cochlea. This agrees exactly with von Bekesy's measurements of the traveling wave discussed in Chapter 5. Thus, even with the recent developments of laser light and Mössbauer techniques, the CM remains (with certain limitations) a useful tool for studying the traveling-wave motion of the cochlear sac to a wide range of intensities and frequencies of stimulation.

Action Potential (AP)

The whole nerve action potential (AP), unlike the other potentials discussed, is not a true cochlear potential, although it can be recorded from the cochlea. The AP is the sum of the action potentials of many individual neurons, which are firing nearly simulta-neously within the auditory nerve. Since stimulation of the individual neurons depends on the shearing forces of the hair cells created by the traveling-wave displacement of the basilar membrane, neurons that innervate the base of the cochlea will be stimulated at an earlier point in time than those at the apex. The time difference is the length of time it takes for the traveling wave to move from the base to the apex (that is, 2.5 to 4 ms, depending on the species and the measuring technique). This situation creates a general asynchrony of discharge among the individual neurons, which terminate at different points along the cochlea. Since each neuronal dis-

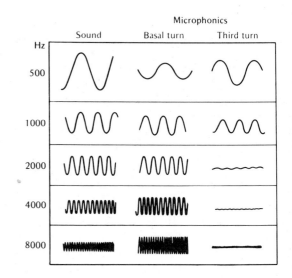

Figure 6.6 Cochlear microphonics recorded differentially from the first and third turns of the guinea pig cochlea. Rows: responses to the various frequencies. Column 1: acoustic stimulus. Columns 2 and 3: CM from turns I and III. For 500 HZ the CM is recorded from both turns; the 500 Hz CM, however, is larger in turn III than in turn I. Also, the 500 Hz CM shifts 180° out of phase between turns I and III because of the time taken by the traveling wave of displacement to reach turn III. For the highest frequency stimulus used (8000 Hz), the response only in turn I indicates that the traveling wave does not reach turn III. *(Adapted from Davis, 1960, by permission)*

charge consists of potentials with both positive and negative values that vary in time, the potentials tend to cancel each other partially when added. At the onset of a click, or of a high-frequency tone burst with a sudden onset, however, only the basal end of the cochlea is stimulated initially, and the discharge of the neurons in the basal turn of the cochlea is synchronous. This almost simultaneous discharge of a large number of neurons in the base is then followed by less synchronous nerve impulses from more apical locations of the cochlear partition. The sum of the initial synchronous discharge of the nerve impulses to an abrupt high-frequency tone burst or click is the part of the AP usually measured. The AP is negative at first and then positive, and it is usually followed by a later negative component arising from the nerves which innervate the more apical portions of the cochlea, and possibly other, more central, sources of potentials. Figure 6.3 shows the waveform of an AP superimposed on the CM.

The most widely used stimulus for AP studies is the click (see Fig. 1.12c for a description of a click). Clicks may be classified as either rarefaction or condensation. In Chapter 2 we discussed the rarefaction and condensation of air molecules. A *rarefaction click* is simply a click stimulus that initially creates a rarefaction of air molecules in front of the tympanic membrane. Thus the initial motion of the tympanic membrane is outward (lateral). The *condensation click* has the opposite initial action, and the tympanic membrane's initial motion is inward (medial). Figure 6.7 shows AP input-output functions for these two types of clicks. The amplitude curves show differences between the two types. Though the reason for the differences between the AP responses for these two types of clicks is not known, these results are often interpreted in terms of an explanation that there are two excitatory mechanisms for the neural response, and they operate in different intensity ranges.

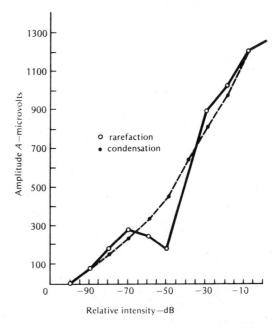

Figure 6.7 Input-output functions showing changes in amplitude of the first peak of the AP to rarefaction and condensation click stimuli. The differences in response to these two stimuli appear to be a function of intensity. *(Adapted from Peak and Kiang, 1962, by permission)*

Within the limitations we have mentioned (that is, the overwhelming contribution of the basal turn) the AP reflects grossly the output of the cochlea. Since the input-output function and waveshape of the AP from a normal cochlea are known, deviations from normative data can be used as indications of cochlear dysfunction. This is particularly important because of our present ability to record the AP from humans.

STRUCTURE OF THE AUDITORY NERVE

In our discussion of the anatomy and physiology of the auditory system, we have established that the basilar membrane performs a type of frequency selectivity via the traveling

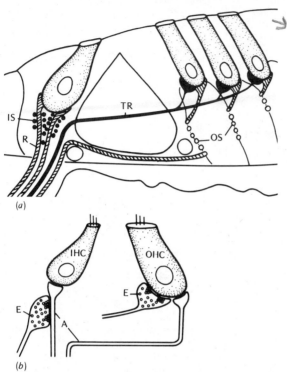

(a)

(b)

Figure 6.8 **6.8a:** Schematic diagram of different groups of nerve fibers in a cross section of the organ of Corti. The afferents (A) are shown lightly shaded; the efferents (E) are shown in black. R: afferent radial fibers which compose 95 percent of the afferent neurons and innervate the inner hair cells; OS: remaining afferent fibers called outer spiral fibers because they follow the spiral of the cochlea before terminating at the base of the outer hair cells; IS: inner spiral fibers which compose 20 percent of the efferent system; these fibers run longitudinally under the inner hair cells; TR: tunnel radial fibers which compose 80 percent of the efferent system. **6.8b:** Schematic diagram of the manner in which the efferents synapse on the afferents below the inner hair cells (IHC). Both types of nerves synapse directly with the outer hair cells (OHC). *(Adapted from Spoendlin, 1973, by permission)*

the efferent system. **6.8b:** Schematic diagram of the manner in which the efferents synapse on the wave in such a manner that hair cells at different locations along the cochlear partition can respond differentially to frequency. Electrophysiological recordings of cochlear poten-

tials reflect this frequency selectivity. Intensity has been associated with the amount of basilar membrane displacement and resultant shearing of the hair cells. Intensity changes are also reflected in the various cochlear potentials. Brief reference has been made to the nerves that synapse with hair cells and carry information about the acoustic stimulus centrally, toward the auditory cortex. If we are to understand how the auditory nerve preserves the frequency and intensity information existing in the cochlea, we must know the pattern of innervation between the nerve fibers and the hair cells as well as the nature of the neural discharges.

The patterns made by the auditory nerve communicating with or innervating the hair cells along the basilar membrane limit the type of encoding that might be possible in auditory nerve fibers. We shall describe two basic types of nerve fibers: afferent and efferent. *Afferent fibers* are sensory nerves that carry information from the peripheral sense organ (in this case the organ of Corti) to the brain. *Efferent fibers* typically bring information from the cortex to the periphery. Basically there are two types of auditory afferent fibers and two types of auditory efferent fibers. The afferent nerve supply consists of (1) *radial fibers* and (2) *outer spiral* fibers. The radial fibers compose about 95 percent of the total number of afferent fibers. As illustrated in Figures 6.8 and 6.9, radial fibers innervate the inner hair cells exclusively, each fiber innervating the base of only one inner hair cell and then leaving the organ of Corti through an opening in the osseous spiral lamina called *habenula perforata* to travel to the modiolus. Figure 6.10 is a transmission electron micrograph showing the path taken by the radial fibers. There are about 45,000 or 50,000 afferent fibers in the cat and 95 percent of them are thought to innervate the 2600 inner hair cells. Thus each inner hair cell may be innervated by 16 to 20 radial

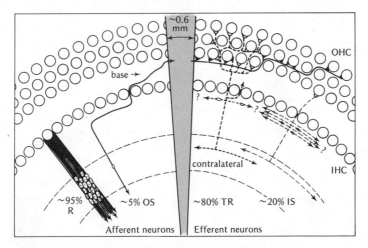

Figure 6.9 Schematic diagram of the innervation pattern of the cat organ of Corti. Left: afferent innervation pattern. About 95 percent of the afferent fibers are radial fibers (R) which innervate only the inner hair cells. About 5 percent of the afferents are outer spiral fibers (OS) which go to the outer hair cells; each fiber innervates about ten outer hair cells basal in direction in relation to the habenula perforata through which it passes. Right: efferent innervation pattern. About 80 percent of the efferent fibers are tunnel radial fibers (TR) which innervate outer hair cells. About 20 percent of the efferents are inner spiral fibers (IS) which run under the inner hair cells but are not thought to synapse directly with the hair cells. *(Adapted from Spoendlin, 1974, by permission)*

fibers, as shown schematically in Figure 6.9. Similar calculations for the human cochlea estimate that an average of eight radial fibers would innervate one and only one inner hair cell. Thus the radial fibers are said to have a many-to-one connection to the inner hair cells. The other 5 percent of the afferent fibers are the outer spiral fibers and are said to have a one-to-many connection as shown in Figures 6.9 and 6.11. In the basal area the outer spiral fibers innervate the outside row of the outer hair cells. As they move in an apical direction they innervate the middle and finally the innermost row of outer hair cells. They then travel further in an apical direction for about 0.6 mm, finally crossing along the floor of the tunnel of Corti between the pillar cells and through the habenula perforata to the modiolus. The involved course of the outer spiral fibers along the base

of the first row of outer hair cells is shown in Figure 6.12. Figure 6.13 shows endings of a number of outer spiral fibers at the base of an outer hair cell. They can also be seen in Figure 6.14. On the average each outer spiral fiber innervates about ten outer hair cells. Thus, the afferent fibers in the VIIIth nerve innervate either one or a small number of hair cells.

The efferent fibers that come to the inner ear from the superior olivary region of the brain stem (see Fig. 7.1) on the same side of the cochlea under consideration are called the *uncrossed olivocochlear bundle,* or UCOCB. That is, UCOCB fibers come from the superior olive on one side of the head to the cochlea on that same side. These 50 to 200 fibers, which enter the cochlea from the modiolus via the habenula perforata, are called the *inner spiral bundle,* which are illustrated in Figures 6.8

modiolus
central core of cochlea

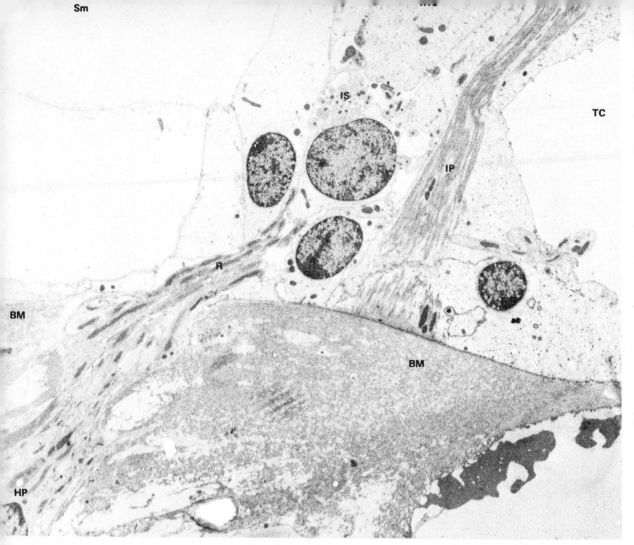

Figure 6.10 Transmission electron micrograph showing the radial fibers (R) entering the habenula perforata (HP) and going toward the base of the inner hair cell (IHC). The fibers of the inner spiral bundle (IS) are also seen in their path below the base of the IHC. For orientation, the following are also labeled: BM: basilar membrane; TC: tunnel of Corti; IP: inner pillar cell; Sm: scala media. *(Chinchilla photograph courtesy of Dr. Ivan Hunter-Duvar, Hospital for Sick Children, Toronto)*

and 6.9, and were also shown in Figure 5.7. Histological evidence indicates that these fibers of the inner spiral bundle synapse with the afferent fibers beneath the inner cells but only rarely synapse directly with the inner hair cells (Fig. 6.8b).

The bundle of efferent fibers that arises from the superior olive on the side opposite the cochlea under consideration is called the *crossed olivocochlear bundle* or COCB. That is, COCB fibers come from the superior olive on one side of the head to the cochlea on the other side of the head. There are only about 500 to 600 total efferent fibers going to the cochlea, and the majority of them (about 400) are the COCB fibers that compose the *tunnel*

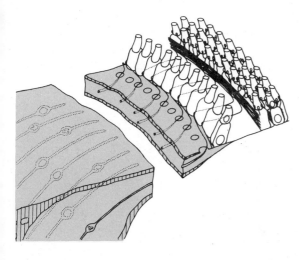

Figure 6.11 Schematic diagram of the outer spiral fibers which constitute the afferent innervation of the outer hair cells. Notice that the nerves innervate the outer and inner hair cells differently. (*Adapted from Spoendlin, 1974, by permission*)

Figure 6.12 Scanning electron micrograph of the first row of outer hair cells (OHC1) and supporting Deiters' cells (D), as seen from the tunnel of Corti with the outer pillar cells removed. At the base of the outer hair cells the fibers of the outer spiral bundle (OS) are seen. The insert shows their interwoven pattern in detail. Note that the Deiters' cells at the base of the first row of hair cells have bulges, rather than the phalangeal processes shown arising from the Deiters' cells beneath the third row of outer hair cells as in Figure 5.6. (*Chinchilla photographs courtesy of Dr. Ivan Hunter-Duvar, Hospital for Sick Children, Toronto*)

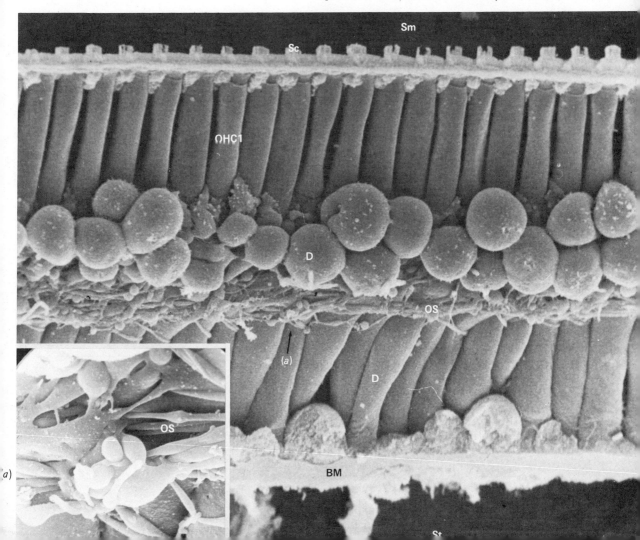

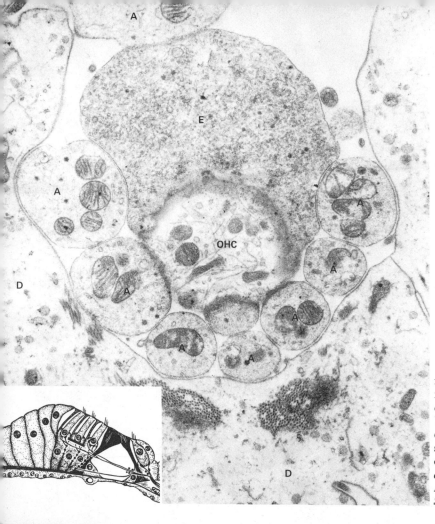

Figure 6.13 Transmission electron micrograph showing many afferent nerve fibers (A) coming from the outer spiral bundle surrounding the base of an outer hair cell. A large efferent nerve ending (E) is also seen. (The insert shows the location of the section; see Fig. 5.3.) *(Chinchilla photograph courtesy of Dr. Ivan Hunter-Duvar, Hospital for Sick Children, Toronto)*

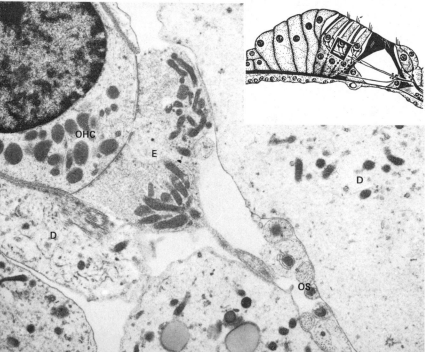

Figure 6.14 Transmission electron micrograph showing an efferent nerve ending (E) at the base of an outer hair cell (OHC). Fibers of the outer spiral bundle (OS) are also seen. (The insert shows the location of the section, perpendicular to that of Fig. 6.13; see Fig. 5.3.) *(Chinchilla photograph courtesy of Dr. Ivan Hunter-Duvar, Hospital for Sick Children, Toronto)*

radial fibers in the cochlea. The tunnel radial fibers come from the modiolus, through the habenula perforata, between the pillar cells, across the upper portion of the tunnel of Corti, and synapse at the base of the outer hair cells. A tunnel radial fiber is clearly seen in Figure 5.5. The synapse of a radial efferent on the base of an outer hair cell is shown in Figures 5.7 and 6.14. The innervation of the efferent tunnel radial fibers on the outer hair cells is most dense in the base and most sparse in the apex. In the first turn the fibers innervate all outer hair cells; in apical turns, however, they fail to innervate the outermost rows of outer hair cells. The VIIIth nerve fiber anatomy may be outlined as follows:

1. Afferent fibers
   a. Radial fibers (R), from inner hair cells
   b. Outer spiral fibers (OS), from outer hair cells
2. Efferent fibers
   a. Uncrossed olivocochlear bundle: inner spiral bundle (IS), from superior olive to cochlea on same side of head
   b. Crossed olivocochlear bundle: tunnel radial fibers (TR), from superior olive to cochlea on other side of head

Both the efferent and afferent fibers are devoid of their insulating myelin sheaths between the organ of Corti and the habenula perforata. The nerve fibers leave the cochlea through the habenula perforata in an ordered manner and are gathered in a twisted bundle within the modiolus. The nerve fibers that innervate the hair cells at the apex are in the middle of the nerve bundle. The fibers from the cochlear turns toward the base make up the outside fibers of the nerve bundle. Figure 6.15 shows a cross section of the cochlea with the apex at the top; the middle of the cross section is the modiolus. The fibers from the apex run down the middle of the modiolus, and those from the other turns of the cochlea form the outside of the nerve bundle. Thus

fibers carrying low-frequency information (from the apex) are in the middle of the VIIIth nerve bundle, whereas high-frequency fibers (toward the base) are on the outside of the bundle. The auditory nerve bundle is joined by nerves from the vestibular system to form the entire VIIIth nerve tract. After the VIIIth nerve leaves the cochlea, its next junction is the cochlear nucleus. The structure of the nervous system central to the cochlea will be discussed in Chapter 7.

There is therefore an orderly connection between the hair cells and VIIIth nerve fibers, and the VIIIth nerve fibers are organized within the nerve bundle. Thus on an anatomical basis we might expect that the discharge patterns of the VIIIth nerve fibers will reflect the frequency and intensity encoding performed by the mechanics of the inner ear.

FUNCTION OF THE AFFERENT AUDITORY NERVE

The hair cell initiates the neural part of the auditory processes. Somehow the mechanical deformation of the hair cell receptor system produces the graded electric potentials discussed earlier (that is, potentials whose magnitude is proportional to the amount of stimulation), which may be referred to as receptor potentials (namely CM and SP). The hair cell then liberates a chemical transmitter, which probably initiates a graded electric potential in the nerve fibers that innervate the base of the hair cell. This graded neural potential is propagated along the nerve fiber to the habenula perforata, where the myelinated portion of the fiber is reached. At that point neural spikes or discharges are produced that travel along the VIIIth nerve to the cochlear nucleus. Since the graded neural response of the unmyelinated portion of the nerve fiber is thought to generate the spikes, it is called a generator potential.

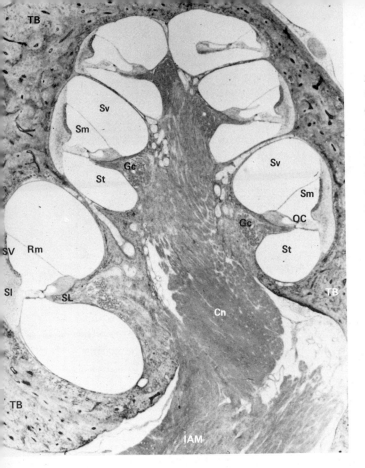

Figure 6.15 Light micrograph of a mid-modiolar section of a cat cochlea. The cochlear nerve (Cn) is seen in the modiolus. Fibers from the apical turns form the center of the cochlear nerve, while the basal turn fibers join with the nerve at its outer edges. The nerve leaves the cochlea via the internal auditory meatus (IAM). *(Photograph courtesy of Dr. Ivan Hunter-Duvar, Hospital for Sick Children, Toronto)*

The electrophysiologist studies the spike discharge patterns of single neurons by amplifying these minute potential changes with electronic devices. The discharge pattern of the neuron initially exhibits a relatively large potential shift. It then remains in an exhausted condition for a short period of time (known as the absolute refractory period) during which no stimulus, however strong, can be effective. The absolute refractory period lasts approximately 1 ms and therefore limits the number of discharges a given nerve

may be capable of delivering per second. After the absolute refractory period comes a period of relative refractoriness during which the ability to respond depends on the intensity of succeeding stimuli. Appendix D explains the physiology of neurons in greater detail. At this point we must be careful to make the distinction between the action potential of an individual neuron and the whole nerve action potential, the AP. The individual neuron's action potential or spike is said to have an all-or-none characteristic. By this it is meant that the amplitude of the neural discharge does not vary with the intensity of the stimulus (that is, it is not a graded response). If the neuron has adequate stimulation, a discharge of a given size will occur, and the impulse will be propagated along the neuron at a given speed. The best analogy is that of shooting a rifle. The bullet leaves the rifle with a given speed and will travel a distance (comparable to the amplitude of the neural discharge) regardless of how hard one pulls the trigger. All that is required is adequate stimulation; that is, the trigger must be pulled with a certain force in order to shoot the rifle. It is an all-or-none situation; either the rifle will shoot or it won't. Similarly, either the individual neuron will discharge or it won't.

Once an electrophysiologist is recording the discharges of a single neuron—or single unit response, as it is often called—he has several methods of dealing with the data. He investigates the characteristics of the neurons by these different methods in an attempt to understand how the relevant aspects (frequency, intensity, and so on) of the acoustic signal are encoded. One way of studying auditory nerve fibers is to determine how the frequency selectivity established by the traveling wave is reflected in the neural discharge pattern. A method of studying such discharge patterns is first to establish what the neuron's discharges are like in the absence of a stimulus and then use that as a pattern against which we can compare various stimulus-evoked discharge patterns. *Spontaneous activity* is the neural activity that occurs in the absence of a stimulus. For single units of the auditory nerve this would be the neural activity occurring in the absence of sound. Since it is virtually impossible to work in complete silence, there is always the possibility that the neural activity observed in the absence of a controlled sound stimulus may be caused by an ambient acoustic stimulation. Thus it is difficult to specify the exact nature and cause of spontaneous activity. For our discussion, however, the neural activity in the absence of sound introduced by an experimenter will have to suffice as our definition of spontaneous activity.

One of the most useful indicators of neural activity is to measure the discharge rate of the single unit. The discharge rate is simply the number of times a unit discharges or "fires" in a given time period. For instance, we know that due to the absolute refractory period the neuron has a 1-ms period after it has discharged before it can discharge again. Thus the maximum discharge rate of a single unit is 1000 times per second. The discharge rate of spontaneous activity in single units of the auditory nerve may range from only a few spikes, or discharges, per minute to more than 100 discharges per second.

Once the spontaneous discharge rate of a neuron has been determined, then the *single neuron threshold* to a particular stimulus can be calculated. The threshold of a single neuron may be defined as the *minimum* stimulus level that will cause an *increase* in the discharge rate above the spontaneous discharge rate. For instance, if we wish to determine the threshold to a 1-kHz sinusoid with a spontaneous discharge rate of 40 spikes per second, we increase the intensity of the 1-kHz sinusoid until the discharge rate is just detectably greater than 40 spikes per second; that in-

tensity will be the threshold. A lower intensity signal will not affect the discharge rate, and a more intense signal may significantly increase the rate of discharge above 40 spikes per second.

Increasing the intensity of the acoustic stimulus and measuring changes in the discharge rate of the single neuron is called calculating an intensity function, or input-output function. One such *input-output function* or *intensity function,* shown in Figure 6.16, depicts a neuron's response to a 4.1-kHz sinusoid. This neuron had a very low spontaneous discharge rate, and its threshold was near 40 dB SPL. This neuron's response shows the typical increase in discharge rate for an increase in stimulus level to about 30 to 40 dB above the neuron's threshold (80 dB SPL in this case), and then the discharge rate remains constant. A nerve's response may be increased over a range of 20 to 50 dB (called the dynamic range) above threshold, after which the discharge rate will remain constant or decrease slightly if stimulus intensity is increased further.

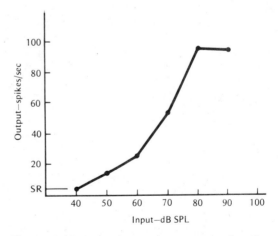

Figure 6.16 Intensity or input-output function for a single neuron. The output of the neuron is plotted in spikes per second as a function of the input intensity (4.1 kHz tone) in dB SPL. SR: spontaneous rate of firing. (Replot of data shown in Fig. 6.18.)

Any single nerve will respond (that is, increase its discharge rate above the spontaneous rate) to many frequencies of acoustic stimulation. Thus we can determine the threshold of a neuron to each frequency over a range of frequencies of stimulation. A plot of the level of stimulation necessary to reach the threshold of a nerve at each frequency in a wide range of frequencies is called a *tuning curve*. Tuning curves for six different units are shown in Figure 6.17. The curves derive their name from the sharp dip, occurring at a particular frequency, which indicates that the neuron is especially sensitive or "tuned" to that frequency of stimulation. Another name for a tuning curve is a *response area*. The name "response area" refers to the fact that the curve denotes the areas of frequency and intensity that will cause the unit to discharge or respond above its spontaneous discharge rate. The frequency that requires the least intensity of stimulation to increase the discharge rate above the spontaneous rate is called the *characteristic frequency* or *CF* of the nerve (occasionally the term "best frequency" is used in this same sense). The CF of the unit is indicated by the lowest point (or dip) in the tuning curve.

Tuning curves are usually drawn with frequency plotted on a logarithmic scale. The higher-frequency side of the tuning curve appears very steep. The lower-frequency side of the tuning curve is less steep and for higher

Figure 6.17 Tuning curves for six single units with different characteristic frequencies. The stimulus level in relative decibels needed to reach each unit's threshold is plotted as a function of the stimulus frequency. Note the steep slope on the high-frequency side of the curve and the shallow slope on the low-frequency side. The bottom three units have higher characteristic frequencies and show low-frequency "tails" which indicate that they are responsive to a wide range of frequencies of stimulation. (*Adapted from Kiang and Moxon, 1972, by permission*)

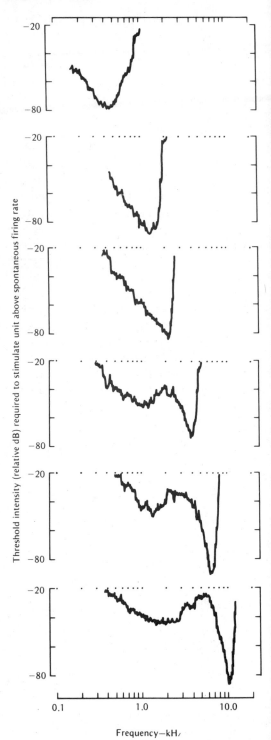

CF units, such as the bottom three in Figure 6.17, a long, low-frequency "tail" is obvious. This means that nerves respond best to their CF, are unlikely to respond to many frequencies higher than CF, and will usually respond to frequencies lower than CF if the stimulation is approximately 60 dB above the threshold at CF.

Another way of looking at the tuning characteristic of single neurons is to plot their discharge *rate* (not threshold) as a function of frequency for a given level (or levels) of stimulation. Such a set or "family" of curves for six levels of stimulation is given in Figure 6.18. The form of these rate discharge functions is like that of inverted tuning curves. From these curves the best frequency (BF) can be determined as the particular frequency that results in the maximum discharge rate for a given stimulus intensity. For single fibers in the auditory nerve the BF is nearly the same for each level of stimulation. When several levels of stimulation are presented, as in Figure 6.18, an intensity function can be calculated from

the curves. If the reader understands the previously explained concept of an intensity function, he or she should try to calculate the intensity function at the BF for the unit shown in Figure 6.18. A comparison with Figure 6.16 will reveal a similarity that is not coincidental.

The data in Figures 6.17 and 6.18 show the response of single auditory nerve fibers to stimuli of different frequencies. These nerve fibers synapse with one hair cell or with a relatively small number of hair cells in a fairly localized region of the cochlear partition. It is therefore not surprising that the pattern of discharge rate reflects the same type of frequency selectivity obtained at one point along the basilar membrane. *That is, the auditory nerve preserves the frequency selectivity found along the basilar membrane. Each nerve fiber could be characterized as revealing a type of band-pass filtering of the acoustic input.* Further studies of auditory nerve discharge rate have shown that fibers located on the outside of the auditory nerve bundle (those that innervate basal hair cells) have high-frequency CFs,

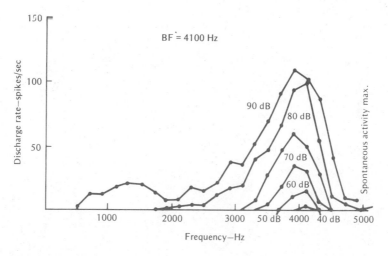

Figure 6.18 Rate of response curves for a single unit at six different intensities. The discharge rate is plotted as a function of the frequency of the tone stimulation. Each curve is generated by holding the level of the stimulus constant and recording the discharge rate for each frequency. The unit has a best frequency (BF) of 4100 Hz. *Adapted from Rose, Hind, Anderson and Brugge, 1971, by permission)*

whereas those toward the middle of the nerve bundle (those fibers that innervate the apex of the cochlea) have low-frequency CFs. This is a further demonstration of the correspondence between the frequency selectivity found in the cochlea and that measured in the eighth nerve.

If we continue to study the auditory nerve fiber, we discover another property of its discharge pattern that might be important for our ability to perceive frequency. Single nerves with CFs below 4 or 5 kHz tend to discharge once per cycle for low-frequency sinusoid stimulation (below 1 kHz). Figure 6.19 shows the type of discharge pattern we might expect in that situation. This type of response is called a *time-* or *phase-locked response,* or a *following response,* since the response appears locked to, or follows, the peaks in the stimulus. Because of the absolute refractory period of the neuron, the unit cannot discharge to every cycle (peak) of a sinusoid near or above 1 kHz, although the fiber could discharge to every other or every third (and so on) cycle of the stimulus. To observe phase locking to these higher frequencies we must resort to a method of data analysis known as *histograms.*

Histograms are graphic displays of a single neuron's response to repeated presentations of a given stimulus. The vertical axis of a histogram is usually some measure of the number of responses. It may be labeled "frequency of responses," "percentage of response," or usually just "number of discharges." The horizontal axis is always time, but it may represent time after stimulus onset or the time interval between successive neural discharges.

Poststimulus time histograms (PST) (or "latency histograms," as they are less frequently called) display the total number of responses at a given location in time to a repeated stimulus. The beginning point in time is usually some point just prior to the stimulus onset, such as 5 ms (see Fig. 6.20). The data shown in Figure 6.20 illustrate typical PST histograms to tone bursts. The greatest number of discharges occur at the onset of the tone burst ("on" effect). The number of discharges decreases rapidly until a constant number of discharges is maintained for the duration of the tone burst. Immediately after the offset of the tone burst the number of discharges in this neuron is zero or near zero

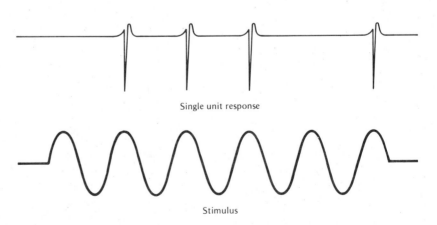

Single unit response

Stimulus

Figure 6.19 Single neuron discharges to a low-frequency stimulus. Top trace: discharge pattern of the single unit. Bottom trace: the low-frequency stimulus. Note that the neuron responds with a discharge to almost every cycle of the stimulus.

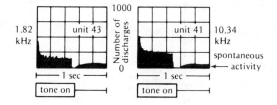

Figure 6.20 Typical PST histograms to tone bursts. For each histogram the tone burst is presented 1200 times. The histogram is started 5 ms before the onset of each tone burst. Each time the unit discharges, the histogram increases vertically at the point in time (on the abscissa) the discharge occurred. On the average, more responses occur at the beginning of the tone burst than at the end. After the tone burst there is a decrease in spontaneous activity. *(Adapted from Kiang, Watanabe, Thomas and Clark, 1965, by permission)*

(less than the spontaneous rate). After a short period of time the number of discharges returns to the normal spontaneous rate. The PST histograms in Figure 6.20 show the number of discharges at each point in time for 1200 presentations of the tone burst stimulus. It should be clear from comparing Figures 6.19 and 6.20 that the PST histogram can reveal response patterns that would never be seen by simply recording discharge rate or studying the response of a unit to each individual stimulus presentation. Figure 6.20 does not show the time-locked synchrony of the discharges to the lower CF tone because the time scale is too large.

Interval histograms provide a method for studying the time interval between each single neural discharge. The horizontal axis of the interval histogram represents the time between neural discharges or the interspike interval. The vertical axis shows the number of interspike intervals that occurred. Thus if an interval histogram has its largest peak at 1 ms, then the time between successive discharges was most often 1 ms. Such an interval histogram is shown in Figure 6.21d in which the stimulus was a 1000-Hz sinusoid of 1-second duration repeated 10 times. Because of the

absolute refractory period of the single neuron, we would not expect an interspike interval of less than 1 ms. Although Figure 6.21d shows that a 1-ms interspike interval occurred more than any other specific interval, it should be pointed out that interspike intervals of 2 to 10 ms were also plentiful. Another point of interest in Figure 6.21d is that the neural discharges occurred at integral multiples of 1 ms. This phenomenon is also true of other frequencies of stimulation, as illustrated by the interval histograms to other pure tone stimuli shown in Figure 6.21. The relationship between the period of the stimulus (and integer multiples of that period) and the interval between discharges is shown clearly in Figure 6.21. This supports the idea that single neural discharges are locked to the cycles of the stimulus at low frequencies, as was shown in Figure 6.19. Some locking of the responses to the cycles of the stimulating frequency occurs up to about 5 kHz. We must remember, however, that this does not indicate that the nerve discharges to every cycle of the stimulus, but it does imply that the nerve discharges to multiple integers of the period of the input up to 5 kHz. *Thus the frequency of low-frequency stimuli could be determined by the phase locking of the auditory nerve to the acoustical vibration in addition to the band-pass filtering characteristics previously mentioned.*

FUNCTION OF THE EFFERENT SYSTEM

The exact function of the efferent system is not understood, but electrophysiological evidence indicates that the system is inhibitory in nature. By electrical stimulation of the crossed olivocochlear bundle and simultaneous measurement of the cochlear potentials and afferent neural activity, investigators have found the following effects: (1) There is a decrease in discharge rate of afferent single

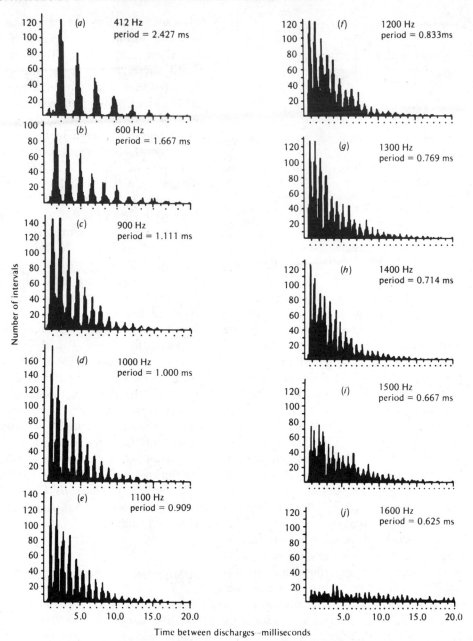

Figure 6.21 Interval histograms showing periodic distributions of interspike intervals to pure tones of different frequencies. The stimulus frequency is indicated in each graph. The intensity of all stimuli is 80 dB SPL, and the tone duration is 1 sec. The responses to ten stimuli constitute the sample on which each histogram is based. (The abscissas plot time in milliseconds between successive neural discharges. Dots below the time axes indicate integral values of the period of each frequency employed.) *(Rose, Brugge, Anderson and Hind, 1967, by permission)*

units in response to acoustic stimulation when the COCB is stimulated. (2) The EP is reduced as a result of COCB stimulation; the reduction of the EP is greatest in the first turn and least in the apical turn. (3) The CM increases slightly in the first turn and shows no measurable effect in the apical turns; the low-frequency CM recorded from the first turn shows more of an effect (that is, increase) than the high-frequency CM from the same turn.

Since there is a reduction in the afferent single-unit discharge rate with COCB stimulation, it should be apparent that the AP will also decrease with COCB stimulation. The

PST Histograms

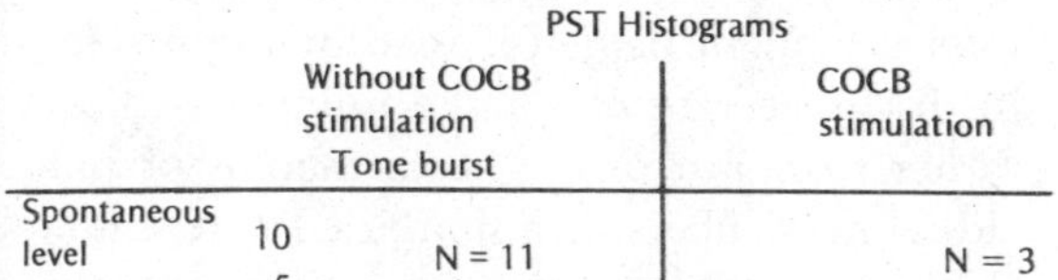

Figure 6.22 Comparison of PST histograms without (left) and with (right) COCB stimulation of an auditory nerve fiber with best frequency at 9.7 kHz. For these histograms ten consecutive presentations of tone bursts, 50 ms in duration, were used. N: total number of nerve impulses sampled during 100 ms. The threshold is used as a reference for sound intensity. Notice that the number of discharges (N) was less when the COCB was stimulated. (*Adapted from Teas, Konishi and Nielsen, 1973, by permission*)

degree of inhibition of the AP produced by stimulation of the COCB can be as large as an equivalent reduction of 25 dB in the intensity of the stimulus. Figure 6.22 shows the decrease in discharge rate of a single unit as a result of COCB stimulation for various levels of acoustic stimulation.

Stimulation of the UCOCB efferents also produces inhibition of the neural responses to sound but no change in CM. Both COCB and UCOCB fibers are thought to be activated by stimulation to the contralateral ear.

What is the efferent system's relationship to "hearing"? We don't know. Behavioral experiments with animals whose COCB had been rendered ineffective by cutting it show that absolute thresholds are not changed. There may, however, be a deterioration in frequency-resolving power in the presence of sustained stimulation.

ENCODING OF FREQUENCY AND INTENSITY

From the information covered in the two preceding chapters we can describe, in a variety of ways, how the auditory system might be able to encode (determine) the frequency and intensity of an acoustic waveform. We have seen that the traveling wave of the basilar membrane vibrates with a maximum amplitude at a place along the cochlea that is dependent on the frequency of stimulation. Thus which hair cells will be sheared maximally depends on the frequency of the stimulus. The afferent VIIIth nerve fibers innervate these hair cells in a systematic fashion, and each nerve fiber is most sensitive to a particular frequency. The individual fibers within the auditory nerve are also organized according to the frequency at which they are most sensitive and the location along the cochlea at which they innervate hair cells. Thus, each place or location within the nerve is responding 'best" to a particular frequency. The nerve is topographically organized according to the tonal frequency that stimulates the auditory system. Thus through the *tonotopic* organization of the VIIIth nerve, the frequency of the input can be determined by which nerve fiber (place) discharges with the greatest relative discharge rate. This way of determining frequency is referred to as the *place theory.* If a location along the cochlear duct is injured or if a portion of the cochlear nerve bundle is destroyed, the sensitivity of the auditory system to certain frequencies will be greatly decreased. These changes are seen as shifts in the absolute behavioral thresholds (see Chapter 10) to particular frequencies of stimulation corresponding to the site of injury. Such data are often cited as evidence for a place theory of frequency analysis.

One can also notice from the data shown in Figure 6.19 and from the interval histograms that auditory nerve fibers also discharge at rates proportional to the period of the input stimulus, when the input frequency is less than approximately 5000 Hz. Thus, it is possible that information is available to the nervous system about stimulus frequency from an analysis of the periodicity of neural discharge rate. That is, the periodicity of the nerve discharges could be used to determine the frequency of an input stimulus. Thus for frequencies of less than 5000 Hz both the place of maximal discharge and the periodicity of discharge pattern can aid the nervous system in determining the frequency of stimulation.

Intensity may be assumed to be encoded by an increase in the discharge rate within the auditory system. This would involve an increase in the discharge rate of a single auditory nerve fiber. Notice, however, in Figure 6.16 that a single neuron's discharge rate will increase only for a relatively small range of intensity change (less than 50 dB). Thus a single neuron's response cannot account for the 150-dB dynamic range of intensity to which we are sensitive. This would imply that intensity might be determined by the increase in discharge rate of a large number of fibers rather than just one. The thresholds of individual nerve fibers with similar CFs are similar (within 20 dB), so the dynamic range that could be covered would still be small relative to the total dynamic range of the ear. Inclusion of discharges from many fibers whose CFs are other than those of the stimulus (see for instance the low-frequency tails of the tuning curves shown in Figure 6.18) may help to account for the wide dynamic range of the ear. However, more research is required if we are to understand the encoding of both intensity and frequency information more completely.

Summary   The electric potentials (CM, SP, AP, and single units) of the inner ear are created as a result of the hydromechanical disturbances. Resting potentials are also present regardless of stimulation (especially EP). The likely sources of these potentials are the hair cells for the CM, the stria vascularis for the EP, and simultaneous discharges of eighth nerve single units for the AP. There are numerous possible sources of the SP. The bandpass filtering characteristics of the traveling-wave motion of the basilar membrane are evident in the responses of these potentials. The type of response recorded is also a function of the recording technique.

There are two types of afferent fibers: radial fibers and outer spiral fibers. The radial fibers make up 95 percent of all afferents. Each radial fiber innervates only one inner hair cell, and each inner hair cell synapses with many radial fibers. The outer spiral fibers compose the other 5 percent of the afferent fibers. They each innervate about ten outer hair cells in an orderly fashion. The responses of the single neurons of the auditory nerve demonstrate that they have a wide range of spontaneous activity. The units' discharge rate increases with an increase in stimulus intensity for a 20–50 dB range above threshold. Single nerves respond to a wide range of frequencies but are most sensitive to one frequency, which is called the characteristic frequency (CF) of a unit. Neurons with high CFs respond to a wider range of frequencies than do units with low CFs. Interval histograms reveal that fibers with CFs below 5 kHz respond to the periodicity of low-frequency stimulation.

The efferent fibers are composed of two types: (1) The tunnel radial fibers compose about 80 percent of the efferents and innervate the outer hair cells. Their innervation density is greatest in the base. (2) The inner spiral bundle represents the other 20 percent of the efferent fibers. It runs under the inner hair cells, but the fibers are thought to synapse predominantly with the afferent fibers rather than the inner hair cells. Stimulating the efferent fibers by electrical stimulation of the COCB results in an increase in the CM, a decrease in the EP, a decrease in single-unit response, and a decrease in the AP. All of these effects are best observed when recorded from the basal end of the cochlea or from single units that innervate the basal end of the cochlea. Place and phase-locking theories are used to account for the neural system's ability to encode frequency. Intensity is thought to be encoded by the amount of neural discharges.

Supplement

It is of historical interest to note that the CM was discovered accidentally by Wever and Bray in 1930. At that time they were recording from the auditory nerve and considered the CM to be a neural potential. This misconception was soon clarified by Adrian (1931) and Saul and Davis (1932).

Von Bekesy (1951) displaced the basilar membrane mechanically and demonstrated that the CM reflected the membrane displacement. Shortly thereafter, Tasaki and Fernandez (1952) introduced the use of the differential electrode technique to cochlear physiology. Several investigators however, have cautioned against the use of the CM in the study of cochlear mechanics unless the investigator is fully aware of the limitations of the recording techniques (see Dallos and Cheatham, 1971). A great deal of literature is available dealing with the CM itself or using it as an investigative tool. The reader who is exposed to further literature in the area will find that one way of studying cochlear physiology is to use CM isopotential curves. These are curves that plot the level of stimulus necessary to maintain a given voltage output of the CM as a function of the frequency of the stimulus. For the reader who is interested in learning more about the CM, including its origin, function, and recording techniques, these articles are informative: Dallos (1969, 1973), Tasaki and Fernandez (1952), Tasaki et al. (1954), Teas et al. (1962), and Weiss et al. (1971).

In recent years minor surgical and nonsurgical techniques have been developed that allow the recording of the AP, and to a lesser extent the CM and SP, from humans. Recording of these potentials from humans is called *electrocochleography.* Placement of the recording electrodes is usually somewhere between earlobe and the cochlea. Because of this electrode placement, the results are similar to the round window electrode experiments reported on animals. The early animal experiments investigating the AP are the basis for human electrocochleography (Teas et al., 1962; Peake and Kiang, 1962). The most sensitive recording location is the *promontory,* which is the bony protruding wall between the oval and round window. The promontory recording requires penetration of the tympanic membrane with a fine needle electrode, the point of which rests on the promontory. This approach to recording cochlear potentials is often called the transtympanic approach. A less severe but less sensitive recording procedure is to place the recording electrode in the external canal. An external-canal electrode may rest against the wall of the canal or the tympanic membrane or it may penetrate slightly the wall of the canal or the annular ligament of the tympanic membrane. Each approach, transtympanic or extratympanic, has its advantages and disadvantages, which are thoroughly discussed in the literature (Simmons and Glattke, 1975; Eggermont et al., 1974; Cullen et al., 1972; Davis, 1976).

With the advent of computer processing of the responses of single auditory nerve fibers has come a mass of new information about the auditory system and a new surge of interest. The responses of single neurons in the auditory nerve can be more complex than we have shown in this chapter. Most of the single-neuron response data have been presented in a fashion that makes them appear consistent with the cochlear mechanics discussed in the previous chapter, but there exist many examples in which it is shown that the neuronal discharges do not reflect the basilar membrane motion in a simple fashion. There is much more information available to the interested reader. The first article reporting responses of single auditory nerve fibers by Tasaki (1954) is an excellent starting point. In 1965 Kiang et al. published a monograph devoted solely to the discharge patterns of single fibers in the cat's auditory nerve. That monograph provides an excellent basis of knowledge for the evaluation of more recent investigations of the auditory nerve fibers, such as: Anderson et al. (1971), Evans (1970a,b, 1972a,b, 1975), Evans and Wilson (1973), Hind (1972), Kiang (1968), Kiang et al. (1970), Kiang and Moxon (1972), Konishi and Nielsen (1973), and Rose et al. (1967, 1971).

The peripheral efferent fibers have proven to be difficult to investigate. The first investigator was Rasmussen (1943), who demonstrated the existence of the efferents followed by others who were interested in tracing the course and innervation of these efferent fibers (Engstrom, 1958; Ishii and Balogh, 1968; Iurato, 1962, 1964; Kimura and Wersall, 1962; Smith and Rasmussen, 1963; Spoendlin, 1966, 1970; and Spoendlin and Gacek, 1963). The physiological significance of these efferent fibers has been studied by many investigators, perhaps most thoroughly by Fex (1968). The results shown in this chapter are based on work by Teas et al. (1972). Behavioral studies of the significance of the efferent system are few, and their results are generally inconclusive. For a review of the efferent system see Eldredge and Miller (1971) and especially Iurato (1974).

Spoendlin's revelation that 90 to 95 percent of the afferent fibers innervate the inner hair cells has dominated the literature in recent years. It was not a well-accepted finding initially, but it has gained acceptance in the scientific community as others replicate his results (Wright and Preston, 1975; Smith, 1972) and as his investigations receive more exposure. Most of the data presented in this chapter regarding the innervation of the organ of Corti by afferent and efferent fibers are based on Spoendlin's (1973, 1974) work.

Wever (1949) suggested the *volley theory* as a way to combine the place and phase-locking theories of hearing. In the volley theory the frequency of low and middle frequencies is determined by the phase locking of neural units to the stimulus. At high frequencies the frequency is determined by the place principle.

In addition to the measures of cochlear and neural activity discussed in this chapter, the term *latency* is used in describing the physiology of the auditory system. Latency defines the time from stimulus onset to the time of cochlear or neural activity. For example, the time from the onset of a click until the occurrence of the AP response is the AP latency. In general, increases in stimulus intensity result in decreases in cochlear and neural latencies. The AP response occurs sooner following stimulation if the click is intense. Figure 6.7 shows differences in AP amplitude between rarefaction and condensation clicks; differences in AP latency also occur for these two types of clicks. Changes in AP latency are often studied during electrocochleography; the latency of the AP response measured during electrocochleography also appears to vary as a function of the spectral content of the stimulus (Davis, 1976). These results and those obtained from comparing PST histograms of single auditory neurons with different CFs to the AP response further demonstrate that the AP response is mostly related to activity occurring in the regions of the cochlea dealing with high frequencies (toward the base).

Before closing our discussion of the peripheral auditory system there are a few summaries of the system that should be cited. Teas (1970) and Goldstein (1968) both have chapters devoted to much of the same materials presented in Chapters 5 and 6 of this text. An issue of the *Journal of the Acoustical Society of America* (vol. 34, no. 9, part 2, 1962) is dedicated to von Bekesy's work. An earlier work is the book by Wever and Lawrence (1954). At a higher level of difficulty are the chapters by Eldredge (1974), Fex (1974), Flock (1974), and Evans (1975) in the *Handbook of Sensory Physiology.* Dallos (1973) has written a complete text devoted to the physiology and biophysics of the peripheral auditory system. Moller (1973a) has edited a symposium text that also contains many articles relevant to Chapters 5 and 6 of this book. Plomp and Smoorenburg (1970) have edited a book on frequency analysis in hearing that includes discussions of much of the material presented in Chapters 5 and 6 and integration of these ideas with material to be presented in later chapters on the psychophysics of pitch. Zwicker and Terhardt (1974) have also edited a text entitled *Facts and Models in Hearing,* which indicates some of the latest attempts to understand the relations between neuronal and psychological realms of audition.

CHAPTER 7
The Central Auditory Nervous System

Anatomy of the Ascending Auditory Pathways
Tonotopic Organization
Single Neuron Responses in the Central Auditory System
Descending Auditory Pathways
Auditory Cortex

The first six chapters discuss the nature of sound, its transmission through the environment, its analysis, how it is collected by the outer ear and transformed into mechanical energy, how the inner ear transforms the mechanical energy into neural impulses, and the nature of the neural impulses that leave the cochlea and travel toward the auditory cortex of the brain.

This chapter deals briefly with the structure and function of the auditory system as it conveys its information from the cochlea to the auditory cortex. It is during this process that the perception of the sound as "hearing" is thought to occur. Later chapters will discuss the relationship of this percept to the physical stimulus. Once again a review of Appendixes C and D will be helpful to the reader who lacks general knowledge of anatomy and physiology.

ANATOMY OF THE ASCENDING AUDITORY PATHWAYS

Figure 4.1 depicted the general anatomy and physiology of the auditory system but not the anatomy of the *central auditory system*. Figure 7.1 illustrates in schematic form the principal

Figure 7.1 Highly schematic diagram of the ascending (afferent) pathways of the central auditory system from the right cochlea to the auditory cortex. No attempt is made to show the subdivisions and connections within the various regions, cerebellar connections, or connections with the reticular formation. *(Based on similar diagrams by Ades, 1959; Whitfield, 1967; Diamond, 1973; Harrison and Howe, 1974a)*

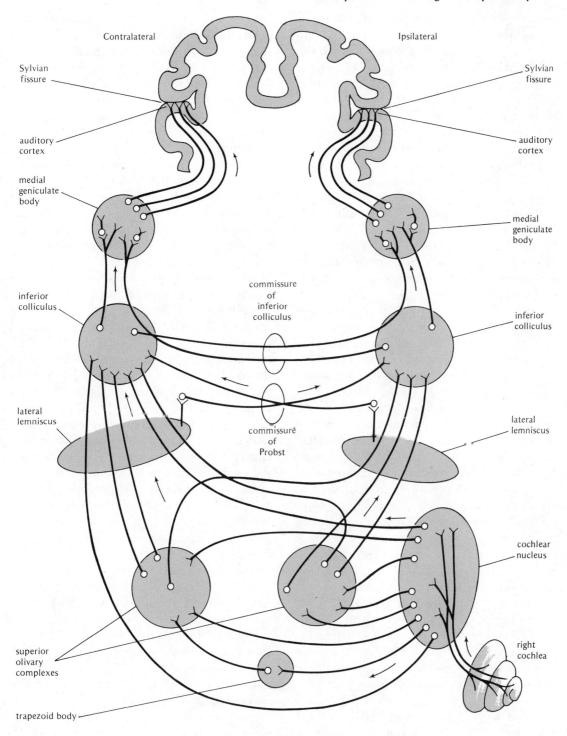

Contralateral

Ipsilateral

Sylvian
fissure

Sylvian
fissure

auditory
cortex

auditory
cortex

medial
geniculate
body

medial
geniculate
body

inferior
colliculus

commissure
of
inferior
colliculus

inferior
colliculus

lateral
lemniscus

commissure
of
Probst

lateral
lemniscus

cochlear
nucleus

superior
olivary
complexes

right
cochlea

trapezoid body

connections of the *ascending* or afferent (from the cochlea toward the cortex) auditory system. A glance at this figure will demonstrate to the reader that the system is intricate. The afferent fibers of the acoustic nerve leave the cochlea and travel to the *cochlear nucleus.* Those fibers *higher* in the system (closer to the cortex) have many pathways, called *tracts,* some traveling *contralaterally* (to the opposite side) and others remaining *ipsilateral* (on the same. side). Furthermore, some fibers may leave one point and go directly to the next, but others may bypass the obvious next point and travel to a higher location. Still others will send *collaterals* or branches to one point as the main tract travels past that point to terminate at a higher location. Because of the complexity of this intricate system of pathways connecting one point to another, it is often convenient to label the fibers according to the number of connections (called synapses) that occur earlier than the region under discussion. The fibers of the acoustic nerve that leave the cochlea are the *primary* or *first-order fibers,* all of which make connections, or synapse, in the cochlear nucleus. The fibers that leave the cochlear nucleus after one synapse are called *second-order fibers.* The fibers that originate after the next synapse are called *third-order fibers,* and so on. Within the central nervous system are *nuclei* at which a group of nerve cell bodies are located. These nuclei should not be confused with the nucleus of a single nerve cell body. Appendix C clarifies the use of many of these terms.

Although the schematic diagram shown in Figure 7.1 appears involved, it is greatly simplified compared to the known complexities of the ascending auditory system. To define as neural elements of the central auditory system all nuclei activated by stimulation of the organ of Corti would impose an impossible task of description. Stimulation of the organ of Corti may trigger neural activity of far-reaching systems, finally causing activity in

muscles and corresponding motor responses. Figure 7.1 represents only the most important afferent connections that are thought to serve the function of hearing per se. Regions that receive an auditory input in addition to inputs from other sensory systems have been excluded. Other information not elaborated in Figure 7.1 are cerebellar connections, the innervation pattern within the various auditory nuclei, and the various types of cell bodies and their interconnections within the auditory nuclei. An additional simplification in Figure 7.1 is that it shows only the tracts for one ear. Obviously we must also consider how the system works when both ears are stimulated.

Figure 7.2 is another simplified schematic illustration showing that the main tracts and nuclei above the cochlear nucleus are stimulated *binaurally* (that is, by both ears). By studying Figure 7.2 we can trace the general pathway of the neural signal from the cochlea to the cortex. After the neural impulses leave the cochlea, they travel to the *cochlear nucleus* where the first synapse is made. From the cochlear nucleus, tracts lead to both the ipsilateral and contralateral *superior olive,* so bilateral representation occurs at this point and above. From the superior olive, neural impulses are transmitted to the *inferior colliculus,* from there to the *medial geniculate body,* and finally to the *auditory cortex.* These are the major nuclei of the central auditory nervous system, although other nuclei exist. Compared to Figure 7.1, Figure 7.2 is a tremendous oversimplification. It is not our purpose, however, to present a detailed account of the anatomy of the central auditory system, but rather to stress the importance of the major nuclei shown in Figure 7.2 and to bring an awareness of the complexity of the auditory nervous system shown in Figure 7.1.

It should be obvious from Figure 7.1 that investigation of both the anatomy and the physiology of the auditory system becomes more involved in the "higher" parts of the

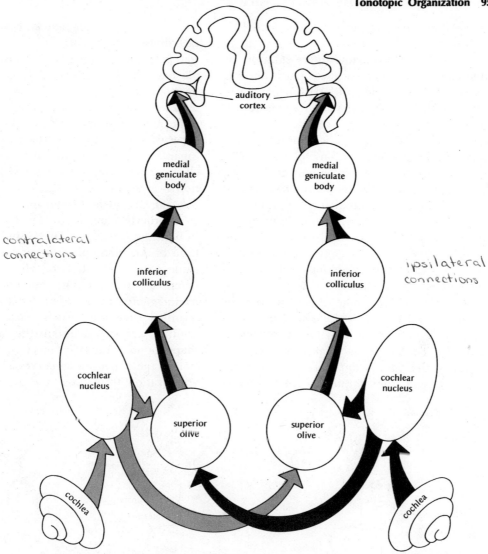

Figure 7.2 Highly schematic diagram of the bilateral central auditory system; the main pathways and nuclei are shown for both cochleas. Bilateral representation from binaural stimulation occurs at the superior olive and in all regions above. *(Based on a similar diagram by Lindsay and Norman, 1972)*

system. To simplify our discussion of the types of electrophysiological responses found in the central auditory system we shall often resort to examples from the "lowest" (nearest to the cochlea) possible part of the system. Frequently the electrophysiology discussed in this chapter will therefore be that occurring in the cochlear nucleus.

TONOTOPIC ORGANIZATION

In Chapter 6 we discussed the concept of frequency being represented by a particular place along the basilar membrane, the place being determined by the location of maximum displacement of the basilar membrane in response to a particular frequency of stimulation. Higher frequencies were represented in the base of the cochlea and lower frequencies in the apex. This spatial representation of frequency along the cochlear partition was maintained by the afferent VIIIth nerve fibers. Fibers with high characteristic frequencies innervated the base of the cochlea and those with low CFs the apex. The maintenance of this spatial representation of frequency throughout the nuclei of the central auditory pathways is referred to as *tonotopic organization*. The test for tonotopic organization is to determine whether there is an orderly spatial representation of fibers with various CFs.

Figure 7.3 shows schematically the projection of the cochlear location and cochlear nerve fibers upon the cochlear nucleus. Upon entering the cochlear nucleus each nerve fiber separates and goes to three separate regions within the cochlear nucleus. The three regions are the *anteroventral cochlear nucleus* (AVCN), the *posteroventral cochlear nucleus* (PVCN), and the *dorsal cochlear nucleus*

(DCN). From this diagram we can see that in each division of the cochlear nucleus the cochlear partition is completely represented from the base to apex. Electrophysiological investigations of the cochlear nucleus confirm this representation by demonstrating that the CFs of fibers within each region duplicate the CFs expected on the basis of the auditory nerve innervation of that region. An example of an electrode penetration from one such investigation is given in Figure 7.4. This figure shows how the CFs of the various units are arranged in an orderly manner from low CF to high CF in both the AVCN and DCN. Similar observations of this tonotopic organization have been made within the superior olive, the lateral lemniscus, the inferior colliculus, and the medial geniculate. Furthermore, tuning curves recorded from the various nuclei of the ascending pathways maintain the same general shape found in the eighth nerve. The preservation of the sharp tuning curves and tonotopic organization throughout the ascending audi-

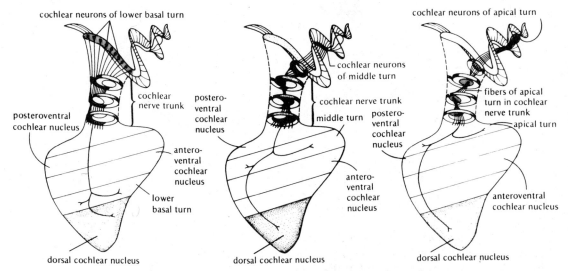

Figure 7.3 Schematic diagrams showing that basal turn (left), middle turn (center), and apical turn (right) auditory nerve fibers innervate different areas of the three main regions of the cochlear nucleus. The spatial separation of frequency from base to apex in the cochlea is reflected in the characteristic frequencies of the fibers that leave the cochlea and is maintained within each of the three main regions of the cochlear nucleus. *(Based on a similar diagram by Schuknecht, 1974)*

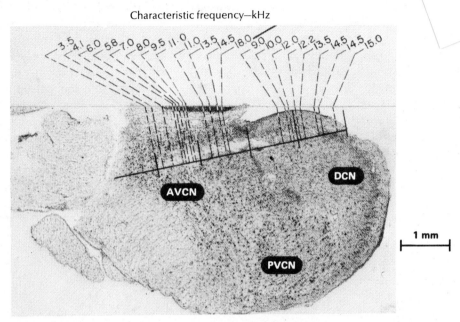

Characteristic frequency—kHz

Figure 7.4 Cross section of the cochlear nucleus showing the track made by an electrode penetration. The characteristic frequencies of neurons recorded from various points within the anteroventral cochlear nucleus (AVCN) and dorsal cochlear nucleus (DCN) show that the spatial separation of frequency is maintained within those two divisions of the cochlear nucleus. (PVCN: posteroventral cochlear nucleus.) This tonotopic organization is maintained throughout the central auditory system. (*Adapted from Rose, Galambos and Hughes, 1959, by permission*)

tory pathway is a strong support for the *place principle* of frequency encoding introduced in Chapter 6.

SINGLE NEURON RESPONSES IN THE CENTRAL AUDITORY SYSTEM

Measures of single-fiber responses used to characterize the discharge patterns of VIIIth nerve fibers are also useful for studying the central pathways. In the VIIIth nerve fibers, spontaneous activity varies greatly in discharge rate from fiber to fiber. The interval histograms of spontaneous activity of various neurons, however, are essentially unchanged regardless of the CF of the unit and its discharge

rate. In the central auditory system this regularity of interval histograms of spontaneous activity is not maintained. Interval histograms of spontaneous activity at these levels are more variable, changing as a response to a variety of nonauditory events, such as the state of alertness.

Single auditory nerve fibers were shown to have intensity functions that produced an increased discharge rate with an increase in intensity over a 20- to 50-dB range. Single fibers from the central pathways generally have a smaller dynamic range than those of the VIIIth nerve. Furthermore, central fibers may show a decrease in discharge rate with an increase in stimulation at high intensities. Thus the intensity function of a central fiber may be similar to that of an auditory nerve fiber or it may be shaped like an inverted U, showing an increase in discharge rate with an initial increase in stimulus intensity and then decreasing at higher intensities. Such intensity functions can be further complicated by simultaneous acoustic stimulation of the opposite ear. Bilateral acoustic stimulation occurs commonly in nature but is difficult to control experimentally in a systematic way.

We pointed out in Chapter 6 that single-unit responses of the VIIIth nerve show phase locking of discharges to the stimulating sinusoid. Phase locking to individual cycles of the tone also occurs in the cochlear nucleus for low-frequency stimuli. In addition, synchronous responses to low-frequency stimuli have been observed in the trapezoid body, the inferior colliculus, and the superior olive. As we investigate higher in the system, however, we find that the relationship between the neural discharges and the period of low-frequency stimuli is less clear.

In Chapter 6 we showed that PST histograms to tone bursts were essentially the same for all fibers of the auditory nerve. In the central auditory system, however, PST histograms to tone bursts may illustrate any number of patterns, as seen in Figure 7.5. The higher-order fibers may respond in the same manner

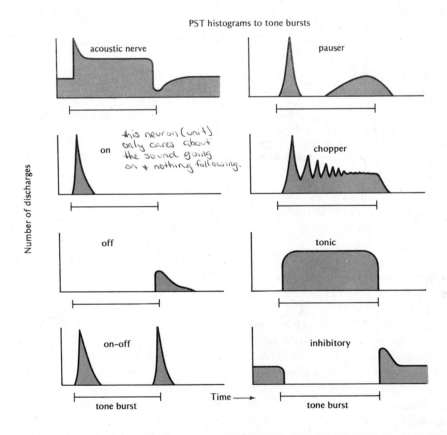

Figure 7.5 Idealized PST histograms to a variety of tone bursts recorded from the central auditory system. The time patterns of responses of the central system are thought to reflect the wide variety of tasks that it must accomplish.

as the primary fibers, or they may produce *"on" responses, "off" responses,* or *"on-off" responses,* or they may exhibit more complex responses such as those called *pausers* or *choppers.* Not all of these patterns can be recorded from every nucleus within the system. On the other hand, one pattern may be recorded from one region within a nucleus and another from a different region within the same nucleus. This wide variety of responses should not be surprising considering the complexity of the system and the variety of tasks it must perform. For instance, we would hardly expect the system to analyze the input signal in a similar manner when performing frequency discrimination, alerting, localization, speech discrimination, and intensity detection.

Poststimulus time histograms to click stimulation for auditory nerve fibers demonstrate either a single peak or a multiple peak depending on their CF. For higher-order fibers PST histograms to click stimuli may be in a variety of patterns. These patterns are not, however, related to the CF of the fiber. The typical PST histogram of low-CF fibers to click stimulation recorded from the auditory nerve fibers is not as prevalent in the responses of higher-order fibers even as "low" in the system as the cochlear nucleus. The lack of multiple peaks related to the CF of the unit (that is, peaks at times equal to 1/CF) is interesting since this temporal information is therefore evidently not usually transmitted beyond the cochlear nucleus in its original form. Figure 7.6 shows a comparison of PST histograms from low-CF fibers in both auditory nerve and cochlear nucleus (AVCN) in response to click stimulation. Such data imply that a simple relaying of information from one low-CF nerve to another does not occur in this part of the cochlear nucleus. Thus even the first nucleus in the central system is complex.

Central sites in the auditory system process information coming from the two ears. Two ears are crucial for our ability to localize

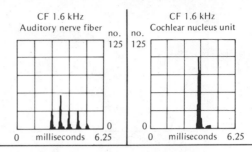

Click rate: 10/sec

Figure 7.6 Comparison of PST histograms to click stimulation for two fibers of the same characteristic frequency (1.6 kHz): auditory nerve fiber (left) and cochlear nucleus fiber (right). Low-CF fibers in the cochlear nucleus typically do not show the modulated pattern related to 1/CF that is characteristic of auditory nerve fibers. The click is presented at time equal to 0. *(Adapted from Kiang, 1965, by permission)*

acoustic events in space. Chapter 12 describes many of the phenomena of binaural (two-eared) hearing. In general, a sound in space will arrive at one ear before it reaches the other ear; the sound is more intense at the ear at which it arrives first. Thus, differences in interaural (between ears) arrival time and interaural intensity are important stimulus variables for binaural processing. Many neurons and nuclei in the ascending pathways have been studied as a function of presenting interaural intensive and temporal differences. The neurons in the superior olivary complex are a good example of the type of neural responses one finds as a result of binaural stimulation. Typically, information from one ear (usually the ear contralateral to the site of the neuron) will inhibit the activity of the neuron when it is receiving information from the other ear (usually the ipsilateral ear). That is, in some cases a stimulus is presented to both ears at the same time and with the same intensity, and very few (if any) neural discharges are recorded from a superior olive neuron. However, for some neurons, as the intensity at one ear is decreased relative to that at the other ear, the neuron will discharge at a higher rate. Some neurons, such as the one

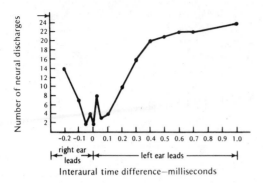

Figure 7.7 Number of neural discharges from a superior olive neuron as a function of the interaural time difference between clicks presented to both ears. Note that as one ear receives the click slightly before the other ear, the neuron increases in number of discharges. *(Adapted from Moushegian, Rupert and Whitcomb, 1972, by permission)*

shown in Figure 7.7, discharge at higher and higher rates as the interaural time difference is varied. Other neurons discharge differentially as a result of a combination of changes in interaural time and intensity. These neurons could indicate the presence of interaural differences and thus provide the neural processing for location or relative location of sounds in space. Neurons in higher centers also discharge differently in response to interaural differences, although their response patterns appear to be more complex than those obtained for neurons in the superior olive.

DESCENDING AUDITORY PATHWAYS

We have seen that the ascending auditory system is very complex anatomically and that electrophysiological responses from the nuclei of the central auditory system are equally complex. One factor contributing to these complexities is the existence of an equally involved *descending system* (efferent), as shown in Figure 7.8. Descending fiber tracts may arise in the auditory cortex or in a variety of nuclei and terminate at other nuclei, espe-

cially in the cochlear nucleus and the olivary complex. Chapter 6 has already discussed part of this system, which consists of COCB and UCOCB fibers arising in the olivary complex and terminating in the cochlea. Those fibers appeared to have an inhibitory action on electrophysiological responses of the cochlea, although their exact function is as yet unknown. As was shown in Figure 7.5, the responses of neurons in the central auditory system vary a great deal. Some of this variation might be due to inhibitory responses of the descending pathways. But the descending pathways cannot be considered a simple inhibitory neural network. For instance, electrical stimulation of a particular segment of the superior olive can cause an increase in discharges in certain cochlear nucleus neurons. Thus, both facilitatory and inhibitory connections might exist within this descending system. Therefore, rather than considering this system as only one that limits the passage of information from "lower" to "higher" levels of the ascending system, a more general view is that the descending auditory pathways represent a control system that varies the routing and hence helps shape sensory input.

AUDITORY CORTEX

As shown schematically in Figure 7.1 the human *auditory cortex* is located in a deep groove or convolution in the brain called the *fissure of Sylvius*. The inaccessibility of the auditory cortex in the primate brain makes it difficult to study. In the cat's brain the auditory cortex is more accessible, and therefore it is often used in research involving the cortex. Figure 7.9 compares the auditory cortex of the cat and the monkey. The cat's cortex is often subdivided into various areas, as illustrated in the figure. The human auditory cortex is more like the monkey's. The bottom diagram is drawn with the Sylvian fissure opened to expose the auditory cortex. The projections to

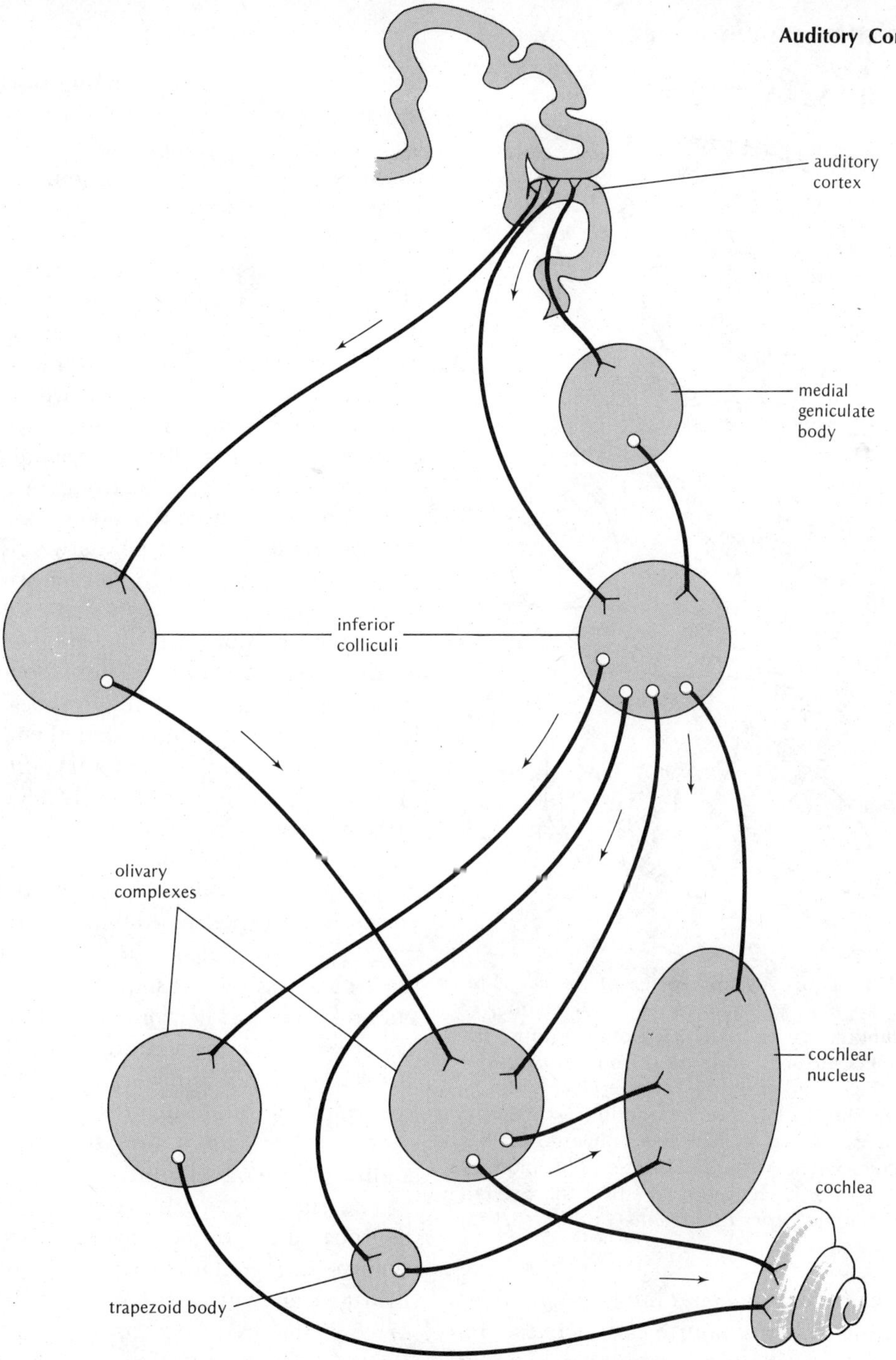

Figure 7.8 Highly schematic diagram of the descending pathways of the central auditory system from one side of the auditory cortex to the right cochlea. No attempt is made to show the subdivisions and connections within the various regions. The complex crossing and bilateral innervation shown for the ascending system in Figure 7.1 is also present in this system. *(Based on a diagram by Harrison and Howe, 1974b)*

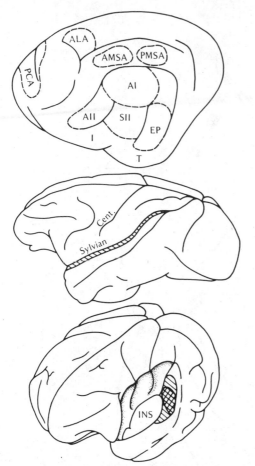

Figure 7.9 Top: Auditory cortex of the cat. The cat auditory cortex, which is easily accessible, is often subdivided into the various regions indicated. The primary auditory regions are AI, AII, SII, and EP. Other areas that receive auditory input are shown. Center: The auditory cortex of the monkey, which is like the human one, lies within the Sylvian fissure. Bottom: The monkey auditory cortex is shown by opening the Sylvian fissure. (*Adapted from Elliott and Trahiotis, 1972, by permission*)

the cortex contain *bilateral* information. Thus each cochlea has an input to each hemisphere.

Early studies of the tonotopic organization of the auditory cortex revealed that frequency maps of the cortex could be made by stimulating small portions of the exposed cochlea and demonstrating a point-to-point projection of the cochlea onto the primary cortex (tonotopic organization). Frequency maps of the cortex could also be made by using tone bursts and recording the resulting activity at the cortex. The studies were made with the animal under deep anesthesia; in some cases local application of strychnine to various areas of the cortex was used to raise the excitability of these cortical areas. Later studies showed that under reduced or no anesthesia no well-defined frequency representation is present in the cortex. However, more recent studies using monkeys have produced consistent results from both anesthetized and awake animals. In these experiments a large number of data points were precisely taken from one animal to determine the locations from which the measurements were made. These data produced reliable frequency maps of the primate cortex. The inconsistencies found earlier may be due to measuring a few points in one animal and then superimposing the results from several animals. The auditory cortex is not so well defined as to allow such superimposition.

From studies of both anesthetized and awake animals evidence now exists that the cortex is organized in columns of cells. Each column is perpendicular to the surface of the cortex and has cells of similar CF. The tuning curves for cortical neurons vary in shape, some being as narrow as those found in the VIIIth nerve and others being broader. This type of cortical organization might allow the auditory system to arrange information for complex auditory pattern recognition.

The time pattern of responses of cortical neurons seems to be especially sensitive to changes in stimulation. One-third of the cortical neurons can be stimulated only by tones of changing frequency or by more complex sounds. Very few units maintain a discharge rate above the spontaneous level for the duration of the stimulus, as was seen in VIIIth nerve fiber discharge patterns. Figure 7.10

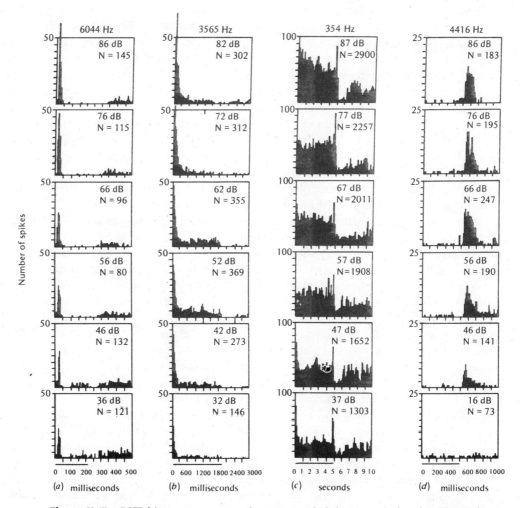

Figure 7.10 PST histograms to tone bursts recorded from cortical units. Bar at bottom of each column: duration of the tone burst. Columns: variations in the patterns caused by changes in frequency. Rows: changes in intensity. Note that most of the units respond to changes (at onset or offset) in stimulation, rather than to the total duration of the stimulus. *(Adapted from Brugge and Merzenich, 1973, by permission)*

shows PST histograms illustrating various discharge patterns of cortical neurons to stimuli at their CFs and at various levels of intensity. Sinusoidal tone bursts do *not* seem to be the appropriate stimuli to investigate the response patterns of all cortical neurons. By using tonal stimuli that vary in their frequency content as a function of time *(frequency-modulated stimuli)*, interesting response patterns have been

detected. Some neurons will respond only to an increase in frequency, others only to a decrease in frequency, and still others only to an increase in frequency of low-frequency stimuli and to a decrease in frequency of high-frequency stimuli. Thus these neurons might underlie the perception of some of the more complex stimuli to which we are sensitive.

Another method of studying the function of

the auditory system is to cut or remove part of it and observe differences in an animal's ability to analyze acoustic stimulation. Typically, animals are trained to make a response that indicates they have detected or recognized some auditory stimulus; a part of the cortex is then removed, and the animal is retested to see whether there is a change in its ability to perform the original task. If so, the missing part of the cortex is assumed to be responsible for the animal's ability to analyze the stimulus for this auditory task. Experiments utilizing such *lesions* and *behavioral techniques* are difficult to summarize because of differences in the site and size of the lesions, the testing techniques, and the nature of the stimulus. Generally, simple tasks are less affected by cortical lesions than are more complex tasks. Pure tone intensity and frequency discrimination tasks (see Chapter 10) may be disrupted after the lesion, but they can be relearned. More difficult tasks based upon patterns (such as order of presentation or localization of a sound in space) suffer more after lesion of the auditory cortex than do simpler tasks. Thus, it appears probable that failure on different types of tasks reflects different deficits in central processing of the stimulus. On the other hand, failure to find a deficit, temporary or permanent, does not necessarily indicate that the lesioned structure did not take part in analysis of the stimulus tested in the normal animal. The animal behavioral studies, in agreement with the electrophysiology, appear to indicate that the cortical centers are organized more to process complex stimulus situations than to encode the basic parameters of the stimulus.

In our discussion of the auditory cortex we have stressed the fact that it is relatively inaccessible and that discrepancies in the data from various investigations can often be attributed to differences in anesthesia. This being the case, responses from the auditory cortexes of awake-behaving animals (especially humans) become extremely significant to the contribution of knowledge about how we hear. A method of recording cortical activity that can be used with awake adult humans is to place electrodes on the scalp and to record variations in electrical activity that occur in conjunction with the presentation of an auditory stimulus. When responses are recorded in this manner, the electrical activity of interest, called the *auditory evoked response* (AER), is often quite small relative to other recorded activity. This activity reflects changes in the *electroencephalogram* (EEG), which is related to acoustic stimulation. By a method known as *signal averaging*, the desired responses, which appear in conjunction with the presentation of an auditory stimulus, can be separated from the unwanted activity. These potentials are usually recorded from the scalp at the center of the top of the head, known as the *vertex*. The AER, a complex response, occurs at the abrupt onset or termination of an acoustic signal. Its waveform has a negative peak about 100 ms after presentation of an appropriate stimulus and a later positive peak. The response is highly variable from person to person, increasing in amplitude and decreasing in latency (time between stimulus onset and response onset) with increases in stimulus intensity. Its variability may even be great from trial to trial for the same subject. Different cortical sources have been postulated to account for the early (about 50-to 100-ms) and later (about 300-ms) components of the waveform. Correspondingly, it has also been suggested that the earlier components are more affected by variations in the acoustic stimulus, whereas the later components are more affected by nonacoustic variables such as attention, espectancy, significance, decision, and contingency.

The waveform in Figure 7.11 shows the auditory evoked response to a 1000-Hz, 30-ms tone presented at 20, 40, and 60 dB SL.

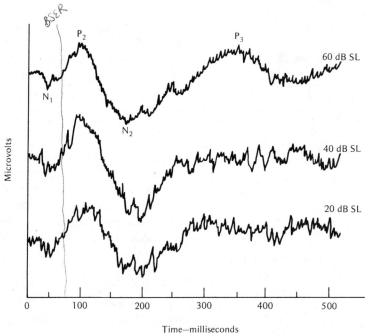

✳ **Figure 7.11** Auditory evoked response (AER) to 64 repetitions of a 1000-Hz, 30-ms tone burst presented at 20, 40, and 60 dB SL. Points N_1, P_2, N_2, P_3 refer to particular points in the waveform (see text). *(Figure courtesy of Dr. Donald C. Teas, University of Florida, Gainesville)*

The AER was obtained by presenting the tone 64 times. The EEG activity following each stimulus presentation was then summed. This method of signal averaging tends to cancel any parts of the EEG activity that are random (not correlated) with respect to the signal and to enhance any EEG activity correlated with the signal. The peaks and valleys at approximately 60, 100, 160, and 350 ms are referred to as N_1 (negative peak), P_2 (positive peak), N_2 (negative peak 2), and P_3 (positive peak 3). These peaks almost always occur in the AER, but their amplitude and time of occurence (latency from stimulus offset) can vary as a function of stimulus variables (for example, intensity) or variables dealing with the attention of the subject.

In Chapter 6 we discussed the recording of the AP from humans. The AP has a latency from stimulus onset of about 1 ms, depending

on the intensity of the stimulus (see Supplement, Chap. 6). The AERs just discussed have latencies of 50 ms or more, depending on which particular response is being measured. The AP is known to be generated by the synchronous firing of the cochlear nerve fibers, and the AER is thought to be a cortical response. Are there electrophysiological responses with intermediate latencies that involve the mediating auditory pathways that can be recorded from humans? The answer *appears* to be yes. The recording of these responses is accomplished with a vertex electrode. These responses are called *brain stem electric (or evoked) responses* (BSER) because they are thought to be generated predominantly by nuclei of the brain stem. Figure 7.12 shows a brain stem evoked potential in response to a click stimulus presented binaurally. The latencies of these responses are from 1 to 8 ms.

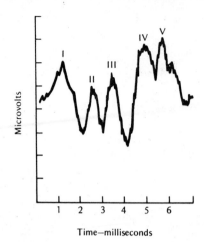

Time—milliseconds

✳ **Figure 7.12** Brain stem evoked potential response (BSER) to a click presented 1000 times binaurally. The response was recorded from the vertex referenced to the right mastoid. Roman numerals represent the labeling of the peaks according to Jewett and Williston, 1971 (see text). *(Recording courtesy of Dr. Donald C. Teas, University of Florida, Gainesville)*

They are low in voltage and require signal averaging to make them "stand out" of the background electrical activity. The source of the first wave, wave 1, is the acoustic nerve. The places where the other potentials originate are not well established, but it is thought that wave II is generated by the cochlear nucleus, wave III by the superior olivary complex, wave IV by the lateral lemniscus (a nucleus between the olivary complex and the inferior colliculus), and wave V (also called P_6) by the inferior colliculus. As normative data are established for these responses and the source or sources for each wave identified, deviations from these norms can be used to detect possible deficiencies in the auditory pathways of the brain stem. Thus the study of electrophysiology of the auditory pathways is slowly producing data for the study and diagnosis of human hearing from the cochlea to the cortex.

In conclusion, it can be said that the central auditory system is anatomically complex, with a variety of ascending and descending pathways. Electrophysiological responses reflect this complexity. Indications are that the auditory cortex is responsible for the analysis of the most complex auditory information received by the auditory system.

Summary In this chapter we have attempted to describe briefly the anatomy and physiology of the central auditory system. The anatomical description was limited to the main nuclei of the ascending and descending pathways and to the auditory cortex in general. Both pathways were shown to have complicated innervation and bilateral representation at almost every nucleus. The interconnections within each nucleus were not discussed in detail, but their existence is evident. The major nuclei of the central auditory nervous system are the cochlear nucleus, superior olive, inferior colliculus, medial geniculate, and auditory cortex. Tonotopic organization was said to be maintained at every level of the system, and tuning curves retained their sharpness at all levels. The descending pathways performed a control function of both a facilitative and inhibitory nature on the incoming information. Time patterns of neurons in the central auditory system, both in the nuclei and the cortex, reflect the anatomical complexities of the nuclei, the pathways, and the cortex. Cells in the superior olive and higher in the system discharge differentially to changes in interaural differences. Auditory evoked responses are a means for obtaining some information concerning central auditory processing.

Supplement   In discussing the anatomy of the system we avoided the detailed anatomy of the various nuclei. Each nucleus contains a number of cell types and inter-connections. For instance, it was stated that tonotopic organizations existed in three areas within the cochlear nucleus. This multiple replication of cochlear topography exists at each of the nuclei. Another measure of the degree of complexity within a nucleus is the *latency of neural transmission* by that nucleus. Latency is the time from stimulus onset to the time the neuron discharges. High-CF fibers in the VIIIth nerve all have approximately the same latency to the onset of a click. The cochlear nucleus latencies are longer and distributed over a much wider time span. Such a wide distribution suggests that many of these neurons are connected by intervening fibers rather than directly connected with auditory nerve fibers. All cochlear nucleus fibers, therefore, should not be considered second order (Kiang, 1965). The variety of response patterns recorded from different regions within each nucleus also suggests different cell types with involved connections both within a nucleus and from the descending pathways. It is undoubtedly the contributions of these various connections, in addition to VIIIth nerve spontaneous activity, that lead to the variety of spontaneous activity found in the central nervous system.

Neurons that discharge to interaural differences have been found in the inferior colliculus (Rose et al., 1966) and in the superior olive of the cat (Moushegian et al., 1967). Some neurons were found that varied their discharge rate to a pure tone on the basis of temporal differences to the two ears, whereas other neurons were found to be sensitive to small differences in intensity.

In recent years investigators have used various procedures to obtain the BSER that occur at latencies of less than 30 ms (some as short as 1 ms) after stimulus onset (Buchwald and Huang, 1975; Jewett et al., 1970) Many stimulus presentations (sometimes more than 3000) are required to obtain reliable results. As we stated, these early latency responses are believed to indicate the synaptic activity of the various sites along the ascending auditory pathway (cochlear nucleus, superior olive, inferior colliculus, and so on). The BSER technique and the electrocochleography procedure described in the Supplement to Chapter 6 offer a means of both studying the central auditory system and revealing abnormalities of the central auditory pathways.

Articles by Benson and Teas (1972), Davis (1968), Donchin and Cohen (1967), and Squires et al. (1975) demonstrate some of the research dealing with the longer latency evoked potentials such as those shown in Figure 7.11.

A system as large and complex as the central auditory system has stimulated a greater body of literature than can be discussed in a short summary. We, therefore, recommend the most recent literature available as the starting point for the reader who wishes to learn more about this system. The *Handbook of Sensory Physiology*, volume V, parts 1 and 2 (Keidel and Neff, 1974, 1975) contains relevant chapters, especially those by Neff et al., Harrison and Howe, and Goldstein and Abeles. This handbook is written at a fairly sophisticated level. Other, older sources may serve as good introductory summaries to supplement the present chapter, such as Whitfield's *The Auditory Pathway* (1967), Mountcastle's chapter on central mechanisms in hearing (1968), and a course summary by Snow and Miller (1975) on the central auditory pathways. Additional general references at more difficult levels can be found in Ades (1959) chapter, various chapters of *Sensory Communication* (Rosenblith, 1959), *The Contributions to Sensory Physiology* (edited by Neff, 1966–1974), and *Sensory Processes at the Neuronal and Behavioral Levels* (edited by Gersuni, 1971).

Listed according to general areas are articles related to the central auditory nervous system: *Anatomy and Physiology of Ascending and Descending Pathways,* see Harrison and Howe (1974a, b), Pfalz (1973), Sando (1965), Whitfield (1968), and Worden (1966); *Cochlear Nucleus,* see Goldberg and Greenwood (1966), Kiang (1965), Kiang et al. (1973), Moller (1973a, b), and Morest et al. (1973); *Superior Olive,* see Goldberg and Brown (1968), Tsuchitani and Boudreau (1966); *Inferior Colliculus,* see Hind et al. (1963), Rose et al. (1966), Van Bergeijk (1962), and Erulker (1975); *Cortical Physiology,* see Brugge and Merzeneich (1973), Evans (1968), Gersuni and Vartanian (1973), Tunturi (1955, 1960), Walzl (1947), and Whitfield and Evans (1965); and *Cortical Lesions,* see Elliott and Trahiotis (1972), Goldberg and Neff (1961a, b), and Trahiotis and Elliott (1970).

CHAPTER 8
Psychophysics: Discrimination Procedures

Classical Psychophysics
Theory of Signal Detection

We have spent a good deal of time describing the acoustic stimulus and the anatomy and physiology of the auditory system. However, we still have little or no information about those changes in the acoustic stimulus to which humans (or other animals) are sensitive; that is, we have not been able to define what an observer can "hear." The firing of a nerve or a group of nerves cannot, according to our present knowledge, provide complete information about "hearing." Somehow we must ask different questions of the observer if we are to investigate his* sensitivity. This involves relying on the observer's behavior—either verbal or nonverbal.

There are two questions to ask the observer: What *can* he respond to? What *does* he respond to? Obtaining answers depends on our

ability to ask the questions properly. We would like to ask the questions in an empirical context.

The field of *psychophysics* deals with the procedures used to ask and to obtain answers to these questions. In its broadest sense, psychophysics is the study of the relationship between psychological and physical aspects of a stimulus. Historically, the methods of psychophysics have centered around two general approaches. One approach focuses on *discrimination*. The observer is presented two or more stimuli—for instance, sinusoids of two different intensities—and then is asked whether the stimuli are different. The discrimination procedures are viewed as an "indirect" means of obtaining an answer to the question: to what can the observer respond? "Direct" meth-

---

* To avoid distracting complexities of wording, we use the masculine generic pronouns in this book, but they should always be understood as meaning "he or she" or "his or her."

ods have also been designed. The late S. S. Stevens believed that an experimeter could obtain a direct estimate of what the observer *does* respond to and, often, what the observer *can* respond to. Thus, the second general class of psychophysical procedures involves directly asking the observer about the stimulus. These are usually called *scaling procedures*. The classical psychophysical procedures and the procedures of the theory of signal detection, which will be described in this chapter, are procedures used to investigate discrimination. The next chapter will deal with such scaling procedures as magnitude estimation and other nondiscrimination psychophysical procedures.

In discrimination tasks the experimenter is interested in obtaining an estimate of the smallest differences in a stimulus parameter (for example, intensity) to which the auditory system is sensitive. That is, to what difference in intensity *can* the observer respond? However, if the experimenter is not careful, he will find out *only* to what difference the observer *does* respond when asked to make the discrimination. The experimenter would like to know to what the observer can optimally respond, instead of to what he just happens to respond at any particular time. Another way of stating the problem is that the experimenter is interested in the observer's *sensitivity* to the stimulus change and not in his ability to respond in the experimental situation (*response proclivity*). The observer might have a particular *bias* toward responding one way, and the experimenter does not want this bias to influence his measure of the auditory system's sensitivity. Thus, using various discrimination procedures, the investigator attempts to arrange the experimental context in such a way that he can measure sensitivity unaffected by response bias (sometimes called criterion for responding or response criterion).

The *scaling* procedures are generally designed to obtain information about various psychological aspects or dimensions. For instance, as the intensity of a sinusoidal sound is changed, what does an observer report? If he responds that its loudness is changing, then scaling procedures attempt to measure how much the loudness changes. When we have obtained the relationship between intensity changes and the observer's report of loudness changes, then perhaps inferences concerning the auditory system's sensitivity can be made.

Before evaluating data concerning the auditory system's sensitivity to sound, we must understand the methods used to obtain these data. If the methods are inappropriate, then the data might reflect only what an observer happened to respond to rather than what his auditory system is actually able to respond to. These concepts are most crucial to understanding audition.

CLASSICAL PSYCHOPHYSICS

Psychophysics is perhaps the oldest area of experimental psychology. Most historians trace its origin to Fechner and his book *Elemente der Psychophysik,* which was published in 1860. Some of the psychophysical methods that originated with Fechner concerned discrimination procedures. Many psychophysicists are interested in measuring the smallest value of some stimulus that an observer can detect. For instance, at 1000 Hz what is the smallest amount of acoustic pressure that an observer can detect? This smallest absolute value (pressure, in this case) is called the *absolute limen* or *absolute threshold*. In addition to investigating the absolute threshold, investigators often study the *difference limen* or *difference threshold*. What is the smallest difference in some stimulus value (for example, pressure at 1000 Hz) that an observer can detect? For instance, if a tone is presented at 1000 Hz and 70 dB SPL, what is the smallest change from 70 dB SPL that the observer can detect?

Both the absolute and difference thresholds

are obtained from discrimination procedures. To obtain the absolute threshold an experiment is performed in which observers discriminate between a stimulus presented with some value of frequency, starting phase, and intensity and a situation in which nothing is presented. The experimenter changes the value of one parameter (such as intensity) until the observer can detect the presence of the stimulus. For the difference threshold two stimuli are presented, differing only in one parameter. For instance, two tones might have slightly different intensities but exactly the same frequency and starting phase. Thus, if the observer can discriminate between the two stimuli, he must be using intensity as his cue for detection.

There are two *basic* classical methods that we will describe: *Method of Limits* and the *Method of Constant Stimuli.* A variation of the Method of Limits, the *Method of Adjustment,* will also be discussed.

Method of Limits

In this procedure the value of a stimulus parameter is successively increased or decreased, and the observer reports whether or not he detected the stimulus. An example of this procedure is shown in Table 8.1 In this case the intensity of a 500-Hz tone is being changed over the range of 9 dB SPL to 19 dB SPL in 1-dB steps. If the experimenter decreases the intensity, the order is presented in a *descending series,* whereas increasing the intensity yields an *ascending series.* After each presentation of the stimulus, the observer responds by saying either "Yes, I hear the tone" (Y symbols) or "No, I do not hear the tone" (N symbols). The experimenter notes on a data

Table 8.1 Method of Limits

Tones from 9 to 19 dB SPL were presented in alternating descending (D) and ascending (A) series in order to compute thresholds for each series. The observer responded either "Yes, I heard the tone" (Y) or "No, I didn't hear the tone" (N). These thresholds (T) are the tonal intensities at which the observer changed his response. The overall mean threshold ($\overline{T}$) is then computed. The column at the far right shows the proportion of "yes" responses for each tonal intensity. These proportions can be used to obtain a psychometric function.

dB SPL (500 Hz)	D	A	D	A	D	A	D	A	D	A	Proportion of "Yeses"
19	Y										
18	Y										1.00
17	Y	Y	Y			Y	Y		Y		1.00
16	Y	Y	Y	Y		Y	Y	Y	Y	Y	1.00
15	Y	N	Y	Y	Y	N	Y	N	Y	Y	0.70
14	N	N	N	Y	Y	N	N	N	N	Y	0.30
13	N	N	N	N	N	N	N	N		N	0.00
12		N		N	N			N		N	0.00
11		N		N				N		N	0.00
10		N		N							
9				N							
	$T=14.5$	15.5	14.5	13.5	13.5	15.5	14.5	15.5	14.5	13.5	
Mean	$\overline{T}=14.5$										

sheet the observer's response to each stimulus. For each series the experimenter determines at what stimulus value the observer changed his response from Y to N (descending series) or from N to Y (ascending series). If the change in response occurs between an intensity of 14 and 15 dB SPL as it did in column 1 of Table 8.1, then the absolute threshold (T) or limen, for that series is 14.5 dB SPL. The experimenter then averages the T values over all of the series to obtain the mean absolute threshold or mean absolute limen. In this case the mean threshold ($\bar{T}$) was 14.5 dB SPL; in other words, at 500 Hz the tone must average 14.5 dB SPL for this observer to say he detected the tone about half the time.

This same procedure can also be used to obtain the difference threshold for a stimulus parameter. In this case the experimenter would present two stimuli differing in some value in both the ascending and descending series. For instance, the 500-Hz tone could be presented at 70 dB SPL followed by a second tone whose intensity might range from 71 dB to 80 dB SPL. The 70-dB tone is the standard stimulus, and the tone of varying intensity is the comparison stimulus. The observer would be presented the 70 dB SPL standard tone and perhaps the 75 dB SPL comparison tone, and he would indicate "Yes, the two tones were different" or "No, the two tones were not different." The procedures shown in Table 8.1 would be used to find the mean difference limen threshold or difference limen.

A careful look at the Method of Limits will reveal that it is limited in obtaining an answer only about the observer's sensitivity; the subject's bias can affect the absolute or difference threshold. For instance, if an observer believes he should respond "yes" only when he hears a loud and clear tone, he will have a higher threshold than will an observer who decides to respond "yes" when he hears anything that sounds like a tone.

A few precautions can help decrease the effects of response bias in the Method of Limits: using both an ascending and a descending series, not telling the observer which series is being presented, randomly starting at different levels of the stimulus, and presenting a different number of stimuli in each series. However, these techniques do not guarantee that the observer's thresholds will be unaffected by his response criterion.

Method of Adjustment

In the Method of Limits the experimenter controls the stimulus parameters, and the subject responds "yes" or "no." If instead we let the subject control the stimulus and adjust some parameter until he can just detect the stimulus, then we have used the *Method of Adjustment*. In the typical Method of Adjustment procedure the subject might be asked to "bracket" his threshold. For instance, he might be asked to turn an intensity knob until he is certain he cannot "hear" a sinusoid (the knob decreases the intensity) and then to turn the knob until he is certain he "hears" the tone (the knob increases the intensity). Next, he is instructed to turn the knob back to where he is *fairly* certain he does not hear the tone, and so on, until he slowly brackets the knob setting at which he can just *barely* hear (or just barely not hear) the tone. This final intensity value is the subject's absolute threshold.

The same procedure can be used to obtain an estimate of the difference threshold. In this case the subject controls a parameter of the stimulus until he can just barely detect a *difference between two stimuli*. The value of the parameter (for example, a knob setting such as intensity) that the subject reports as yielding the *just noticeable difference* between the two stimuli is used to determine the difference threshold.

Von Bekesy adapted the Method of Adjustment procedure to test absolute threshold. In the *Bekesy method* the subject hears a tone that continuously changes in intensity. If he pushes a button, the tone's intensity decreases (becomes softer), as long as the button is pushed; if he releases the button, the tone's intensity continuously increases (becomes louder) as long as the button is released. The subject is instructed to push and release the button in such a manner that the tone remains at a just barely detectable level, or is so that he continues to just barely hear the tone. Eventually, the subject adjusts the intensity to a level at which he pushes, then releases, then pushes, the button. The intensity of the tone changes very little since the tone is just audible. The threshold is determined by computing the average intensity of the tone after the subject has pushed and released the button many times. Quite often the frequency of the tone is slowly changed as the subject is responding. Thus we can obtain a continuous record of the subject's absolute threshold to intensity as a function of frequency.

Both the Method of Adjustment and the Bekesy method are prone to influences from the subject's bias. Not only can the subject change his threshold by varying his criterion for "hearing," but the response manipulations can also affect the thresholds. The subject can adopt a habit of turning knobs or pushing buttons that is directly related to the stimulus presentation. These habitual responses can affect the threshold. One way to reduce the possibility of large influences on threshold due to subject bias is for the experimenter to also change the stimulus parameter that the subject is manipulating. For instance, if the subject is changing intensity in order to "bracket" his absolute threshold, the experimenter can also occasionally vary the intensity of the stimulus. This forces the subject to make an additional large change in his response and to pay close attention to the task. The final threshold estimate, of course, must include the intensity values introduced by the experimenter. Although this helps reduce the effect of subject bias on threshold in these two adjustment procedures, it does not eliminate the bias. These methods do, however, offer the advantage of allowing the experimenter to estimate threshold quickly; for this reason they are convenient tools for obtaining thresholds in a clinical situation. The fact that they are prone to error associated with subject bias makes the adjustment procedure less well suited for laboratory situations in which very accurate threshold estimates are often required.

Method of Constant Stimuli

Another way to analyze the data from the Method of Limits is to tabulate for each value of the stimulus parameter the number of times (or proportion of times) the observer says "Yes, I detected the stimulus." This tabulation appears in Table 8.1 at the far right. At 15 dB SPL the observer said "yes" seven out of ten times, or 70 percent of the time. A *psychometric function* is shown in Figure 8.1, in

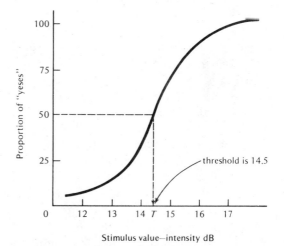

Figure 8.1 Psychometric function relating proportion of "yes" responses to stimulus value (intensity in decibels). A threshold is obtained by noting the intensity (14.5 dB SPL) that yields a 50 percent proportion of "yes" responses.

Table 8.2 Method of Constant Stimuli

The data sheet for 45 trials out of 100 in which the signal level ranged from 12 to 18 dB SPL and the observer responded either "Yes, I heard the tone" (Y) or "No, I did not hear the tone" (N).

Trial	1	2	3	4	5	6	7	8	9	10	11	12	13	14	15
dB SPL	18	12	18	16	14	12	12	16	14	13	15	12	15	18	13
Response	Y	N	Y	Y	Y	N	N	Y	N	N	Y	N	N	Y	N

Trial	16	17	18	19	20	21	22	23	24	25	26	27	28	29	30
dB SPL	17	17	15	13	13	18	14	12	16	16	16	18	14	12	13
Response	Y	Y	Y	N	Y	Y	N	N	N	Y	Y	Y	N	N	N

Trial	31	32	33	34	35	36	37	38	39	40	41	42	43	44	45
dB SPL	17	16	15	13	17	12	16	18	15	13	17	18	16	14	12
Response	Y	Y	Y	N	N	N	Y	Y	Y	N	Y	Y	Y	N	N

which is plotted the proportion of "yes" responses versus intensity. In general, a psychometric function is a plot relating a measure of the observer's performance (such as proportion of "yes" responses) to some value of a stimulus parameter (such as tonal intensity).

The Method of Constant Stimuli is designed to obtain a psychometric function directly from an observer's responses. The experimenter chooses five to ten values of a stimulus parameter, for instance seven values of intensity between 12 and 18 dB SPL of a 1000-Hz tone, and then presents each value approximately 100 times (in the example this would make 700 total trials). The stimuli are presented in a random order, such as that shown in Table 8.2. The observer is asked to indicate on each trial "Yes, I detected the tone" (Y) or "No, I did not detect the tone" (N). The experimenter then tabulates, as in Table 8.3, the proportion of times the observer said "yes" for each stimulus value. These data are then used to plot a psychometric function.

This procedure can be used to obtain a psychometric function for an estimate of an absolute threshold (the procedure just described) or for an estimate of a difference threshold. The procedure for obtaining the difference threshold can be the same as that just described except that each trial consists of two stimuli: for instance, a 70-dB SPL 1000-Hz tone and a 71- to 76-dB SPL 1000-Hz tone. The observer reports either "Yes, the two tones are different" or "No, the two tones are not different." The psychometric function is then a plot of the proportion of "yes" responses versus the difference (in decibels) between the two stimuli associated with each response proportion.

The estimate of either the absolute or difference threshold is obtained from a point on a psychometric function, as shown in Figure 8.1. Some arbitrary value of the proportion of "yes" responses is chosen. Usually this value

Table 8.3 Method of Constant Stimuli

An example of the proportion of times the subject *might* have responded "Yes, I heard the tone" for the seven tonal intensities shown in Table 8.2

Tone Presented (dB SPL)	Proportion of "Yeses"
18	100/100 = 1.0
17	99/100 = .99
16	90/100 = .90
15	80/100 = .80
14	68/100 = .68
13	20/100 = .20
12	0/100 = 0.0

is 50 percent of the total range possible for the proportion of "yes" responses. The psychometric function is then used to obtain that value of the stimulus parameter that would yield the 50 percent value for the proportion of "yes" responses. In Figure 8.1 that value is 14.5 dB SPL, and thus 14.5 dB SPL is labeled *the absolute threshold or absolute limen.*

Notice that in the Method of Limits the mean threshold is also the same value that we would have obtained had we plotted the psychometric function (see Fig. 8.1). That is, the threshold is the intensity value for which the observer would have said 50 percent of the time "Yes, I detect the stimulus." It is also important to note that the absolute or difference threshold is therefore an arbitrary number; if the experimenter decided to use the 80 percent point on the psychometric function, the threshold would be greater.

Over the past 100 years a great deal of attention has been given to the concept of sensory thresholds. Is there one value of intensity that represents the auditory system's threshold to a 1000-Hz tone? If so, the implication is that if this threshold intensity is exceeded by even a tiny bit, the observer will always report that he "heard" the tone. If the threshold intensity is not reached (even if the intensity is only 0.5 dB too low), then the observer would never report "hearing" the tone. This type of behavior is almost never observed in a subject, and thus the threshold concept is not easily accepted today. This fact has been explained in terms of a variable or slightly fluctuating threshold. However, a subject may say "Yes, I detect a tone" when in fact no tone was presented. Thus in modern psychophysics the argument concerning the actual existence of a threshold is moot.

The Method of Constant Stimuli has one large advantage over the Method of Limits in that the experimenter can get an estimate of the observer's bias in the experiment by including "catch" or "blank" trials in the sequence. That is, occasionally the experimenter presents no stimulus to the observer. The observer does not know this has happened, and so he still responds either "yes" or "no." If he has a bias toward either response, then the proportion of "yes" responses on the blank trials will reflect this bias. There are procedures in which the threshold obtained in the Method of Constant Stimuli is "corrected" to take into account the subject's bias. These methods have proved unsatisfactory over the years in that "catch" trials can only indicate the presence of a bias. If this is the case, then the experimenter might decide not to use a particular subject or can hope that his bias does not change over time. If the bias does change, then, of course, the threshold will change, not because of a change in sensitivity but only because of a change in bias.

The classical procedures are therefore still affected by response bias. In most experimental contexts instruction, experience, and feedback can be used to control the effect of bias. Thus in most experiments the data probably reflect the effect of sensory events more than of bias. We shall now study a psychophysical procedure in which a measure of sensitivity is obtained that does not change as a function of the observer's response criterion.

THEORY OF SIGNAL DETECTION

After World War II psychologists began investigating auditory detection of stimuli in the same way engineers had studied the detection of signals by machines (that is, radar detecting an airplane). From this work came the *theory of signal detection* (TSD).

The TSD procedure is similar to the Method of Constant Stimuli. The experimenter might present 100 trials to the observer; 50 trials contain a tone and 50 trials contain nothing (like the "catch" trials). The observer responds on each trial either "Yes, a tone was presented" or "No, a tone was not presented." Of course, only half the trials contained a tone.

There are four possible combinations of stimulus presentations and observer's responses: the stimulus is presented and the observer can say "yes" (a *hit*); the stimulus is presented and the observer can say "no" (a *miss*); the stimulus is not presented and the observer can say "yes" (a *false alarm*); and the stimulus is not presented and the observer can say "no" (a *correct rejection*). The proportion of times the observer had a hit, false alarm, miss, and correct rejection is entered in a *response table,* as shown in Table 8.4. In the theory of signal detection the values of the stimulus parameters remain constant for the full 100 trials; then another 100 trials are presented in which another value of a stimulus parameter (for example, intensity) is used. In one experiment there might be four or five response tables, each one representing the results from presenting a different intensity.

The more intense the stimulus, the easier it is for the observer to detect the tone, and so his hit proportion will increase and his false alarm proportion will decrease (correct rejections must increase). That is, he will detect the

tone more often when it is presented and correctly state "no" when the tone is not presented. The observer might be told to change his response bias. That is, in case 1 he could be told to say "yes" only when he is absolutely sure that he heard the tone; in case 2 he could be told to say "yes" even if he is not sure he heard the tone. In this situation the tone will not become "easier to hear," but the observer will say "yes" more in case 2 than in case 1. Thus the hit proportion will be larger in case 2 than in case 1 since the observer is simply saying "yes" more often in case 2. The false alarms must also be larger in case 2 than in case 1 since the false alarms also represent the "yes" responses. Therefore, changes in sensitivity, *when the response criterion of the subject does not change,* cause hits to increase and false alarms to decrease, whereas changes in bias, *when sensitivity does not change,* increase (or decrease) both hits and false alarms. Four examples of these types of stimulus-response tables are shown in Table 8.5.

We can illustrate these effects in what is called a *receiver operator characteristic* (ROC) curve, as shown in Figure 8.2. Each data point in the ROC curve is taken from the corresponding hit and false alarm proportions of

Table 8.4 Stimulus-Response Table

The stimulus-response table for one stimulus and one response criterion is shown. The stimulus was presented 50 times and the stimulus was absent 50 times. The observer responded "yes" 40 times and "no" 60 times.

		Observer's Response		
		"Yes"	"No"	
Stimulus Present		hit (30/50)	miss (20/50)	50 trials
Stimulus Absent		false alarm (10/50)	correct rejection (40/50)	50 trials
		40 responses	60 responses	100 trials and responses

Stimulus Presentation

Table 8.5   Four Stimulus-Response Tables

Four stimulus-response tables are shown. The top two tables show the results for a high-intensity tone and the bottom two tables represent the data for a low-intensity tone. The two left-hand tables represent a response bias toward saying "yes"; the two right-hand tables show data for a response bias for "no." These data are used to plot the ROC curve in Figure 8.2.

High Intensity (upper curve)

"Yes" (or "A") Response Bias				"No" (or "B") Response Bias		
	"Yes"	"No"			"Yes"	"No"
Stimulus Present	90%	10%		Stimulus Present	70%	30%
Stimulus Absent	30%	70%		Stimulus Absent	10%	90%
	$P(C) = 80\%$				$P(C) = 80\%$	

Low Intensity (lower curve)

"Yes" (or "A") Response Bias				"No" (or "B") Response Bias		
	"Yes"	"No"			"Yes"	"No"
Stimulus Present	75%	25%		Stimulus Present	55%	45%
Stimulus Absent	45%	55%		Stimulus Absent	25%	75%
	$P(C) = 65\%$				$P(C) = 65\%$	

Table 8.5. If we vary (or the observer varies) the bias of an observer, then the data points will fall along curves like the two shown in Figure 8.2. Notice that as you follow one curve from the lower left to the upper right (point B to point A) the false alarms and hits increase. This is what should happen if bias is being altered and sensitivity is not changed. The difference between the two curves represents the observer's sensitivity to the difference in the intensity of the tone. For any two similar points (A or B) on the two curves, the hit rate for the upper curve is greater than that for the lower curve. In general, changes in response criterion will move the hits and false alarms along one curve, whereas changes in sensitivity will yield a point on another curve in the ROC space. Therefore, the *ROC curve enables us to separate bias effects from sensitivity effects.* Notice that the area under the upper curve is larger than the area under the lower curve, and this area cannot change as a function of bias. *Thus the area under any ROC curve is a measure of sensitivity, which is unaffected by response bias.*

Another measure of sensitivity is computed by using this equation:

$P(C) = $ (hit proportion) $\times$ (proportion of times signal presented) $+ (1 - $ false alarm proportion) $\times$ (proportion of times signal not presented)   (8.1)

If the signal is present half the time and no signal the other half, then

$$P(C) = \frac{p(\text{hit}) + (1 - p(\text{false alarm}))}{2}$$

That is, percent correct $P(C)$ is similar to the area under the ROC curve although $P(C)$ is slightly affected by response bias. Other

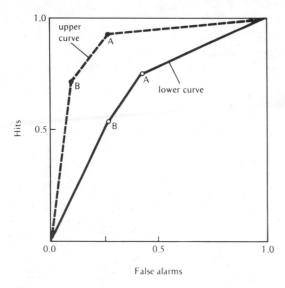

Figure 8.2 Receiver operator characteristic (ROC) curves for two different intensities (upper curve: high intensity; lower curve: low intensity). The points (A or B) along either curve reflect changes in response bias, not in sensitivity. (The four points are taken from the data in Table 8.5.)

measures are derived from the TSD procedure that depend only on sensitivity and not on response bias.

A psychometric function can then be derived using the area under the ROC curve. For each value of a stimulus parameter (such as intensity) we obtain a response table; the response table is used to plot a point on the ROC curve. Numerous points allow us to draw the ROC curve that is used to compute an area. The area and thus the measure of sensitivity will not change as a function of response criterion. Thus as the stimulus intensity changes, the area under the ROC curve will vary between 50 percent and 100 percent, and the psychometric function will be similar to that obtained with the other psychophysical methods. We can then use the midpoint of this function (in this case 75 percent) to estimate a threshold in the same way as in the Method of Constant Stimuli. Psycho-

metric functions for $P(C)$ can also be obtained in essentially the same manner.

In all three psychophysical procedures the first and most important function that is obtained is the psychometric function. After the psychometric function is derived, then an estimate of the threshold is obtained. The value of the threshold is arbitrary since the choice of a value of the observer's performance (that is, $P(C)$) was arbitrary. Thus the thresholds are a function of both the stimulus and of the level of the observer's performance. This can be extremely important if the psychometric function is shallow—that is, if $P(C)$ does not vary considerably as a function of changes in the stimulus parameter. In this case changes in the value of $P(C)$ required to define threshold can lead to a large change in the resulting threshold.

We have discussed three types of discrimination procedures used in psychophysics. The TSD method appears to be the "best" in that its measures of performance are relatively unaffected by response bias. In practice, however, the difference obtained among the three procedures when the observers are highly trained is very small. The disadvantage of the TSD method is the amount of time required to obtain a threshold.

We shall next examine a technique that combines some of the advantages of both the Bekesy method and the TSD method.

Adaptive Procedures

The adaptive procedures have been designed to take advantage of the ability of TSD to use false alarm rates in the estimate of threshold as well as the speed at which thresholds can be estimated by the Bekesy method. In general a subject will be presented two observation intervals per trial. The signal to be detected (for an estimate of absolute threshold) is presented in either the first or the second observation interval, and no signal is presented in the other interval. The subject is to decide whether the tone was presented in the first or in the second interval. There are two ways for him to be correct and two ways for him to be incorrect. He can be correct in saying the stimulus was presented in the first interval, or he can incorrectly report that the stimulus was presented in the first interval. He can correctly report the stimulus found in the second interval, or he can incorrectly report the stimulus in the second interval. In these procedures the value of the stimulus parameter changes toward easier detection if the subject was incorrect, and the parameter is changed to make the detection more difficult if the subject was correct. For instance, if the subject is correct twice in a row in identifying the interval in which the tone appeared, the tone's intensity might be decreased by 2 dB. Whenever the subject makes an incorrect identification, the intensity of the tone increases by 2 dB. After a time the tone's intensity will reach a level at which the subject is making about as many correct as incorrect identifications. This intensity is then calculated as the threshold. Notice that, unlike in the Bekesy method, it is whether or not the subject is correct in determining the occurrence of the stimulus that controls the signal level. In the Bekesy method the stimulus level was changed if the subject "thought" he did or did not hear the stimulus. The adaptive procedure is less prone to bias than the Bekesy method since the adaptive procedure changes the intensity according to a subject's responses on catch-type trials (when the subject was incorrect).

In the adaptive procedure two observation intervals were presented per trial. This is usually called the *two-alternative, forced-choice* method. When one observation interval is presented per trial the procedure is called a *single-interval* procedure. Both of these methods are commonly used in TSD procedures.

Summary Psychophysical procedures have been devised that allow the experimenter to use an observer's behavior to determine to what stimuli the observer can and does respond. The discrimination procedures are used to measure the auditory system's sensitivity, but the results are often confounded by response bias. These procedures generate psychometric functions that measure the absolute or difference thresholds. The three classical procedures—the Method of Limits, Method of Constant Stimuli, and Method of Adjustment (including the Bekesy method)—are more prone to the confounding of response bias than is the modern method, the theory of signal detection (including the adaptive procedures).

Supplement   As was stated in the introduction to this chapter, psychophysics is one of the oldest areas of experimental psychology. Many books and articles have been written on psychophysical procedures. The chapters on psychophysics by Trygg Engen in Volume 1 of *Woodworth and Schlosberg's Experimental Psychology* (3rd ed.), edited by J. W. Kling and L. A. Riggs (1972), offer an excellent review of the application of the classical methods.

The application of the classical methods to the study of difference thresholds can be more involved than the examples discussed in Chapter 8. The subject can be asked, for example, to decide whether one stimulus is "louder," "the same," or "softer" than another stimulus. In this case the comparison stimulus would be presented at intensity values higher, the same as, or lower than a standard intensity stimulus. The determination of the difference thresholds includes obtaining a psychometric function for both the "louder" and "softer" responses and using "the same'" responses as catch trials. These procedures and others are described in detail in the chapters in Volume 1 of *Woodworth and Schlosberg's Experimental Psychology,* edited by Kling and Riggs (1972). Von Bekesy in 1947 introduced his technique for measuring thresholds.

The distinction between sensory capability and response proclivity is an important difference. C. S. Watson (1974), in his chapter in B. Wohlman's *Handbook of Psychology,* provides an excellent discussion of this issue.

TSD was discussed briefly in this chapter. The theory offers a variety of ways of obtaining estimates of sensitivity that are not influenced by bias. The theory of signal detection is best explained in *Signal Detection Theory and Psychophysics* by D. M. Green and J. A. Swets (1974). A briefer, but excellent, review is supplied by Egan and Clarke (1966) in their chapter in *Experimental Methods and Instrumentation in Psychology,* edited by J. B. Sidowski. The theory of signal detection has provided three impacts on hearing: (1) a model for how the auditory system detects signals in the background of noise, (2) a new and more powerful psychophysical procedure than the classical methods, and (3) an alternate view to the threshold theory (sometimes called quantal theory) of sensation.

Another way of developing the logic behind the separation of bias and sensitivity is by assuming that the subject is using some aspect of the stimulus environment to make a decision as to whether or not the sound was presented. Let us label this aspect of the environment the decision variable (for example, it might have to do with the acoustic pressure in the room). We shall also assume that when no sound is presented, there is still some probability that the observer will sample a value of the environment (for example, a high pressure) that will lead him to say that the sound was presented. Likewise, when the sound is presented, there is some probability that the observer will sample a value of the environment (for example, a low pressure) that will lead him to say that no stimulus was presented.

However, high values of the decision variables are more likely to occur if a sound is presented and low values are more likely to occur if no sound is given. Figure 8.3a shows a way to represent these assumptions, with normal distributions representing the probability of occurrence of values of the decision variable given that no signal was presented (no signal curve) and given that a signal was presented (signal curve). Thus, if on one trial the subject sampled decision variable Y, this value has a higher probability of occurring (B) if the signal was presented than if the signal were not presented (A). Thus, in this case the subject might choose to respond, "Yes, a signal was presented."

Figure 8.3b represents a subject who decided to say "yes" if the decision variable had a value greater than P (the criterion point) and to say "no"

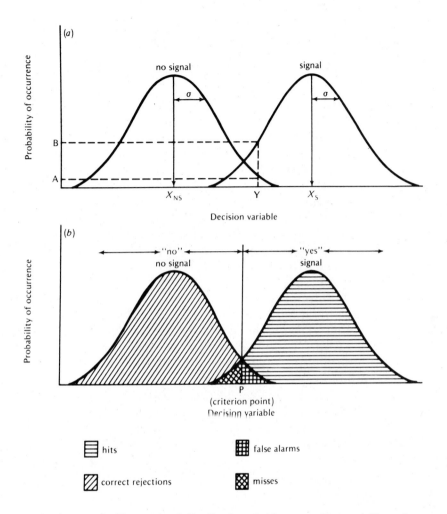

Figure 8.3 Two normal distributions (with means X_{NS} and X_S and common variance σ) of the probability of occurrence of values of a decision variable, given no signal $(_{NS})$ and signal $(_S)$ presentations. **8.3a:** Subject may sample a decision value, Y, which would yield a higher probability of occurrence if a signal were present (B) than if no signal were present (A). **8.3b:** Areas under the normal distributions corresponding to hits, false alarms, correct rejections, and misses for a criterion point placed at P.

when the decision variable had a value less than **P**. Notice that the probability of saying "yes" and being correct that it was present is represented by the area under the signal curve and to the right of the criterion point, the vertical marked area. Recall that this probability is a hit. The rest of the probabilities in the stimulus response tables can also be obtained in Figure 8.3b. Thus these two probability curves could be constructed from the values obtained from a stimulus-response table.

If the subject changes his bias, he merely changes the location of the criterion point. Changes in sensitivity move the signal distribution further away (to the right) of the no-signal distribution. *Therefore any measure of the separation between the two distributions will describe sensitivity, and it will be unaffected by response bias* since changes in response bias does not affect the placement of the distributions. We measure the separation between the two distributions by subtracting the mean of the no-signal distribution (X_{NS}) from the mean of the signal distribution (X_S) and dividing by the standard deviation (σ). This difference is labeled d'. Thus $d' = (X_S - X_{NS})/\sigma$. Tables of d' for various values of hits and false alarms can be obtained from Appendix I of Swets' (1964) book *Signal Detection and Recognition by Human Observers*. A more detailed discussion of d' and the ROC curve is contained in Egan's (1975) excellent book, *Signal Detection Theory and ROC Analysis*. d' is a very common measure of sensitivity when the TSD procedure is used. Like the area under the ROC curve it changes only with changes in sensitivity and not with changes in response bias.

It should be emphasized that although the area under the ROC curve does not change with bias, $P(C)$ can be affected by bias. Dennis McFadden (1970), in his article "Three Computational Versions of Proportion Correct for Use in Forced-Choice Experiments," describes the types of changes in $P(C)$ that result from changes in subject bias. In all cases, however, $P(C)$ varies far less as a function of bias than does the probability of a hit. Robinson and Watson (1972), in Volume 2 of *Foundations of Modern Auditory Theory*, describe ways of designing an auditory experiment using the theory of signal detection.

There are a variety of adaptive procedures. The one described in this chapter is discussed in an article by Harry Levitt (1971), "Transformed Up-Down Methods in Psychoacoustics." This article describes other methods and reviews the conditions that must be met before these adaptive methods can be used.

CHAPTER 9

Psychophysics: Scaling and Other Procedures

Indirect Scaling
Direct Scaling
Matching Procedures

In Chapter 8 we described methods for determining the smallest detectable difference between two stimuli. Quite often other information about auditory processing is required. For instance, an instructor might be speaking too softly and you would like him to speak twice as loud. It is easy to determine what actually is twice as intense by physically measuring the pressure or energy of the sound and then increasing it until the physical measure has doubled. But what is our measure of loudness? Loudness is a subjective quality. That is, if the instructor doubled the pressure at which he was speaking, the pressure would increase by 6 dB, but this increase would not be judged as a doubling in loudness. If the instructor were speaking at 50 dB SPL and he used a microphone and amplifier to speak at 100 dB SPL, this would be con-

siderably more than a doubling of loudness. Since sounds have both subjective and physical properties, we require some rule or function that would relate a subjective attribute (loudness) to a physical measure (pressure). Some of the subjective attributes of sound will be discussed in more detail in Chapter 13. The present chapter is devoted to a brief description of some of the methods used to measure these subjective aspects of sound. We shall discuss three basic types of psychophysical procedures: *indirect scaling, direct scaling,* and *matching*.

INDIRECT SCALING

Fechner's theories led to the development of indirect scaling methods. Fechner believed that the difference threshold or the *just noticeable difference* (jnd) between two stimuli could be used to obtain the relationship between a subjective attribute (loudness) and a physical stimulus parameter (pressure). He based much of his argument on Weber's studies. In the early 1800s Weber observed that our ability to distinguish between two weights depends on their *relative* masses. We have all observed that it is easy to distinguish between a 1-pound and a 2-pound weight, but not so easy to differentiate a 100-pound weight from a 101-pound weight even though both pairs of weights differ by 1 pound. Weber found that the difference between two weights which could just be detected was proportional to the value of the smaller weight that the subject had to lift while making the comparison. That is, if the jnd for a 1-pound weight was 0.1 pound, then the jnd for the 100-pound weight was 10 pounds. Fechner stated this relation in equation form:

$$\frac{\Delta S}{S} = \text{constant} \qquad (9.1)$$

where ΔS is the just noticeable physical difference in some stimulus value and S is the smaller of the two values being discriminated. The ratio $\Delta S/S$ is called the *Weber fraction*. Fechner believed that each ΔS was equal to one unit of a subjective measure, that is, the just noticeable difference (jnd). Let us say that ΔS at 100 units of pressure was 10 units; thus, a change of 10 units of pressure is equal to a change of one subjective unit of loudness. Since Fechner thought that the Weber fraction was a constant, as the intensity S increases, the units of ΔS must increase proportionally. Thus, if at 100 units 10 units were a jnd (10/100), then at 1000 units of pressure the jnd must be equal to 100 units of pressure (100/1000). But at this level (1000 units) 100 units of pressure also equals one subjective unit of loudness. Therefore, a greater and greater change in intensity is required for one

subjective unit of loudness as the overall intensity S increases. From this idea, Fechner derived the *Fechner relation:*

$$P = K \log S \qquad (9.2)$$

where P is the psychological or subjective unit, S the physical unit, log the logarithm, and K a proportionality constant.

To determine how much intensity is required to double the loudness of a sound, we decide by how much pressure S must change so that $K \log S$ (that is, P) would increase by a factor of 2.

Fechner's two assumptions were (1) that all jnd's could be summed to produce a scale of the subjective sensation, and (2) that any jnd is one unit along a scale of that subjective attribute. However, these two assumptions, as well as the Fechner relation, have not held up well to experimental testing. Although his ideas were not precisely correct, Fechner did introduce the notion of scaling and showed the importance of both the jnd and the Weber fraction. From his work other methods of obtaining scales relating P (subjective attribute) to S (physical stimulus) have been derived. These methods aim to obtain the scale empirically rather than to use only a formula, as Fechner suggested. Although the scales are formed from experimental data, the experimenter is assuming the existence of a subjective scale for the stimulus he is measuring which he can obtain by the proper analysis of the experimental data. Three of these methods —pair comparison, stimulus rating, and ranking method—are briefly described in the following paragraphs.

Pair Comparison

In pair comparison the subject is presented ten or more stimuli in groups of two (that is, in pairs) and is asked to compare them along some dimension. For instance, which tone is louder, A or B? The stimuli are then ordered from the loudest (in this case) to the softest. In some instances, of course, there will be some reversals or inconsistencies in the ranking. That is, a subject might have considered tone A louder than tone B and tone B louder than tone C, but ranked tone C louder than tone A. The scale is therefore formed by using many subjects to make the paired comparisons. Then the proportional data for each comparison are used. That is, 90 percent of the subjects might have stated that A was louder than B, and only 50 percent stated that B was louder than C. The scale of loudness is obtained by noting that A and B are further apart in loudness than B and C since more people judged A louder than B than judged B louder than C. From this type of information a scale of loudness can be developed.

Stimulus Rating

The basic idea of the stimulus rating procedure is for the subject to rate each stimulus on a scale of, for instance, from 1 to 100. How loud is stimulus A if 100 is loud and 1 is soft? The mean ratings for each stimulus are then calculated. The scale is derived by ordering the stimuli according to their rating. Two stimuli close together in rating are considered close together in loudness.

Ranking Method

A subject is presented ten or more stimuli and asked to rank them in some order. For instance, he is presented ten tones and is asked to rank them from loudest to softest. Again, many subjects are used in order to form the scale. The mean rank for each stimulus is then tabulated. Thus, stimulus A might have been ranked on the average, 1.5, stimulus D, 2.0, and stimulus F, 3.5. The scale of loudness is derived by noting that A must be closer in loudness to D, than D is to F since the differ-

ence in the mean ranking between A and D was smaller than between D and F.

DIRECT SCALING

The indirect scaling methods require the experimenter to obtain group data and then to infer from these data the scale that relates the subjective attribute to the physical stimulus. S. S. Stevens in the late 1930s demonstrated that reliable and valid scales of subjective attributes could be obtained if the experimenter directly asked the subject about the stimulus. For instance, the experimenter would ask the subject to choose a number corresponding to the loudness of a tone. The numbers chosen by the subject directly become the subjective units of the scale.

Over the past 40 years many direct scaling procedures have been developed to obtain these judgments of magnitude. Some of the methods are described in the following paragraphs.

Magnitude Estimation

Observers are instructed to assign numbers to a particular attribute of a stimulus. For instance, the intensity of a tone might be varied, and the observer indicates by using numbers how loud each intensity appears. The subject is usually instructed to make his judgments relative to some standard stimulus and to assign numbers according to ratios. The standard intensity may be labeled 100, and if the stimulus the observer is listening to appears twice as loud as the standard, he should assign it the number 200. The magnitude estimates form the subjective scale.

Ratio Comparisons

An observer is presented a standard stimulus that changes along some dimension (intensity) and is asked to adjust another (comparison) stimulus value in this dimension so that it appears, say, half or twice as much along the subjective attribute as the standard stimulus. For instance, a 500-Hz tone is presented at 60 dB SPL; the observer is given another 500-Hz tone whose intensity he can control. He then adjusts the comparison tone so that it sounds half as loud as the standard tone. The scale is developed by the experimenter by assuming that a tone judged half as loud as a second tone would have a scale value half that of the second tone.

Cross-Modality Matching

The observer is given control of one stimulus and is asked to match one attribute of it so that it equals the value along another dimension of a stimulus controlled by the experimenter. For instance, the observer might have control of the intensity of a light, and the experimenter is varying the intensity of a tone. The observer is asked to adjust the intensity of the light so that it is as bright as the tone is loud. The physical measure of light intensity in this case is used as the subjective scale.

Although these procedures may seem unusual, they do provide reliable and valid data. When the data are plotted as the logarithm of the magnitude of the subjective measure versus the logarithm of the stimulus value, the data are almost always fit by a straight line. For instance, in a magnitude estimation procedure of loudness, if the results are plotted as the log of the magnitude estimation numbers versus decibels of intensity (the decibel is the log of intensity), then data such as those shown in Figure 9.1 are obtained. As shown, the data are fit by a straight line. The fact that a straight line fits data that are plotted on log-log coordinates means that the magnitude estimate is related to the stimulus

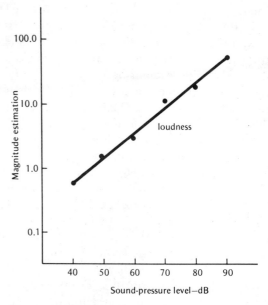

Figure 9.1 Data obtained from a magnitude estimation experiment. The magnitude numbers (on a log scale) are plotted against the sound-pressure level in decibels (also a log scale). The data are fit by a straight line, which implies that the magnitude numbers (subjective loudness) are related to intensity by a power function. *(Adapted from Stevens, 1975, by permission)*

dimension by a *power function*. Considerable work in scaling is concerned with the properties of power functions.

The power function is given by

$$P = kS^n \qquad (9.3)$$

where P is the subjective unit, S the physical unit, k the proportionality constant, and n the power variable. Stevens has shown that the power function fits the scaling data better than the Fechner relation. He has measured the power function for many different stimuli and attributes. By knowing the power function we can compute such information as the number of decibels required to double the loudness of a 1000-Hz tone at 70 dB SPL.

Notice that if in equation (9.3) we take the logarithm of both sides of the equation (see Appendix B for the use of logarithms), we have

$$\log P = n \log S + \log k \qquad (9.4)$$

In equation (9.4) $\log k$ is still a constant and $\log P$ is now linearly related to $\log S$. That is, if we plot $\log P$ versus $\log S$ we generate a straight line, as in Figure 9.1. The slope of this line is the number n, or the power variable. Thus we can easily estimate the power variable by plotting the scaling results on log-log coordinates and obtaining the slope of the straight line that is fit to the data. The power value is often used in relating the psychological aspects to the physical aspects of any stimulus.

Thus scaling can be used to obtain answers about observers' judgments of acoustical events. We have only briefly described the area of scaling, but interest in scaling covers a great deal more than the contents of this chapter.

MATCHING PROCEDURES

Many variations of the discrimination and scaling procedures have been developed to study auditory function. A variation often used is the matching procedure.

In the matching paradigm two stimuli are presented to the observer, and he is asked to match their equality along some stimulus attribute. For instance, a 500-Hz tone might be presented at 40 dB SPL, and the subject is asked to adjust the intensity of a 1000-Hz tone so that the two tones (500 and 1000 Hz) sound equally "loud." Or a subject might be presented a complex stimulus, such as a complex waveform consisting of the sum of three sinusoids (700, 800, and 900 Hz). The subject could then be asked to adjust the frequency of a second stimulus, which is a pure tone, so that the pure tone sounds equal in "pitch" to that of the complex waveform.

With the matching procedures the two waveforms to be matched usually differ in many physical dimensions, and the subject is asked to adjust one of these physical dimensions in order to make a subjective match. One should remember that two waveforms that differ in many physical dimensions but are equal in physical intensity or physical frequency may not sound equal in the subjective domains of loudness and pitch. Loudness and pitch are subjective measures that are *not* perfectly related to their physical counterparts, intensity and frequency. We shall see in Chapter 13 that there can be large differences between physical and subjective measures.

The matching procedures allow the experimenter to decide which aspect of a stimulus makes it appear equal according to some subjective attribute to another stimulus. Thus, although tones of different frequencies might have equal physical intensities, they are not all equally loud. Matching procedures allow one to determine how much change in intensity is required to make the various tones sound equal in loudness.

The matching procedures are most often used to measure subjective attributes of physical stimuli. The intent is similar to that of the scaling procedures. The matching procedures, however, are also similar to the method of adjustment in that subjects adjust a comparison stimulus so that it is judged "equal" to the standard stimulus. In general, the method of adjustment is used to describe situations in which the standard and comparison stimuli differ *only* in the physical dimension that the observer is adjusting, whereas in the matching procedure the stimuli may vary in many dimensions in addition to the one the observer is adjusting.

Summary Two basic methods are used to obtain scales that relate subjective attributes of sound to physical measures. These methods and their procedures are:

1. Indirect scaling
   a. Pair comparison
   b. Stimulus rating
   c. Ranking method

2. Direct scaling
   a. Magnitude estimation
   b. Ratio comparisons
   c. Cross-modality matching

The Weber law, Fechner relation, and power function are relations important in determining scales according to these various procedures. Matching procedures are also used to determine the values for subjective attributes of sound.

Supplement   The word "psychophysics" was originally derived to cover those areas of psychology in which investigators attempted to obtain scales of subjective attributes. E. G. Boring's (1942) book *Sensation and Perception in the History of Experimental Psychology* offers an excellent history of the development of psychophysics.

Trygg Engen's chapter on "Scaling Methods" in Volume 1 of *Woodworth and Schlosberg's Experimental Psychology* (edited by Kling and Riggs, 1972) offers a good review of the methods of direct and indirect scaling. In addition, Marks' (1974) book *Sensory Processes* and S. S. Stevens' (1975) book *Psychophysics* present in-depth views of direct scaling and the power function. Watson's (1974) chapter in Wohlman's *Handbook of Psychology* provides an excellent discussion of the difference between discrimination procedures and scaling procedures.

When determining a scale an experimenter usually uses one of at least four types of scales. That is, he uses one of four types of ways to assign numbers to objects, or events, or subjective attributes: (1) Nominal scales, which are used for classification. For instance, number 88 is a tackle on the football team while number 9 is the quarterback. (2) Ordinal scales, which simply arrange objects in order. For instance, 1 is less than 4, which is less than 10, and so on. (3) Interval scales, in which the assigned numbers differ in successive order by a constant interval. For instance, 1, 2, 3, 4, . . . is an interval scale in which the interval is 1, and 2, 4, 6, 8, . . . is an interval scale in which the interval is 2. (4) Ratio scales, in which the assigned numbers differ in successive order by a constant ratio. For instance, 10, 100, 1000, 10,000, . . . is a ratio scale in which the ratio is 10. The decibel scale is formed from a ratio scale. The indirect scales are usually ordinal or interval scales, whereas the direct scales are ratio scales. The book *Mathematical Psychology: An Elementary Introduction*, by Coombs, Dawes, and Tversky (1970), offers an introductory study of measurement and scaling theories. This book and others on measurement theory emphasize the importance of using careful methods when attempting to obtain a scale of a subjective attribute.

CHAPTER 10
Auditory Sensitivity

Threshold of Audibility
Duration
Differential Sensitivity
Frequency Discrimination
Intensity Discrimination
Temporal Discrimination

THRESHOLD OF AUDIBILITY

Perhaps the first question to ask about the auditory system concerns its absolute sensitivity to frequency, starting phase, and intensity. When answers to these questions are obtained for sinusoidal stimuli, then the results might form a fairly complete picture of the absolute sensitivity of the auditory system to any stimulus since all acoustical stimuli can be defined in terms of sinusoids. As we shall see in this and the following chapters, however, the problems are not that simple.

When a pure tone is presented to one ear, the auditory system is actually *insensitive* to starting phase. This does not mean, as Helmholtz suggested, that the *auditory system* is phase-insensitive. For instance, if two sinusoids of different frequencies are added together, the perceived quality of the sound will vary as the

starting phases of the sinusoids are varied. Also, as was mentioned in Chapter 1, if a sinusoid is presented to both ears and there is a change in the interaural (between-ears) phase difference, then the observer reports a change in the perceived location of the tone.

We can determine auditory sensitivity to frequency by determining the intensity required for an observer to detect the presence of a sinusoid at each of many frequencies. There will probably be very low and very high frequencies to which, no matter how intense the sinusoid, the system is insensitive. These frequency limits would then define the bounds of the auditory system's sensitivity to frequency. The curve relating the smallest intensity required for detection to the frequency of the tone is called *threshold of audibility* (sometimes called an audiogram).

The threshold of audibility is obtained in

the laboratory in the following manner. For each frequency tested a psychometric function is obtained using one of the psychophysical procedures. The psychometric function relates the observer's performance to the intensity of the sinusoid. Figure 10.1 demonstrates the results from this part of the experiment. Next, the threshold is determined for each frequency by choosing a performance level, such as 75 percent, for $P(C)$. The thresholds of audibility are plotted as the threshold in decibels versus frequency, as in Figure 10.2. If a subject has a low threshold at one frequency, we can also describe his behavior by stating that he is very sensitive at that frequency. Thus "high sensitivity" and "low threshold" can be used to describe the same set of data. Figure 10.2 shows the results from a variety of experiments in which the thresholds were measured. The intensities of the tones were originally expressed in decibels relative to 1 dyne/cm² of pressure. These numbers are shown on the left axis. After the thresholds were determined, the approximate intensity required to detect the 1000-Hz tone was calculated. This level was labeled zero dB on the *sound pressure level* (SPL) *scale* (that is, 0 dB SPL equals 0.0002 dyne/cm² of pressure). The right axis was constructed so that the intensity is in decibels of sound pressure level, or dB SPL. Remember also that the threshold of audibility describes

the intensities required for some arbitrary level of performance (that is, $P(C)$). Thus thresholds of audibility as determined in the laboratory or clinic are a function both of frequency and of the level of the observer's performance.

The thresholds of audibility have been obtained in two types of experimental environments. In one case, headphones are placed on the observer, and the thresholds are obtained; this procedure is called the *minimal audible pressure* (MAP) approach. In order to determine exactly what intensity is arriving at the ear from the headphone, a calibration procedure must be used. As we mentioned in Chapter 3, membranes and speaker cones act as low-pass filters. Since most headphones contain membranes that provide the vibrating surface that transmits the sound, they act as a low-pass filter. In addition to obtaining the characteristics of the headphone, we must also determine what pressure the headphone will exert at the tympanic membrane. Recall that pressure is force per unit area. Thus if a headphone is placed at the external auditory meatus, we must determine the pressure being generated in the volume between the headphone and tympanic membrane. It has been calculated that this volume averages 6 cubic centimeters (6 cm³). Thus, the headphone can be calibrated by measuring the pressure it ex-

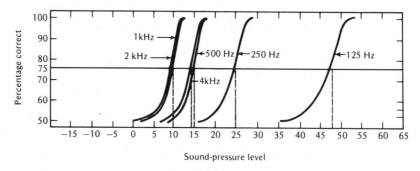

Figure 10.1 Psychometric functions obtained for six tones. The thresholds are obtained at a $P(C)$ of 75 percent. (*Adapted from Watson, Franks and Hood, 1972, by permission*)

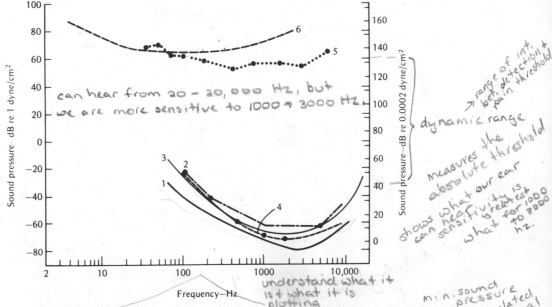

Figure 10.2 Threshold of audibility curves from four studies (1–4) and estimates of the maximum intensity limits of audibility from two studies (5–6). Curves 1 and 3: from Sivian and White (1933). Curve 1: minimum audible field (MAF). Curve 3: minimum audible pressure (MAP). Curve 2: MAP American Standard Association standard (1951). Curve 4: American National Standards Institute standard (1969). Curve 5: Wegel's (1932) threshold of "feeling" estimate. Curve 6: von Bekesy's (1936a) threshold of "tickle" estimate of the upper limit of audibility. The large dots are from Watson, Franks and Hood's (1972) study shown in Figure 10.1.

erts into 6 cm³ of volume attached to the headphone. An object with a volume of 6 cm³, sometimes referred to as a 6-cm³ (or 6-cc) coupler, is attached to the headphones. The pressure in the coupler is measured in decibels (usually dB SPL) at each frequency, with the intensity into the headphone presented at the previously measured threshold intensity for that frequency. The pressure values obtained from the coupler at each frequency will then be the thresholds (in dB SPL) for those frequencies.

The use of the 6-cm³ coupler also allows us to obtain the filter characteristic of the headphone. A sinusoid is presented to the headphone at different frequencies but always at the same input intensity. The pressure in the coupler is then measured. If this pressure

changes as a function of changes in frequency, then the headphone is acting as a filter or resonator, and the pressure at the output of the phone will not be the same for all input frequencies. The amount of pressure change allows the exact characteristics of the filtering action of the headphone to be determined.

The other method for obtaining tonal thresholds is called the *minimal audible field* (MAF) approach. In this case a loudspeaker is used instead of a headphone, and again a calibration procedure is required. The observer's thresholds are determined with the threshold expressed in terms of the intensity at the input to the loudspeakers. The subject is then removed from the laboratory, and a small calibrated microphone is placed where he was seated. The experimenter then presents the same frequencies and intensities used to determine the thresholds. A calibrated microphone then determines the actual pressures (in dB SPL) at the location of the ear, and these numbers are used to describe the thresholds of audibility.

Figure 10.2 illustrates the differences between the measurements taken with an MAP and an MAF procedure. Notice that the MAP procedure tends to give higher thresholds than the MAF procedure. *Part* of this difference is due to the fact that the MAP procedure measures pressures analogous to those at the tympanic membrane, whereas the MAF procedure measures pressures analogous to those at the external auditory meatus. (Remember that there is amplification between the external auditory meatus and the tympanic membrane.)

Although determining the audiogram appears rather straightforward, it is demanding in terms of the instrumentation required. The main obstacle the instrumentation must overcome is the remarkable sensitivity of the auditory system. The fact that we can detect tones over a range of frequencies from 20 Hz to 20,000 Hz requires very good loudspeaker or headphone systems. Zero dB SPL corresponds to 0.0002 dyne/cm², which is an extremely small amount of pressure. At this pressure and at a signal frequency of 1000 Hz the tympanic membrane is vibrating through a total distance approximately that of the diameter of a hydrogen atom. Zero dB SPL is within 20 percent of the pressure that would be exerted by the random motion of air molecules colliding with one another. Only in recent decades has equipment been made that can reliably produce the tones required to obtain an audiogram.

The sensitivity of the auditory system also causes threshold measurements to be highly variable because small amounts of uncontrolled noise will affect the detectability of the tone. Threshold variability also can be a result of the subject's detection criterion. For instance, if a subject is asked to just detect the tone, the thresholds in Figure 10.2 are obtained. If, however, he is asked to respond only when he hears a "tonal" quality, then higher thresholds would be found, since a higher intensity is required for a sound to be identified as having a tonal quality.

The thresholds of audibility define the smallest amount of pressure to which the auditory system is sensitive. What about limits in terms of the most pressure the auditory system can tolerate? The upper curves in Figure 10.2 show different ways to obtain this upper limit. We can ask the subject to indicate when he "feels" the sound, when he experiences pain, when he feels a tickling sensation, and so on. All of these are indications that the sound pressure is reaching a maximum. This maximum limit appears to be approximately 150 dB SPL, and it remains relatively unchanged as a function of the frequency content of the stimulus. Thus, the dynamic range (difference between threshold in dB SPL and the maximum limit in dB SPL) of the auditory system is a function of frequency; it is approximately 150 dB at 1000 Hz but only 60 dB at 20 Hz.

The auditory system, therefore, is sensitive to approximately a 20,000-Hz range of frequencies and a 150-dB range of intensities. Thus humans are sensitive to a remarkably large frequency and intensity range, as well as to extremely small pressure levels.

DURATION

One variable that was not specified in the procedures used to obtain tonal thresholds is the duration of the sinusoid. From a number of points of view we would expect that the longer a sound lasts, the easier it is to hear. For the thresholds of audibility shown in Figure 10.2 the tones had a duration of more than 500 ms.

When time (T) is involved in the measurement of intensity, we must be careful in noting whether the intensity is expressed as power (*P*) or energy (*E*). Remember that

$$P = \frac{E}{T} \qquad (10.1)$$

In order to describe the auditory system's sensitivity to duration, the experimenter can keep either the power or the energy of the signal constant (but not both) as he changes its duration. Of course, if energy is maintained constant, then the power of the signal must change as the duration changes; equation (10.1) is used to determine the energy of the signal.

Figure 10.3 shows the thresholds for different frequencies as a function of the duration of the signals. In this figure *power* was changed as the signal duration was varied. That is, for each duration a psychometric function was obtained in which performance of the observer

was related to the power of the signal. Then for each duration the threshold in power was determined from the psychometric functions and plotted in Figure 10.3.

Notice that at durations greater than approximately 250 to 500 ms the threshold in units of power for various tones does not change; for durations greater than about 250–500 ms, the tone does not become easier to detect. However, as the tone's duration is made shorter than 250 ms, the power of the tone must be increased in order for the observer to detect the tone. This increase is *approximately equal to 8 to 10 dB of power increase for each tenfold decrease in the duration of the tone.* This in turn means that the signal energy is remaining approximately constant for a constant level of the observer's performance, although this effect is slightly dependent on the frequency of the sound. That is, equation (10.1) states that energy will remain constant

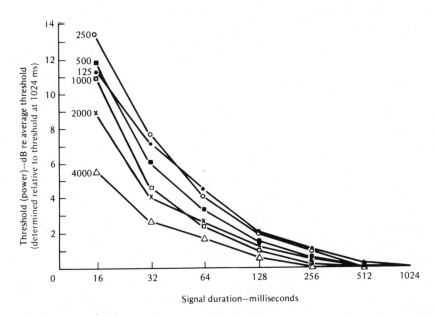

Figure 10.3 Thresholds in *power* for six tonal frequencies (ranging from 125 to 4000 Hz) displayed as a function of tonal duration. The values—that is, the intensity scores—are calculated and plotted in relation to the thresholds obtained at 1024 ms. *(Adapted from Watson and Gengel, 1969, by permission)*

if, as duration decreases, power increases. In other words, if $P = E/T$, then $\log P = \log (E/T)$, or $10 \log P = 10 \log E - 10 \log T$. (See Appendix B, rule 2.) Therefore $10 \log E = 10 \log P + 10 \log T$. Thus for a tenfold change in duration, power must also change tenfold to keep energy constant. For the data shown in Figure 10.3 it is important to realize that *duration is expressed in relation to 1 second*. Therefore, a change from 1 second to $\frac{1}{10}$ of a second (100 ms) is a change of $\frac{1}{10}$ or, in logarithms, ($10 \log \frac{1}{10}$) or -10. So as duration becomes shorter (less than 1 second), the power must become larger if energy is to remain constant. For example, if a 500-ms tone has a power of 80 dB, then the energy of the 500-ms tone is 77 dB; that is,

$$10 \log E = 10 \log P + 10 \log T$$
$$E \text{ in dB} = P \text{ in dB} + 10 \log T$$
$$= 80 \text{ dB} + 10 \log \frac{500 \text{ ms}}{1000 \text{ ms}}$$
$$= 80 \text{ dB} - 3 \text{ dB} = 77 \text{ dB}$$

If the duration is changed from 500 ms to 50 ms and energy remains 77 dB, then

$$77 \text{ dB} = P \text{ in dB} + 10 \log \frac{50}{500}$$
$$= P \text{ in dB} - 10 \text{ dB}$$

or

$$P \text{ in dB} = 87 \text{ dB}$$

Thus, the power of the 50-ms tone must be 10 dB higher than the 500-ms tone if energy is to remain constant.

Between approximately 10 ms and 500 ms the energy of the signal must remain approximately constant for constant performance by the observer. This is shown in Figure 10.4, in which the threshold in *energy* for the 1000-Hz tone is plotted as a function of time. The difference between Figure 10.4 and Figure 10.3 is that the vertical axis has been changed from power to energy. In Figure 10.3 and 10.4 the change in threshold is expressed relative to that obtained at 1024 ms; as the duration decreased, the power shown in Figure 10.3 had

to be increased. In Figure 10.4 the energy had to be decreased as duration decreased in order to obtain just detectable tones. The fact that the auditory system is sensitive to energy over the approximate range of 10 to 500 ms is often referred to as the *constant-energy* or *temporal integration* property of the auditory system.

Once the duration of a sinusoidal signal decreases below 10 ms, then much more power is required for detection than is needed to keep energy a constant. It appears that the auditory system is not a constant-energy detector below 10 ms. In Chapter 1 we showed that a tone that is turned on and off spreads its energy over a large frequency region. As the duration of the tone becomes shorter and shorter, this frequency region over which the energy is spread becomes larger and larger. Thus for very short-duration tones (less than 10 ms) the frequency region over which the energy of the tone is spread becomes so large that not all of the energy is contributing to its detectability. Since there is some energy at fre-

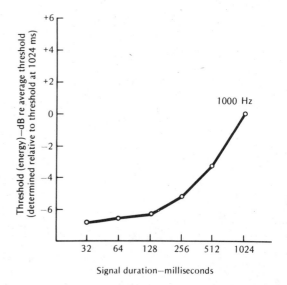

Figure 10.4 Threshold in *energy* for the 1000-Hz tone of Figure 10.3 plotted as a function of tonal duration. The values are determined in relation to the threshold obtained at 1024 ms.

quencies to which the ear is insensitive, there will be *less* energy in the region where the ear is sensitive. This in turn means that the total power or energy of the tone must be increased so that enough energy is in the auditory system's frequency region of sensitivity for the tone to be detected.

Therefore the duration of the signal used to establish tonal thresholds is important. If it is longer than approximately 500 ms, the thresholds represent intensity in power; if the signal is between 10 and 500 ms, the thresholds reflect approximately constant energy; for signals whose durations are less than 10 ms the spread of energy makes the determination of thresholds difficult.

DIFFERENTIAL SENSITIVITY

Although the threshold of audibility defines the frequency and intensity range of the auditory system, it does not describe our sensitivity to *changes* in intensity and frequency. Recall from Chapter 8 that psychologists have investigated differential sensitivity for approximately as many years they have studied absolute sensitivity. The Weber fraction is:

$$\frac{\Delta S}{S} = \text{constant} \qquad (10.2)$$

where ΔS is the just noticeable physical difference in some stimulus value and S is the smaller of the two values being discriminated. Psychoacousticians have attempted to determine whether the Weber fraction for the intensity and the frequency of sinusoids is a constant and, if so, over what range of intensities and frequencies.

Extreme care must be taken in studying differential sensitivity. As mentioned previously, not all of the energy of a tone is at the tonal frequency if the tone is very short or if it is turned on and off abruptly. This same spread of energy also arises if either the frequency, intensity, or phase of an ongoing tone is suddenly changed. Thus we cannot simply study

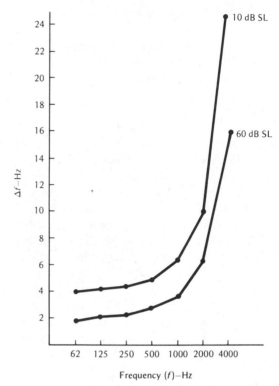

Figure 10.5 Value of Δf required to discriminate a change in frequency from a standard tone (f in Hz) for two intensities, 10 and 60 dB SL (from Fig. 10.6).

differential sensitivity by changing the intensity or frequency of an ongoing tone and asking an observer if he detects the change. The observer will probably hear the change because he detects a click resulting from the spread of energy rather than an intensity or frequency change. Riesz (studying intensity) and Shower and Biddulph (studying frequency) used elaborate techniques to control the spread of energy in order to study differential sensitivity. Although simpler techniques have been used, the data obtained by these investigators are representative of the differential sensitivity of the auditory system.

FREQUENCY DISCRIMINATION

Figure 10.5 shows the value of Δf (frequency difference) required to just discriminate a change in frequency from a given frequency f. The data are plotted as Δf versus f, with the various curves representing different intensities. These data represent the values of the difference threshold (Δf) for frequency. That is, psychometric functions in which the observer's performance was related to various frequency differences could be obtained, and then the difference threshold for frequency calculated from the psychometric functions.

As can be seen, the value of Δf increases as f increases above about 1000 Hz. This increase is about enough to maintain the Weber fraction for frequency, $\Delta f/f$, constant. This can be seen in Figure 10.6, in which the Weber fraction ($\Delta f/f$) is plotted as a function of f. Notice that over a wide range of frequencies and intensities this fraction is constant at approximately $\Delta f/f = 0.005$. This means that at low frequencies Δf can be as small as 2 Hz.

(For instance, if f is 400 Hz, then $\Delta f/400 = 0.005$, so $\Delta f = 400 \times 0.005 = 2$ Hz.)

INTENSITY DISCRIMINATION

Figure 10.7 demonstrates the value of ΔI *in dB* required for the observers to detect a difference in intensity from the initial intensity value I. The value of ΔI is plotted as a function of I, and the different curves represent the results using different frequencies. Although Riesz did not use psychometric functions, the data in Figure 10.7 could come from psychometric functions in which the observer's performance was plotted as a function of intensity differences for each value of I. ΔI is the difference threshold for intensity.

Notice that the auditory system is sensitive to approximately a 0.5-dB change in intensity

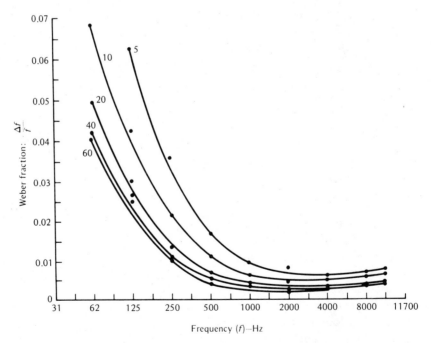

Figure 10.6 Weber fraction, $\Delta f/f$, plotted as a function of frequency (f in Hz). The five curves represent five sensation levels; the 10-dB SL and 60-dB SL curves represent the data shown in Figure 10.5. (*Adapted from Shower and Biddulph, 1931, by permission*)

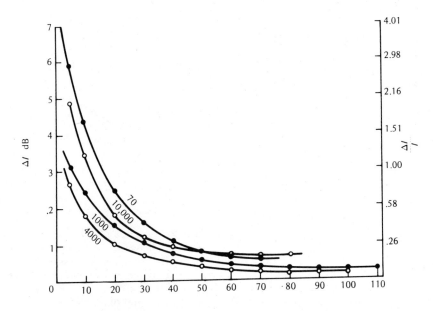

Figure 10.7 Weber fraction for intensity, ΔI in dB, on the left axis; $\Delta I/I$, not in dB, on the right axis as a function of the intensity, I, in dB SL. The curves represent four different frequencies. ΔI in dB, on the left axis, is also the difference threshold for intensity. See Supplement. *(Adapted from Riesz, 1928, by permission)*

across a broad range of frequencies and intensities. The fact that ΔI expressed in decibels is a constant as a function of I implies that $\Delta I/I$ for pressure, energy, or power (or the Weber fraction) is a constant. This results from the fact that the logarithm (decibels) of a ratio (such as the Weber fraction) is equal to a difference between the divisor and dividend of the ratio (see Appendix B, rule 2). Thus, a constant ratio (Weber fraction) yields a constant logarithm difference (constant decibel difference). There are different terms that can be used to describe the results from an intensity discrimination experiment: (1) the results can be plotted as in Figure 10.7 on the left-hand axis as ΔI in dB versus I in dB, (2) as $\Delta I/I$ (not in dB) as in Figure 10.7 right-hand axis, or (3) as ($\Delta I + I$) in dB versus I in dB as in Figure 10.8. Each one of these plots appears quite different, but all display exactly the same data.

In general, then, the Weber fraction for intensity and for frequency is approximately a constant for a wide range of frequencies and intensities. It is important, however, to recog-

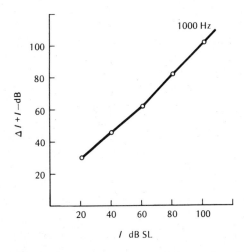

Figure 10.8 Values ($\Delta I + I$), in dB, as a function of I in dB SL. The data are from the 1000-Hz curve shown in Figure 10.7.

nize the disparity between the constancy of the Weber fraction and the data. That is, the fact that for many conditions the Weber fraction is not a constant indicates that auditory processing is more subtle than could be described by a simple Weber fraction relationship.

TEMPORAL DISCRIMINATION

If we asked a subject to detect the difference between a 50-ms sinusoid and a 60-ms sinusoid, additional variables besides duration would be present that might aid the subject in his detection of a difference. Recall from Figures 10.3 and 10.4 that since tones of different durations sometimes have different thresholds, the 50- and 60-ms tones might appear different in loudness. Also, the spectrum of pulsed tones depends on the duration of the tone (Chapter 1); thus the two tones differ in spectra. These two additional variables (loudness and spectrum) make the study of temporal discrimination difficult.

Modern investigators, including Abel and others, have attempted to avoid these problems by presenting the subject with what they call acoustic markers. One stimulus could consist of the following: a tone might come on for 170 ms and be followed 10 ms later by the same 170-ms tone. The other stimulus might be two 170-ms, tones separated by 20 ms instead of by 10 ms. The subject's task is to decide whether these two stimuli are different. If they are judged to be different, then one assumes that the auditory system can detect this 10-ms *difference* between the markers.

The data in Figure 10.9 show the results from Abel's experiment. At various separations of T milliseconds between the two tonal markers, the value of the additional amount of time ($\Delta T_{0.75}$) required for a P(C) of 75 percent is shown for the condition when the markers were 1000 Hz and 85 dB SPL. Thus,

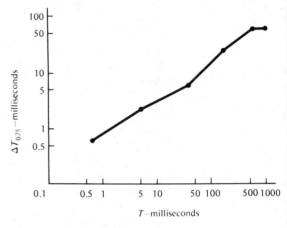

Figure 10.9 Value of $\Delta T_{0.75}$ (change in temporal separation between two markers) required for a P(C) of 75 percent as a function of T (standard separation between two markers). The ability to make a temporal discrimination decreases with increasing temporal differences. (*Adapted from Abel, 1972, by permission*)

as duration increases, we require a greater and greater change in duration in order to make a temporal discrimination. Although $\Delta T_{0.75}$ increases as a function of T, it does not increase at a rate such that $\Delta T_{0.75}/T$ (Weber fraction) equals a constant. Notice that at T equal to approximately 0.5 ms, $\Delta T_{0.75}$ is also approximately 0.5 ms, so the Weber fraction is 1.0. At 500 ms of T, the value of ΔT is 50 ms, so the Weber fraction is 0.1.

Although these results, as well as those of other investigations, show that the difference in time required for temporal discrimination increases as the standard time increases, there is a great deal of variability as to the exact nature of the temporal relationships. Much of this variability is a result of the loudness and spectral problems mentioned. Knowledge of temporal discrimination and acuity is important for a complete understanding of auditory processing. However, our knowledge to date has been limited by the fact that other aspects of auditory perception often change when we vary the temporal characteristics of a sound.

Summary The threshold of audibility describes the auditory system's sensitivity to intensity and frequency and was historically used to define SPL. The thresholds are measured either in an MAF or an MAP paradigm, both of which involve a calibration procedure. The duration of the tone used to determine absolute threshold is crucial. If the duration is between approximately 10 and 500 ms, its energy must remain approximately constant for a constant level of detection by the observer. For durations 500 ms or longer the power must be held constant, whereas for durations shorter than 10 ms, much more energy is required for tonal detection since short duration tones are affected by spread of energy. The data from subjects detecting differences in frequency obey, to a first approximation, the Weber-Fechner law, with $\Delta f / f$ equaling approximately 0.005. The Weber fraction also applies approximately to discriminations of differences in tonal intensity. In this case only a 0.5-dB difference is necessary for reliable discrimination performance. Temporal discrimination is difficult to study due to loudness and spectral changes associated with changing duration.

Supplement

Measures of auditory sensitivity have existed since the early part of the twentieth century. The first thorough study of the threshold of audibility was conducted by Sivan and White (1933). Since that time thresholds and the methods used to measure them have become standardized by both the American National Standards Institute (ANSI), formerly the American Standards Association (ASA), and the International Standards Organization (ISO). See Table 10.1 for these thresholds. Since the description of the MAP and MAF calibration procedures in this book is incomplete, the ANSI or ISO standards should

Table 10.1 Thresholds of Audibility

Frequency (hertz)	Thresholds (decibels SPL) [a]		
	ASA, 1951	ISO, 1964	ANSI, 1969
125	54.4	45.5	45.0
250	39.5	24.5	25.0
500	24.0	11.0	11.5
1000	16.5	6.5	7.0
1500	16.5	6.5	6.5
2000	17.0	8.5	9.0
3000	16.0	7.5	10.0
4000	15.0	9.0	9.5
6000	17.5	8.0	15.5
8000	21.0	9.5	13.0

[a] These thresholds are MAP measurements.

be consulted before the MAP or MAF calibration procedures are used. ANSI and ISO standards can be obtained from the American National Standards Institute, 1430 Broadway, New York, N.Y. 10018. Von Bekesy (1936a) used the "tickle" threshold and Wegel (1932) the "feeling" threshold to measure the highest levels of intensity the ear can tolerate. Watson, Franks and Hood (1972) used TSD procedures to compare psychometric functions and response bias with data obtained for the ISO and ANSI standards.

J. W. Hughes (1946) was one of the earliest to study the effect of duration on threshold. Watson and Gengel (1969) provided an update of these temporal integration data. Garner (1947) was among the first to demonstrate the effect of spectral energy spread on auditory thresholds when the duration of a tone is short. Leshowitz and Wightman (1971) have continued to study energy spread associated with short-duration signals and auditory thresholds.

The curve relating signal power to signal duration over the range of 10 to 500 ms can be expressed as follows:

$$10 \log P + a \, 10 \log T = C$$

where P is power, a the slope constant obtained from a curve like Figure 10.3, T signal duration, and C a constant. The slope constant a usually has a value of less than one. Thus, there is not a perfect 10-dB increase in power for each tenfold decrease in duration, but more like an 8- to 9-dB increase for each tenfold decrease in duration. This function is often referred to as the temporal integration function. Green, Birdsall, and Tanner refined this equation in a paper published in 1957.

McGill and Goldberg (1968) continued the study of intensity discrimination and Weber's fraction that began with Riesz (1928); likewise, Jesteadt and Bilger (1974) continued the study of frequency discrimination begun by Shower and Biddulph (1931).

Abel (1972) studied temporal discrimination, and Green in 1971 provided a review of temporal phenomena in his article "Temporal Auditory Acuity."

The research cited in this chapter is only a small sample of the work in the area of auditory sensitivity. All of the references mentioned in Chapter 14 contain additional references on auditory sensitivity.

In discussions of intensity discrimination we can measure intensity in nondecibel or decibel units of power, energy, or pressure. Care must be exercised in the use of these different units to describe an intensity discrimination experiment. For instance if a tone has 4 watts of power and another tone has 8 watts of power the two tones differ by 4 watts. But their difference in decibels is *not* 10 log 4 watts. Decibels are the logarithms of the *ratio* of two powers (the smallest over the largest). So, in this case, the difference in decibels is 10 log (8 watts/4 watts) = 10 log 2 = 3 dB. (See Appendix B.) Another example of the use of decibels in intensity discrimination experiments is in describing the Weber fraction. Suppose in the foregoing example that $\Delta I = 4$ watts. Then the Weber fraction in power is $\Delta I / I$ or 4 watts/4 watts or 1.0. But ΔI in dB or the difference in decibels between the two stimuli is 10 log (8 watts/4 watts) = 3 dB. Notice that this is the same as

$$10 \log \left(\frac{I + \Delta I}{I} \right)$$

which equals

$$10 \log \left(1 + \frac{\Delta I}{I} \right)$$

So we could obtain ΔI in decibels from the Weber fraction by:

$$\Delta I \text{ in dB} = 10 \log \left(1 + \frac{\Delta I}{I} \right)$$

$$= 10 \log \left(1 + \frac{4 \text{ watts}}{4 \text{ watts}} \right)$$

$$= 10 \log \ (1 + 1)$$

$$= 10 \log 2$$

$$= 3 \text{ dB}$$

Thus the numbers on the left-hand side of Figure 10.7 were obtained by adding 1 to the $\Delta I/I$ ratios on the right-hand side of Figure 10.7 and taking

$$10 \log \left(1 + \frac{\Delta I}{I} \right)$$

CHAPTER 11
Masking

Tonal Masking
Beats
Combination Tones and Aural Harmonics
White Gaussian Noise
Noise Masking
Temporal Masking
Auditory Fatigue

Sounds in our environment rarely occur in isolation; most stimuli occur either simultaneously or close together in time. The study of masking is concerned with the interaction of sounds. The experimenter is interested in the amount of interference one stimulus can cause in the perception of another stimulus. A change in stimulus threshold is the typical measure of the amount of interference produced. Tonal masking, for instance, deals with the change in tonal threshold associated with the interference, or masking, produced by another tone.

TONAL MASKING

The two stimuli in the intensity discrimination experiment described in Chapter 10 differ only in that one is more intense than the other. The more intense stimulus can be generated in one of two ways: the tone's intensity can be increased from I to $(I + \Delta I)$ (this was the procedure assumed for the intensity discrimination experiments); or two stimuli can be added together to produce the more intense tone. If two tones (tone A and tone B) are added to produce the more intense tone, tone A would have an intensity of I in decibels and tone B would have an intensity such that when it was added to tone A the summed intensity in decibels would equal: $I + \Delta I$ in dB (recall that when two stimuli of equal amplitude, frequency, and phase are added, the summed power increases by 3 dB). Thus the data from the intensity experiment could be plotted as the intensity of tone B required for the subject to determine that it was added to tone A versus the intensity of tone A. That is, as the intensity of tone A is increased, the intensity of tone B must also increase in order for the subject to detect a difference between tone A and the summed intensities of tones A and B. For instance, if tone A is 50 dB SL, then tone B must be 44 dB SL to be detected when it is added to tone A (from Fig. 10.7). In this situation it is apparent that the intensity required for tone B to be detected in the presence of tone A is well above the absolute threshold of tone B.

The fact that the intensity of tone B must be raised above threshold due to the presence of tone A is often described as tone A *masking* tone B. That is, the shift in threshold of tone B due to the presence of an interfering stimulus (tone A) is called masking. The interfering stimulus is the *masker* (tone A), and the stimulus to be detected is the *signal* (tone B).

This nomenclature might seem unnecessary to describe the data dealing with intensity discrimination, but if the two tones were of different frequencies, then it seems appropriate to discuss the interference (masking) of one sinusoid (signal) caused by the simultaneous presence of another sinusoid (masker). This procedure of tonal masking would also provide additional information about frequency discrimination. That is, the data on Δf tell us only that two tones must differ in frequency by a certain amount if they are to be discriminated. We do not know, however, to what extent the two tones are interacting. That is, are two tones that are discriminable entirely independent? If so, then the auditory system would be able to discriminate between the two tones no matter how intense either tone was. This would represent an extremely fine ability of the nervous system to determine the frequency content of auditory events.

We might guess that there is probably a great deal of interaction or masking between two stimuli whose frequencies do not differ very greatly. In order to study this type of masking Wegel and Lane performed a *tonal masking* experiment. They asked observers to detect the presence of stimuli of different frequencies while an 80-db SL (80 dB above the observer's absolute threshold), 1200-Hz tone provided masking. That is, subjects were presented one of two stimuli: either the 80-dB SL, 1200-Hz masker or this masker plus the signal at a different frequency. The intensity of the signal was adjusted until the subject could just barely discriminate a difference between the two stimuli. Thus the threshold of the signal was measured as a function of the signal's frequency. The data are shown in Figure 11.1 as the threshold of the signal (expressed in dB SL) versus the frequency of the signal. The signal threshold is often referred to as the *masked threshold* to differentiate it from absolute threshold. The line at 1200 Hz represents the masker frequency, and the top of the line signifies that the masker intensity was 80 dB SL. Any signal whose intensity is greater than that indicated by the curve can be detected in the presence of the 1200-Hz masker, or conversely any signal whose intensity is less than that indicated by the curve (under the curve) has been masked by the 1200-Hz masker. Notice that (1) the greatest amount of masking occurs when the signal and masker are of the same frequency, (2) signals with frequencies greater than the masker are very effectively masked, and (3) signals whose frequencies are less than the masker can be detected at very low sensation levels. Thus, these data indicate that a *masker of a given frequency masks higher-frequency signals more than it masks lower-frequency signals.*

Before we can conclude that tonal masking data indicate how the auditory system resolves frequency, we should note that at high intensities and in certain frequency regions, *beats* and *combination tones* were reported by Wegel and Lane. That is, the observers were detecting auditory phenomena in addition to the masking of one tone by another.

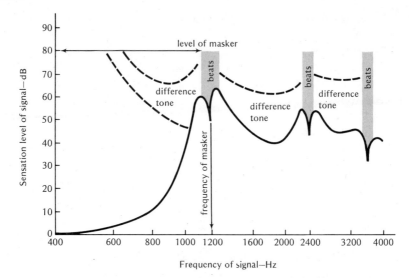

Figure 11.1 Masked threshold of signal in dB SL as a function of signal frequency in Hz with a 1200-Hz, 80-dB SL masker. The figure indicates that in addition to detecting the masker and the signal, the observer can also detect beats and nonlinear difference tones. *(Adapted from Wegel and Lane, 1924, by permission)*

BEATS

Beats and combination tones are reflections of two *different* properties of the auditory system. Beats indicate that the auditory system does not have infinitely accurate frequency-resolving power and that it discerns differences in the time waveform of the stimulus when its frequency-resolving capabilities are exceeded. Combination tones result from the fact that the auditory system is nonlinear. Thus, beats show that the auditory system is not a perfect filter, and combination tones indicate the nonlinear properties of the analyzing capability of the auditory system.

Figure 11.2 shows the time waveform made by the addition of two sinusoids of the same intensity but of different frequencies. In Figure 11.2a the frequencies are greatly different; the period between points A and B represents one frequency, and the period between points C and D the other frequency. In Figure 11.2b the frequency difference between the two tones is small. Notice that the sinusoidal

vibrations look like one pure tone; however, the general shape of the time waveform oscillates at a very low frequency. That is, it appears as a sinusoid whose overall intensity is going up and down at a low rate. The general shape of the waveform is referred to as the *envelope of the waveform* (the dotted line in Figure 11.2b), which itself has a certain frequency. In fact, if tone one has a frequency f_1 and tone two has a frequency, f_2, and the amplitudes of the two tones are equal, then the frequency of the envelope is $(f_2 - f_1)/2$, and the frequency of the sinusoid that lies within the envelope is $(f_2 + f_1)/2$.

For the case shown in Figure 11.2a an observer will hear two separate frequencies, whereas for the waveform shown in Figure 11.2b the observer will hear one frequency, $(f_2 + f_1)/2$, which waxes and wanes in loudness at a rate equal to $f_2 - f_1$. That is, for Figure 11.2b the observer hears a tone that *beats in loudness*. Usually two tones must be close together in amplitude and their frequency difference must be less than 50 Hz in order

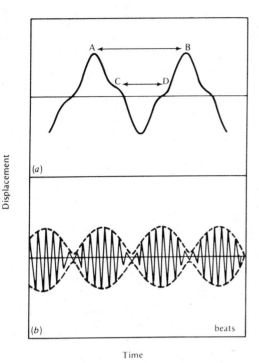

Displacement

(a)

(b)   beats

Time

Figure 11.2 Time domain waveform for the addition of two frequencies. 11.2a: large frequency difference between the tones; 11.2b: small frequency difference between the tones; 11.2b also shows beats, with the envelope of the waveform shown as a dashed line.

for the beating effect to occur. Thus, the shaded area in Figure 11.1 indicates that when the signal was close in frequency to the masker, its intensity was great enough that the observer heard beats that indicated the presence of the signal. Notice that beats were also reported at harmonics (2400 Hz and 3600 Hz) of the 1200-Hz masker. We must better understand nonlinearities before we can account for the presence of these beats at the harmonics of 1200 Hz.

COMBINATION TONES AND AURAL HARMONICS

As was discussed in Chapter 3, combination tones occur when a nonlinear system is pro-

vided with an input consisting of the *sum of two or more sinusoids.* If a nonlinear system is excited with a *single frequency,* then energy will occur at the higher harmonics of the input frequency. When a pure tone of one frequency is presented to the auditory system at a high intensity, observers report hearing tones at that frequency and tones at frequencies equal to harmonics (usually the first two or three harmonics) of the frequency presented. These audible higher harmonics are called *aural harmonics,* and their presence indicates that the auditory system is nonlinear. Figure 11.1 shows that at 2400 Hz (the second aural harmonic of the masker frequency, 1200 Hz) and at 3600 Hz (the third aural harmonic of the masker) the signal frequency is beating with the masker harmonics. In other words, the intense 80-dB SPL, 1200-Hz masker has produced aural harmonics at 2400 and 3600 Hz. When the signal frequency is close to those of these aural harmonics, the beating occurs *between the signal frequency and that frequency produced by the nonlinear properties of the auditory system (the aural harmonics of the intense masker).*

In addition to the aural harmonics produced by the nonlinearity of the auditory system, combination tones are present when the signal and masker are presented simultaneously. The two types of combination tones heard in this experiment were the primary and secondary difference tones. The frequency of the primary difference tone is equal to the difference in frequency between the masker and signal. The frequency of the secondary difference tone (sometimes called the *cubic difference tone*) is produced by the difference between twice the masker frequency minus the signal frequency, or twice the signal frequency minus the masker frequency. (See Appendix A.) The auditory system also is capable of producing *summation tones* at high intensities, although in the tonal masking experiment observers reported hearing only the difference tones. Recall from Chapter 3 that if the input to a nonlinear system is composed of two sinusoids with frequencies f_1 and f_2 (f_2 greater than f_1), then, in addition to the frequencies f_1 and f_2 and their higher harmonics, the nonlinear output will contain energy at frequencies equal to $mf_1 \pm nf_2$, where $m = 1, 2, 3, \ldots$ and $n = 1, 2, 3, \ldots$. Thus, the primary difference tone is $f_1 - f_2$, and the secondary or cubic difference tone is $2f_1 - f_2$ (or $2f_2 - f_1$). The summation tones are $f_1 + f_2$, $2f_1 + f_2$, or $2f_2 + f_1$. Wegel and Lane's pure tone masking experiment shows that subjects do detect difference tones.

By studying the amplitudes and phases of the aural harmonics and combination tones, we can derive a good description of the type of nonlinear device the auditory system might be. Knowing this, we can make additional predictions of the auditory system's processing of information. (Difference tones are also discussed in Chapter 13.)

Although Wegel and Lane's experiment indicates how two tones of different frequencies interact, the presence of beats and nonlinear tones makes a precise understanding of this interaction impossible. What is required is a stimulus whose frequency content we can change but that will reduce the effects of beats or combination tones when we use it to study the auditory system. One such stimulus is white Gaussian noise. We shall next describe the characteristics of this noise and how it has been used to probe the sensitivity of the auditory system.

WHITE GAUSSIAN NOISE

"Noise," as used here, means a sound whose instantaneous amplitude varies over time in a random manner. When the noise is described as "Gaussian," the instantaneous amplitude (displacement) varies in its probability of occurrence according to the normal or Gaussian distribution. A normal distribution of amplitude fluctuations is shown in Figure 11.3. The distribution shows that the mean amplitude is zero (on the average the instantaneous amplitude of the noise at any moment in time is zero), and that the higher or lower the amplitude, the less probable it is that it will occur at any moment in time.

"White" noise indicates that all frequencies

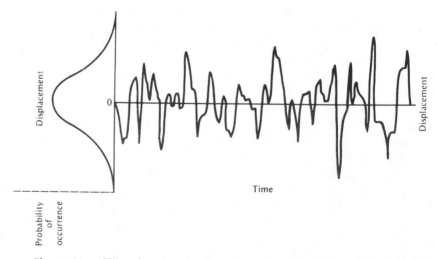

Figure 11.3 Time domain of a Gaussian noise. The value of the instantaneous amplitude (displacement) has a normal or Gaussian probability of occurrence, as shown on the vertical axis.

between some limits are present at the same level; that is, the noise has a continuous and flat power spectrum. This spectrum is shown in Figure 11.4 (see also Fig. 1.12f). Here the *average power* (average rms amplitude) is shown as a function of frequency for the white Gaussian noise. This random noise has a random distribution of phases for each frequency.

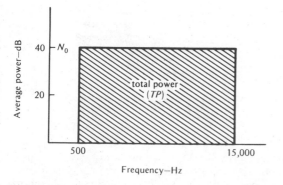

Figure 11.4 Schematic diagram of amplitude spectrum of a "white" noise. The total power (*TP*) of the noise is the summed intensity of all the sinusoids in the noise. N_0 is the spectrum level or the average noise power per unit bandwidth, that is, the average power in a band of noise one cycle wide.

There are two measures of intensity for a broadband noise (that is, noise composed of a wide range of frequencies): (1) *total power* and (2) *noise power per unit bandwidth,* often called *spectrum level,* or N_0. Total power of the noise is what most measuring instruments calculate, and it can be viewed as the sum of the intensities of all the sinusoids in the spectrum of the noise. This is approximately equal to the area (height × width or, in this case, bandwidth × intensity) of the spectrum shown in Figure 11.4. The energy at frequencies far away from the frequency region of interest often will have no bearing on auditory perception. For instance, if the noise has frequencies at 30,000 Hz, it is unlikely that these frequencies affect the auditory system. In this

case the spectrum level of the noise is used. The spectrum level is the intensity measured in a band of noise 1 Hz wide. Since the noise intensity varies, the spectrum level is the average noise power in a band of noise 1 Hz wide. This can be represented by the height of the spectrum in Figure 11.4. Thus, if the total power (*TP*) and the bandwidth (*BW*) of white noise are known, then the spectrum level (N_0) can be calculated. The procedure is analogous to finding the height of a rectangle (N_0) when the area (*TP*) and width (*BW*) are known: $N_0 = TP/BW$ or, in decibels, N_0 in dB $= TP$ in dB $- 10 \log BW$. (See Fig. 11.4 for a description of the use of *TP* and N_0). Thus it is important to specify which measure of noise intensity is being used to describe the intensity of a white Gaussian noise: total power or noise power per unit bandwidth. For example, if a noise has a measured total power of 80 dB SPL as measured by a meter and a bandwidth of frequencies of 10,000 Hz, then total power is 80 dB SPL, but N_0 is 40 dB SPL:

$$N_0 \text{ in dB} = TP \text{ in dB} - 10 \log 10,000$$

therefore

$$N_0 \text{ in dB} = 80 \text{ dB} - 40 = 40 \text{ dB}$$

NOISE MASKING

Since white noise can contain a wide range of frequencies, we would expect it to mask tones of many different frequencies. Hawkins and Stevens performed a masking experiment using a broadband white Gaussian noise to mask a pure tone stimulus. The frequency of the pure tone signal was varied, and the masked threshold of the signal was measured. The data from this experiment are shown in Figure 11.5. There are two important aspects of these data. First, as the intensity of the noise increases, the threshold of the pure tone depends less and less on the tone's frequency. That is, at a noise spectrum level of 0 dB the

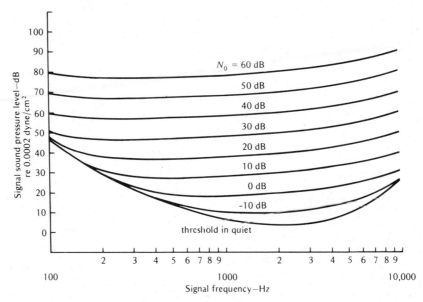

Figure 11.5 Masked threshold for signals in dB SPL as a function of signal frequency in Hz with a broadband white Gaussian noise providing masking. The intensities of the noise masker in N_0 or spectrum level in dB are shown by the curves. The bottom curve represents the thresholds of audibility. *(Adapted from Hawkins and Stevens, 1950, by permission)*

signal threshold changes from 30 to 18 dB SPL between 200 and 1000 Hz. This change in signal threshold is only from 40 to 39 dB SPL when the noise spectrum level is 20 dB. With no noise present, the audiogram shows that the threshold for a tone depends to a large extent on the tone's frequency. However, as the noise background level is increased, the *masked threshold* for the pure tone is less dependent on the frequency of the tone. The second important aspect of these data is that above an N_0 of approximately 20 dB, an increase in the spectrum level of the noise means that the signal level must also be increased by the same amount for the signal to be detected. Modern data suggest that over a wide range of intensities and frequencies the signal *energy* must be 5–15 dB more intense than the spectrum level of the noise for the signal to be detected.

In these masking experiments the ratio of the signal energy to the spectrum level of the noise is used to describe the masked threshold. The *signal-to-noise* ratio (E/N_0) is expressed as the energy of the signal (E) per noise power per unit bandwidth (N_0). In decibels the signal-to-noise ratio equals the signal energy minus the spectrum level. The data from the noise masking experiments suggest that E/N_0 must be approximately 5–15 dB for the signal to be detected.

Hawkins and Stevens used a very broadband noise in their experiment. The data from Wegel and Lane, however, suggested that those frequencies near that of the signal are important in determining masking. Thus we might expect that as the noise was passed through a narrower and narrower band-pass filter (that is, a narrower and narrower band of noise is providing the masking), the detection of a tone whose frequency was in the center of the passband would become easier since there is less total noise power. Conversely, one expects that a signal whose frequency was not in the passband of the filter would be very easy to detect since there would be no energy in the masker at the same frequency as the signal frequency.

Fletcher performed such an experiment in 1940 and made some assumptions about the frequency region of the noise that would be effective in masking the tone. He assumed that some sort of "internal filter" was centered around the frequency of the signal and that the *total noise power* coming through that internal filter determined the amount of masking for the signal. That is, the detection of a tonal signal is determined by the amount of total power present in a narrow range of frequencies. This narrow range of frequencies is the internal filter. Figure 11.6 shows this idealized internal filter schematically for two noise spectra. In Figure 11.6a

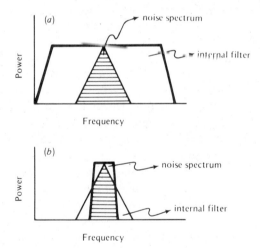

the noise spectrum is much broader than the passband of the internal filter, and hence there should be the maximum amount of masking since there is the maximum amount of total power coming through the filter. In Figure 11.6b the spectrum of the noise is narrower than the passband of the internal filter, and hence the signal should be easier to detect than in the case shown in Figure 11.6a since there is less than a maximum amount of noise power coming through the filter. Fletcher called the internal filter the *critical band*, since the frequencies within the passband of the internal filter were critical for masking.

In Fletcher's experiment the threshold of the signal whose frequency was in the center of the filter remained the same while the noise was passed through narrower and narrower band-pass filters until the passband of the filter reached a critical frequency difference. As the spectrum of the noise was made narrower (with N_0 held constant) than this critical frequency difference, the level of the signal required for detection was decreased. That is, since the signal became easier to detect, its intensity had to be decreased to obtain an estimate of the masked threshold. Fletcher's data, however, were too variable to obtain accurate measures of this critical frequency difference and hence of the critical band. Greenwood performed a similar, but not identical, experiment to Fletcher's and obtained the data shown in Figure 11.7 as the closed circles. Figure 11.7 shows estimates of critical bands obtained in a noise masking experiment at four different center frequencies of the signal (closed circles).

Fletcher made another observation concerning the critical band: when the spectrum of the noise was broad (the internal filter contained the maximum total noise power), the power of the just detectable masked signal (the signal at masked threshold) was equal to the total power contained within the critical band (that is, internal filter). When Fletcher

Figure 11.6 Schematic diagram of the "internal filter" (the triangle). **11.6a:** Broadband noise "produces" maximum power at the output of the internal filter. **11.6b:** The bandwidth of the noise is less than the bandwidth of the internal filter; thus there is less power at the internal filter than in 11.6a. There is more masking for a signal whose frequency is at the center of the internal filter for the broadband noise (11.6a) than for the narrowband noise (11.6b).

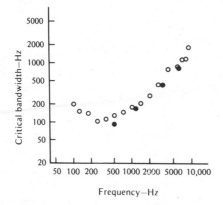

Figure 11.7   Critical bandwidth *(CBW)* as a function of frequency at the center of the band. Closed circlels (Greenwood, 1961) are based on masking by narrow bands of noise. Open circles are the critical ratio estimates of Hawkins and Stevens (1950) multiplied by 2.5. *(Adapted from Scharf, 1970, by permission)*

performed his experiments, he maintained a constant spectrum level of the noise as he narrowed the noise spectrum. This fact, together with Fletcher's observation, makes it possible to predict the width of the critical band without performing the band-narrowing experiment. Equation (11.1) states Fletcher's observation concerning the relationship between masked signal power (P_S) and power of the noise in the critical band (P_{NCB}):

$$P_S = P_{NCB} \tag{11.1}$$

since $P_{NCB} = N_0 \times CBW$ (see the preceding description of noise), where N_0 is noise spectrum level and CBW is an estimate of the critical bandwidth. We may now solve for CBW. Since $P_S = N_0 \times CBW$, then $CBW = P_S/N_0$. Expressed in decibels,

$$10 \log CBW = P_S \text{ in dB} - N_0 \text{ in dB}$$

This estimated critical bandwidth is often referred to as the *critical ratio*. The data from the Hawkins and Stevens experiment can be used to form an estimate of the critical ratio. For example, at 1000 Hz the Hawkins and

Stevens data (Figure 11.5) show that at a noise masker intensity of 40 dB (N_0) the signal power (Hawkins and Stevens' thresholds were measured in power) had to be 58 dB SPL (P_S). Thus, from equation (11.1),

$$\begin{aligned}10 \log CBW &= P_S \text{ in dB} - N_0 \text{ in dB}\\ &= 58 - 40 = 18\end{aligned}$$

or

$$10 \log CBW = 18$$

from which we obtain a value of 63 Hz for CBW (see Appendix B). Notice that 63 Hz is smaller than the critical band estimate shown in Figure 11.7, which was obtained by Greenwood. If we multiply the CBW estimates obtained from the Hawkins and Stevens experiment (Fig. 11.5) by 2.5, we obtain estimates of the critical ratio that agree very well with the data obtained by Greenwood and others. The results of multiplying the values of CBW estimated from Figure 11.5 (the Hawkins and Stevens results) by 2.5 are shown in Figure 11.7 as the open circles. Thus CBW estimates are multiplied by 2.5 in order for the critical ratio estimate of the width of the internal filter to agree with direct critical band measures.

The concept of the critical band has been used often in psychoacoustics. Many experiments and stimuli have been used to define it more accurately and to test the notion that such bands actually exist. For instance, the critical band and critical ratio measure only the bandwidth of the internal filter; many experimenters are also interested in the shape (for example, the roll-off) of the internal filter. The pure tone masking experiment of Wegel and Lane has been viewed by many acoustical scientists as an experiment intended to measure the width and shape of the critical band. But due to the presence of beats and combination tones this procedure has made that estimate impossible. Thus the noise-type experiments provided a better stimulus to study the critical band. The critical band estimates are also consistent with the original intent of the Wegel and Lane experiment of measuring more accurately the frequency-selectivity (not necessarily filtering) properties of the auditory system.

TEMPORAL MASKING

In the masking experiments already discussed, the masker and signal have occurred *simultaneously in time*. There are many acoustical events in which two stimuli follow one another in time. For instance, in music the notes usually appear sequentially in time, and in speech words appear in sequence. Psychoacousticians have, therefore, studied the effect of one stimulus on another occurring before or after the first stimulus to determine the amount of masking provided for a signal that occurs before or after the masker.

Figure 11.8 is a schematic diagram of the stimulus conditions used in studies of temporal masking. There is a masker (the rectangle) and signals or *probe tones* (the arrows), which can occur at different times relative to the masker. At the point labeled A the signal lies temporally in the middle of the masker, representing the *simultaneous masking* conditions we have already studied. When the sig-

nal is presented near the beginning or end of the masker, *backward fringe masking* or *forward fringe masking* occurs. When the signal precedes the masker in time, the condition is called *backward masking,* and when the signal follows the masker in time, the condition is *forward masking.*

Some masking of the signal is caused by the masker in the temporal conditions shown in Figure 11.8. Various stimuli have been used in temporal masking studies (tones, noises, speech, clicks), and the results shown in Figure 11.9 demonstrate the salient data from these experiments. More masking occurs in the fringe conditions than in the simultaneous situation, with the backward fringe providing more masking than the forward fringe. Forward masking of a stimulus can take place when a temporal difference between the two stimuli is between 75 to 100 ms, and backward masking occurs up to 50 ms. Thus, the amount of backward masking declines more quickly as a function of temporal separation of the signal and masker than does the amount of forward masking. These temporal masking data provide interesting questions concerning how the nervous system might be encoding temporal events. The backward masking condition is especially interesting since in this case the threshold of a signal can be affected by a stimulus that comes on after the signal has gone off. At present there are no clear explanations for these temporal masking results.

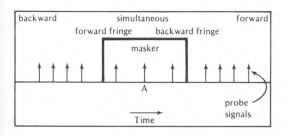

Figure 11.8 Schematic diagram of temporal positions of probe signals in relation to a pulsed masker. Signals can occur before the masker (backward masking), during the time of the masker presentation (simultaneous masking), or after the masker (forward masking). Forward and backward fringes also produce masking.

AUDITORY FATIGUE

The results summarized in Figure 11.9 represent conditions in which the masker was of moderate intensity and duration. A long-term effect, called *auditory fatigue,* occurs when subjects are presented intense stimulation for long periods of time. This effect is not really masking but a loss in hearing sensitivity following exposure to loud stimuli. The sound a

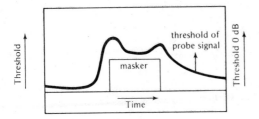

Figure 11.9 Schematic diagram of the relative change in signal threshold as a function of the temporal position of the probe signal in relation to the masker.

person is exposed to is often called the fatiguing stimulus, and the threshold of a test tone is obtained following the offset of this fatiguing stimulus. Because of the temporary shift in threshold this loss in hearing is referred to in terms of the *temporary threshold shift* (TTS). The shift in threshold can linger under some severe conditions for days. An anal-

ogous situation in vision is the loss in sensitivity experienced upon leaving a bright place (like the beach on a sunny day) and going into a dark place (like a movie theater next to the beach). There is a 30- to 40-minute delay before visual sensitivity returns to normal.

Figure 11.10 is an example of the data obtained in temporary threshold shift experiments. In this experiment subjects were exposed to a 115-dB SPL (total power) white Gaussian noise for 20 minutes. At the times indicated on the various curves the thresholds of the subjects were tested at the frequencies shown on the horizontal axis. The change in threshold is calculated relative to the thresholds obtained before the subject was exposed to the noise. Notice that even after one day there can still be a 10-dB loss of hearing.

Auditory fatigue has been studied as a function of many parameters of the fatiguing and

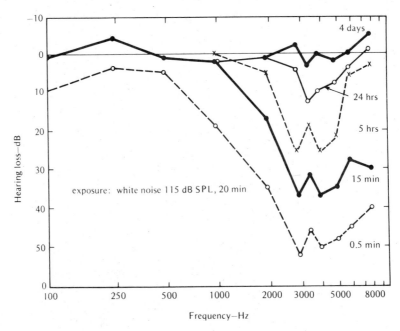

Figure 11.10 Amount of hearing loss in dB as a function of signal frequency with a 20-min, 115-dB SPL white Gaussian noise as the fatiguing stimulus. The curves represent temporary threshold shifts (TTS) measured at various times after the noise was turned off. There is still some hearing loss 24 hours after exposure to the noise. *(Adapted from Postman and Egan, 1949, by permission)*

test stimulus. In general, the amount of TTS increases for increases in the intensity and duration of the fatiguing stimulus. There is probably a trade between the duration and the intensity of the fatiguing stimulus in terms of the amount of TTS that may be produced. That is, a short-duration stimulus must be more intense to cause the same amount of TTS as a long-duration and less intense fatiguing stimulus. The exact nature of this trading is of some dispute. Some scientists believe that approximately a 3-dB intensity decrease for each doubling of duration is required to maintain the amount of TTS constant. If the intensity is decreased by 3 dB each time the duration is increased twofold, then the energy of the fatiguing stimulus remains constant (see Chapter 10). Other investigators believe that approximately 5 dB must be decreased from the intensity of the fatiguing stimulus each time it is doubled in duration to obtain a constant amount of TTS.

Quite often the amount of TTS is measured at a particular time after the cessation of the fatiguing stimulus and comparisons among different conditions are made for these estimates of TTS. In this case one may label the amount of TTS as $TTS_{2\ min}$, $TTS_{20\ min}$, or the like to indicate when the threshold of the test tone was measured. $TTS_{2\ min}$ is often used, since it is an estimate of the maximum threshold shift a fatiguing stimulus might produce.

If the intense noise persists for too long or is too intense, then one's loss of hearing might never recover, and one's threshold might never return to normal. In this case a person would experience *permanent threshold shift* (PTS). Many investigators hope to learn more about PTS by studying temporary hearing loss and TTS. That is, many people today are exposed to sound levels that lead to permanent hearing loss (PTS). It is difficult, if not impossible, to study PTS in the laboratory. Hence there is considerable interest in TTS, which can be studied in the laboratory since the threshold shifts are only temporary. Many scientists hope that by studying TTS they might be able to determine how intense sound affects man and thereby make it possible to prescribe ways to protect man from harmful sound exposure.

Summary   Masking of a tonal signal by a tonal masker has been used to study the interaction of sounds occurring simultaneously and to probe the frequency selectivity of the auditory system. The results indicate that low-frequency tones mask high-frequency signals more than high frequencies mask low frequencies. However, due to the presence of beats and combination tones the exact relationship between tonal signal threshold and tonal masker frequency is difficult to determine. Beats indicate that the auditory system has a limited frequency-resolving power, but that it can follow the amplitude of the input stimulus. Combination tones indicate the extent to which the auditory system is nonlinear. When white Gaussian noise is used as a masker for tonal signals, the ratio of signal energy (E) to masker intensity or spectrum level (N_0) required for masked threshold is approximately 5 to 15 dB as the spectrum level of the noise or the frequency of the signal are varied over a considerable range. Critical bands and critical ratios are used to estimate the bandwidth properties of the frequency-resolving capability of the auditory system. Fringe masking and forward and backward masking are used to determine the interaction of sounds not occurring simultaneously. Auditory fatigue can yield long-term temporary threshold shifts (TTS). In severe situations TTS can become permanent.

Supplement   Masking and auditory fatigue have been reviewed in many books. A recent survey can be found in chapters by Jeffress, Elliott and Fraser, and Scharf in Volume 1 of *Foundations of Modern Auditory Theory* (edited by J. V. Tobias, 1970). The relationship between intensity discrimination and tonal masking was described by Miller (1947) and by McGill and Goldberg (1968). Wegel and Lane published their study of tonal masking in 1924. The problems involved in the detection of a tonal signal by means of a tonal masker (Green, 1969) and a narrow-band noise masker (Egan and Hake, 1950; Greenwood, 1961, 1972) have also been reported. Beats, nonlinearities, as well as spread of energy associated with turning the signal or masker on and off make it difficult to use tonal or narrow-band noise masking to study the frequency processing capabilities of the auditory system.

The works of Smoorenburg (1972) and Hall (1975) are a part of the recent literature involving nonlinearity of the auditory system. The cubic difference tone $(2f_1 - f_2)$ has been studied by many investigators since it appears to be the most prominent combination tone that exists as a result of the nonlinear properties of the auditory system. Riesz (1928) was one of the first to study beats.

Hawkins and Stevens' classical study of noise masking was completed in 1950. Ten years earlier Fletcher (1940) had described the concept of the critical band. Hawkins and Stevens first showed the relationship between critical band estimates and the critical ratio calculations. A more detailed discussion of this relationship can be found in the chapter by Scharf (1970). The theory of signal detection (see Green and Swets, 1974; Swets, 1964) led to many studies aimed at discovering how the auditory system processes a signal and noise in a detection experiment. Jeffress' (1964) paper, "Stimulus-Oriented Approach to Detection Theory," demonstrates the extent to which these theories have developed.

The work by L. L. Elliot in the late 1950s and 1960s (see Elliot, 1962) demonstrates the type of work completed in forward and backward masking. Green (1969) and Leshowitz and Cudahay (1972) have studied forward and backward fringe masking in detail. The work of W. D. Ward (see his 1968 paper) provides a large number of studies of temporary threshold shift. This and other works, especially the books by Kryter (1970) and Henderson et al. (1976), are helpful in explaining the effects of noise on people.

CHAPTER 12
Binaural Hearing

Localization
Lateralization
Binaural Masking

LOCALIZATION

Only one ear is required to process information about the frequency and intensity content of acoustic events. In order to *locate* stimuli in the real world, however, we must depend to a large extent on the binaural (two ears) auditory system. To understand the stimulus cues responsible for our localization abilities, picture a person sitting in a room listening to a sound source without moving his head. In Figure 12.1 we demonstrate the temporal and intensive information arriving at the person's ears that can be used to locate stimuli in the *azimuth* plane (the plane formed by any circle around the head; *range* describes how far an object is from the head). Notice that in Figure 12.1 the stimulus travels a shorter distance to the right ear than to the left ear. Hence it will arrive at the right ear earlier than at the left ear; this yields an *interaural time difference* in arrival of the

sound at the ears. Recall that the speed of sound in air is a constant, independent of frequency. Thus the interaural temporal difference for any frequency is the same for a particular stimulus location, whereas the interaural phase difference will vary according to the frequency of the stimulus. That is, if a tonal sound with a frequency of 1000 Hz (a period of 1 ms) arrives at the right ear 0.5 ms after it has reached the left ear, the tone at the right ear is half a period (or 180°) out of phase with the tone at the left ear. Now if a 500-Hz sinusoid (a period of 2 ms) arrives this same 0.5 ms later at the right ear than at the left ear, there is only one-quarter of a period (or 90°) phase difference between the two ears. Thus, two different tones (1000 and 500 Hz) having a 0.5-ms interaural time difference produce different interaural phase differences.

There is also an *interaural intensive difference* for the condition shown in Figure 12.1 due to two aspects of the binaural system.

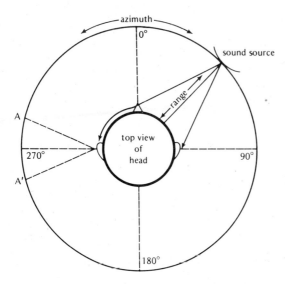

Figure 12.1 Schematic diagram of a sound source on an azimuth plane around the head. Distance of the sound from the ears is the range. Sound sources at symmetrical locations A and A' would produce the same values of interaural time and interaural intensity at the two ears.

First, since the stimulus arrives at the right ear before it reaches the left ear, it is more intense at the right ear (inverse-square-law relationship.) However, the difference in intensity caused by only this aspect of the inverse-square law produces extremely small interaural intensive differences. Second, like any other large object, the head can produce a sound shadow (see Chapter 2) if the object's size is close to the wavelength of the stimulus. Since wavelength is directly proportional to frequency, the interaural intensive difference caused by the sound shadow depends on frequency. The higher the frequency the shorter the wavelength and thus the greater the sound shadow (caused by the head) in establishing the interaural intensive difference. Thus large interaural intensive differences exist at high frequencies.

Figure 12.2 shows the interaural temporal difference measured at the ears for a stimulus located at different azimuth angles. Also in Figure 12.2 we see the interaural intensive difference for different azimuth angles and frequencies. Notice that the interaural temporal difference is regular and varies from 0 to 0.65 ms, whereas the intensive difference varies considerably over the range from 0 to 20 dB. The binaural auditory system therefore could determine the location of a sound coming from, say, the right side by noting that the right ear received the sound first and that the stimulus was more intense at the right ear.

Knowing only the physical magnitudes of the interaural intensive and temporal differences does not enable us to predict how well an observer can locate stimuli in space. Figures 12.3 and 12.4 represent the data from an experiment by Mills in which he asked blindfolded observers to make discriminations between the location of two small loudspeakers each placed approximately 100 cm from the observer's head. As is shown in Figure 12.3, Mills called the smallest angular separation between the two loudspeakers that the observer could just detect the *minimal audible angle* (MAA). Thus, the MAA in degrees of angular separation was measured as a function of the frequency of the sinusoid. The various curves on Figure 12.4 represent various azimuth positions at which the discriminations were made. That is, the curve labeled 0° means that the loudspeakers were directly in front of the observer, whereas the curve labeled 75° means that the loudspeakers were placed 75° toward one ear (the speakers were to the side of the observer). Notice that the observer required larger and larger angular separation between the loudspeakers in order to detect a difference in loudspeaker location (MAA) as they were moved from directly in front of the observer toward one ear (the observer's head was held stationary). In other words, the observer can detect location differences better when the sound is in front of him than when it is toward one side. Of course, in

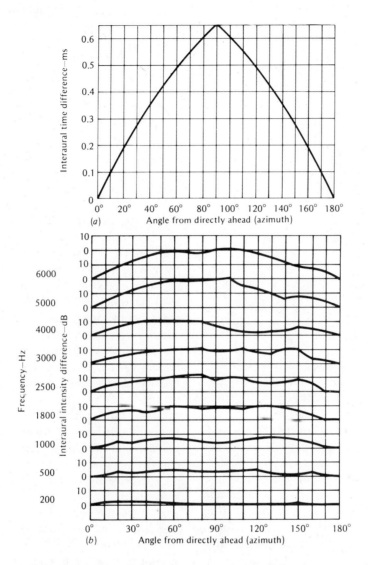

Figure 12.2   12.2a: Values of interaural time difference (ms) measured at different azimuth angles (see Fig. 12.1). **12.2b:** Values of interaural intensity difference (dB) measured at different azimuth angles and frequencies. *(Adapted from Fedderson, Sandel, Teas and Jeffress, 1957, by permission)*

the real world this poses no severe limitation since a person can generally move his head so that the sound source is in front of him.

The other interesting aspect of these data is that for any azimuth location of the loudspeakers, the MAA is smallest for low and relatively high frequencies and largest for middle and very high frequencies. Stevens and Newman had noticed earlier that observers made many mistakes in locating sound sources when their frequency content was in the middle-frequency range. (Notice from Fig. 12.1

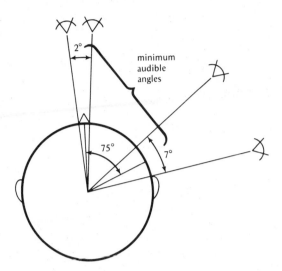

Figure 12.3 Schematic diagram of minimum audible angles (MAA) measured directly in front of the observer and 75° toward one side of the observer. *(Adapted from Yost, 1974, by permission; data from Mills, 1972)*

that a sound source at positions A and A' produces the same interaural differences in time and intensity; thus, as Stevens and Newman found, observers make the most mistakes when the sound comes from symmetrical positions such as A and A'.) Stevens and Newman believed that this middle-frequency region represented those frequencies for which the interaural temporal difference was too large and the interaural intensive difference too small to be used as cues for location. They concluded that there were two cues for determining location: the interaural temporal difference, which provides information for low-frequency stimuli, and the interaural intensive difference, which provides location information at high frequencies. These two cues do not provide as clear information in the middle-frequency range.

The sound shadow effect demonstrates why the physical interaural intensive difference is small at low frequencies and hence why ob-

servers would have trouble using interaural intensity as a cue at low frequencies. That is, the interaural intensive difference due to the head sound shadow decreases as the frequency decreases (wavelength increases). An explanation of why the interaural temporal difference might provide location information at only low frequencies is diagramed in Figure 12.5. Assume that the low-frequency tone shown in the top panel was presented so that it arrived at the right ear first. Thus, the sinusoid arriving at the two ears would appear in time as shown in 12.5a and b. The difference in the timing pattern at the ears could be used by the auditory system for determining that the sound source was toward the right ear. In these panels we assume that the period (time between peaks) of the sinusoid was 0.6 ms (a 1666-Hz tone). From Figure 12.2 we can see that the maximum time difference between stimuli arriving at the ears when the source is placed directly opposite one ear is approximately 0.6 ms. Suppose a sinusoid had a frequency of 1666 Hz (and thus a period of 0.6 ms) and that the sound source was presented opposite the right ear so that the maximum temporal difference between the two ears is 0.6 ms. The 1666-Hz sinusoid would appear at the two ears as in sections a and b of Figure 12.5. Notice now that although the 1666-Hz sinusoid is on the right side and the first period of the left and right waveforms are displaced, the waveforms are identical thereafter (as at point A). Thus except for the first period there is no difference between the stimulation at the two ears, so the observer might assign the sound to a location in front since stimuli that are directly in front of the observer produce no interaural temporal differences. In this case the judgment is incorrect since the stimulus was presented opposite the right ear. Thus for this frequency and this interaural time difference an *ambiguous temporal cue* would exist for locating the sound

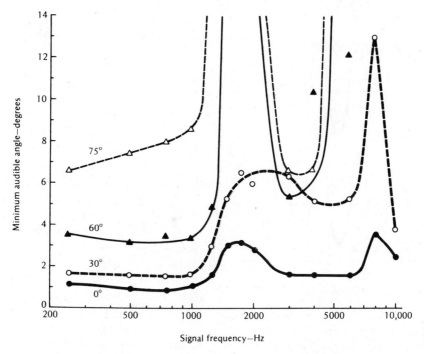

Figure 12.4 Minimum audible angle (MAA) in degrees of azimuth as a function of tonal frequency. The curves show the MAA measured at four different azimuth locations. *(Adapted from Mills, 1972, by permission)*

source. This confusion would not exist for frequencies less than 1666 Hz, but it does occur for those of 1666 Hz and greater.

This is an apparent explanation for why interaural time would not provide accurate location information at high frequencies. Wallach, Newman, and Rosenzweig made another observation about the interaural temporal difference and sound localization. They observed that even in rooms where there are many reflections off walls, floors, and so on, we are still able to localize acoustic events accurately. The reflections cause a complicated pattern of stimulation at the ears. These investigators, therefore, questioned how the auditory system could assimilate these conflicting cues in order to determine stimulus location accurately. They performed an experiment showing that

it is the first wavefront arriving at the ears that establishes the location of the stimulus. That is, the auditory system processes the first wavefront that arrives and suppresses the localization information in later wavefronts coming from the echoes and reflections. Wallach, Newman, and Rosenzweig called this phenomenon the *law of the first wavefront* or the *precedence effect*. The data of these investigators cast doubt on the validity of previous explanations as to why high-frequency tones produce confusing interaural temporal differences. In Figure 12.5, although the later peaks present confusing information, there is no doubt concerning stimulus location if we simply look at the first peak arriving at each ear. By using only the first positive peak in each sinusoid we can determine that the stim-

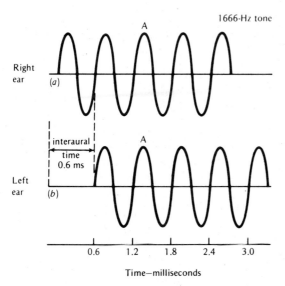

Figure 12.5 1666-Hz tone presented from the right side of the observer. 12.5a: sinusoid arriving at the right ear; 12.5b: sinusoid arriving at the left ear. There is a 0.6-ms interaural temporal difference which equals the period of the 1666-Hz tone. At point A the waveforms are in phase.

ulus arrived at the right ear before it reached the left ear. Thus, the first wavefront might indicate the sound source to be at the right, whereas the later waves indicate the stimulus to be at center. However, this does not explain why the interaural temporal difference is a cue only at low frequencies, as Stevens and Newman suggested. Thus it is not clear how interaural time might be used by the auditory system.

The localization experiments are difficult to use in studying these interactions since the precedence effect will always exist in the free field. It is also impossible to separate the variables of interaural time from interaural intensity since both differences always coexist in localization experiments. One simple way to avoid the confusions present in the free field is to present the stimuli through headphones. Through headphones the experimenter can present only an interaural temporal difference or only an interaural intensive difference and thereby control the binaural variables.

LATERALIZATION

When a tone is presented to an observer by means of headphones, the observer will, under the appropriate conditions, perceive an image that lies within his head and whose location moves as a function of changes in interaural temporal and intensive differences. To differentiate the perception of the internal (or intercranial) image that occurs with headphones from the external image associated with external sound sources, we use the term *"lateralization"* to describe the former and *"localization"* for the latter. The image formed from binaural presentations is sometimes referred to as a *fused image* since the observer reports hearing one image as if the sound sources arriving at both ears were fused. An observer will not perceive a fused image if the interaural temporal difference or the interaural frequency difference is too large. If the interaural temporal difference is larger than approximately 2 ms, the observer will report hearing two images, one at each ear. Also, if the two ears receive independent sinusoidal signals differing greatly in frequency, the observer perceives two images, one at each ear, and he can identify both frequencies.

Jeffress and Taylor have shown that a fused image in a lateralization experiment moves toward the ear that receives the stimulus first or receives the more intense stimulus in the same manner that an external image is perceived more toward the ear that receives the sound first (and therefore receives the more intense sound). Thus, a lateralization procedure appears appropriate for studying the effects of interaural temporal and intensive differences on the locating abilities of the auditory system.

Figure 12.6 shows the results from an experi-

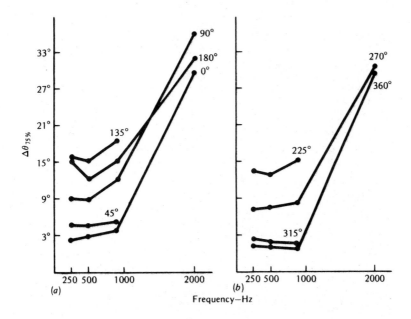

Figure 12.6 Value of $\Delta\theta$ (interaural phase difference change) required for a $P(C)$ of 75 percent discrimination as a function of frequency (Hz). The curves show the values of the standard interaural phase difference (θ). **12.6a:** θ less than 180°; **12.6b:** θ greater than 180°. As θ changes from 0° to 180° and from 360° to 180°, the value of $\Delta\theta$ increases. *(Adapted from Yost, 1974, by permission)*

ment by Yost in which he presented simple tones at different frequencies and varied the interaural temporal (actually interaural phase) difference. These results show, as had those of Jeffress and Taylor, that as the interaural phase difference increased toward 180°, the fused image moved toward the ear that received the tone first (leading in time). As the interaural phase difference exceeded 180°, the image moved from the ear that received the tone last (lagging in time) toward the middle of the head; a tone presented with no interaural difference was perceived toward the middle of the head or at *midline*. This image was placed in different perceptual positions within the head by introducing an interaural phase difference. Assuming that the image was at some location due to a given interaural phase difference, the additional amount of

interaural phase difference the observer required to detect a change in the perceived location of the fused image was determined. The amount of additional phase difference required for detection was called $\Delta\theta$, plotted in Figure 12.6 as a function of the frequency of the tones. The various curves represent the initial interaural phase difference introduced such that for phase differences less than 180° the image was located on the left side of the head (the data in Fig. 12.6a) and for phase differences greater than 180° the image was on the right side of the head (Fig. 12.6b).

Two aspects of these data are important. First, notice that for any initial phase difference, the amount of $\Delta\theta$ required for detection remains constant to approximately 900 Hz and then increases. This indicates that at frequencies greater than 900 Hz, interaural phase is a poor cue for detection (for frequencies above 2000 Hz investigators have been unable to move the fused image as a function of changing the interaural phase difference). This agrees with Stevens and Newman's prediction that interaural time is not a usable cue for localization of high-frequency sinusoids. This same result has also been obtained in lateralization experiments in which the interaural temporal difference, instead of the interaural phase difference, was varied (for instance, varying the time at which the tone is actually turned on at each ear). Thus, the binaural system does not use interaural time at high sinusoidal frequencies in order to localize sound.

The second interesting aspect of these data is that as the image is moved toward one side of the head by introducing phase differences close to 180°, the amount of additional interaural phase difference required to discern a change in perceived location ($\Delta\theta$) also increases. This is consistent with Mills' finding that observers are *less* sensitive to changes in sound source location when the source is toward one, ear than when it is directly in front. The interaural phase difference contributes to this difference in location sensitivity.

The observation of Stevens and Newman concerning the interaural temporal difference and frequency appears correct. That is, the interaural temporal difference is usable only for localization of low-frequency sinusoids (below approximately 1500 Hz). These data also show that the lateralization experiment does allow the study of binaural hearing in a way similar to the localization experiments.

What about the role of interaural intensity in lateralization? Mills' data, shown in Figure 12.7, demonstrate that the amount of interaural intensive difference required to detect a change in the position of a fused image from midline (the case when there is no interaural difference present) is approximately the same independent of the frequency of the tone (except in a mid-frequency region). This does not

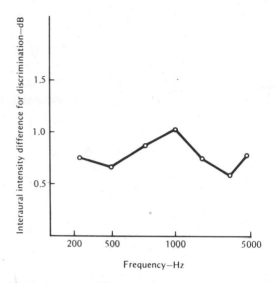

Figure 12.7 Values of interaural intensity required for lateralization detection plotted as a function of frequency. *(Adapted from Mills, 1960, by permission)*

mean that in localizing a sound in the free field the interaural intensive difference does not change as a function of frequency. This relationship is determined by the physics of sound and the size of the head (the sound shadow). That is, even though an observer *can* detect a 2-dB change in interaural intensity at 200 and 2000 Hz with headphones, this 2 dB of interaural intensive difference will not occur in the free field at 200 Hz. The physical interaural intensive difference at 200 Hz is much smaller than 2 dB. Thus at 200 Hz the observer will not be presented a large enough intensive difference in the free field to use for localization. This fact of physics together with the observations concerning interaural temporal discriminations indicates that Stevens and Newman were right in assuming that *interaural time is the more important cue for localization at low sinusoidal frequencies and interaural intensity the more important cue at high sinusoidal frequencies.*

The binaural system is remarkably sensitive

to changes in interaural time and intensity. Figure 12.6 shows that the observer could detect a change of 3° of interaural phase. At 1000 Hz this phase difference corresponds to a 0.01-ms change in interaural time. The data from lateralization experiments have shown that the auditory system is sensitive to temporal differences equal to 10 one-millionths of a second (10 microseconds).

Recall from Chapter 7 that many cells within the central auditory nervous system respond differentially to changes in interaural temporal and intensive differences. Also in Chapters 6 and 7 we showed that the discharges of VIIIth nerve fibers were phase-locked to the periodicity of low-frequency stimuli. The fact that interaural temporal differences are a cue for localization at only low frequencies suggests that the phase locking might be crucial to understanding how the nervous system processes interaural temporal information. If the phase-locked activity of the nervous system is responsible for encoding interaural temporal differences, this would explain why interaural time is a cue only at low sinusoidal frequencies and hence would provide an answer to the dilemma we described earlier concerning why interaural time was a cue only at low sinusoidal frequencies.

BINAURAL MASKING

In the preceding section we described the auditory system's sensitivity to changes in interaural time and intensity, which are principally used to locate stimuli in space. Is the binaural system capable of performing other tasks related to localization? Licklider, using speech signals, and Hirsh, using tonal signals, observed another phenomenon. They found that the threshold for a signal masked by noise was lower when the noise and signal were presented in a particular way to both ears. In these experiments the subjects first determined

their tonal thresholds when both the noise and tonal signal were presented *equally to both ears*. When the tonal signal was removed from one ear, and thus the noise was at both ears and the signal at only one ear, the signal was easy to detect, and therefore the intensity of the tone had to be reduced in order to obtain masked thresholds. Subsequently, many investigators have studied the improvement in detection associated with presenting stimuli to both ears. A certain nomenclature has been developed to describe the various types of binaural configurations of signal and noise.

monotic: stimuli presented to only one ear
diotic: identical stimuli presented to both ears
dichotic: different stimuli presented to the two ears

In general, investigators have found that the masked threshold of a signal is the same when the stimuli are presented in a monotic or diotic condition. However, if the masker and signal are arranged in a dichotic situation, then the signal has a lower threshold than in either the monotic or diotic conditions. There are several ways to present the signals (S) and maskers (M) in a dichotic or diotic manner; again, a set of symbols is used to describe these stimulus conditions.

S_0:   signal presented binaurally with no interaural differences
M_0:   masker presented binaurally with no interaural differences
S_m: signal presented to only one ear
M_m: masker presented to only one ear
S_π: signal presented to one ear 180° out of phase with the signal presented to the other ear
M_π: masker presented to one ear 180° out of phase with the masker presented to the other ear

For the binaural conditions described above, the signal or masker is identical in all dimensions except that denoted by a subscript.

Thus:

monotic: M_mS_m
diotic: M_0S_0
dichotic: $M_0S_\pi, M_0S_m, M_\pi S_\pi, M_\pi S_0, M_\pi S_m$

In order to compare detection in one binaural condition with that in another, the data are usually presented as the difference between the signal level required for detection (masked threshold) in a monotic condition and that required in a diotic or dichotic condition. That is, the signal level required for detection in the relevant diotic or dichotic conditions is subtracted from the signal level required for detection in the M_mS_m condition (monotic condition). Such a difference when expressed in decibels is called a *masking-level difference* (MLD) or a *binaural masking-level difference* (BMLD).

The tabulation below shows the type of improvement in detection provided by dichotic presentation of maskers and signals (MLD). These data represent approximately the maximum MLD obtained when the masker is a continuous white Gaussian noise and the signal is a pulsed sinusoid of low frequency and long duration (greater than 100 ms).

Interaural Condition Compared to M_mS_m	MLD
$M_mS_\pi, M_0S_0, M_\pi S_\pi$	0 dB
$M_\pi S_m$	6 dB
M_0S_m	9 dB
$M_\pi S_0$	13 dB
M_0S_π	15 dB

Figure 12.8 describes the MLD obtained between the M_0S_0 condition and the M_0S_π condition as a function of signal frequency. Notice that as the frequency of the signal increases, the MLD decreases. That is, the difference in the signal intensity required for detection (MLD) between the dichotic condi-

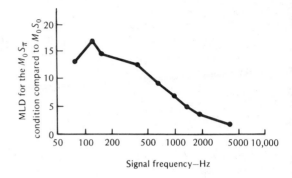

Figure 12.8 Difference in masked thresholds (in dB) between M_0S_π and M_0S_0 conditions (MLD) plotted as a function of signal frequency. *(Adapted from Webster, 1951, by permission)*

tion (M_0S_π) and the diotic condition (M_0S_0) becomes smaller as the signal frequency increases (notice that the MLD never goes to zero; the signal is always easier to detect in the dichotic case than in the diotic case).

The fact that the MLD decreases as a function of frequency has suggested to many psychoacousticians that the MLD might be related to the interaural differences of time and intensity, especially to the interaural temporal difference. When the stimulus condition is dichotic, there are differences in temporal and intensive information between the stimuli arriving at the ears. However, in the diotic condition there are no interaural differences. It is therefore logical to assume that these interaural differences result in the improvement in detection in the dichotic condition.

The MLD has been studied for a wide range of stimulus parameters and listening conditions. In general, the detection of a signal is improved for dichotic presentations, but investigators have not yet demonstrated that other auditory abilities such as discrimination (that is, measures of ΔI or Δf) are improved by presenting stimuli dichotically. The study of the MLD has provided valuable information concerning binaural processing.

Summary   In a localization situation interaural time is the relevant cue for stimulus location at low frequencies, and interaural intensity is the cue at high frequencies. The *precedence phenomenon* stresses the importance of the first wavefront in determining stimulus location. In the lateralization procedure the stimulus is presented through headphones. The location of the fused image in a lateralization experiment is dependent on interaural time for low-frequency tones and on interaural intensity at all frequencies. Signals and maskers presented in dichotic stimulus configurations have lower thresholds (MLDs) than signals and maskers presented in either diotic or monotic configurations.

Supplement   Mills (1972), Jeffress (1972), Durlach (1972), Green and Henning (1969), and Green and Yost (1975) have all reviewed localization, lateralization, or binaural masking in recent years. Feddersen, Sandel, Teas, and Jeffress (1957) measured the actual interaural temporal and intensive differences in subjects and around spheres. W. Mills' (1956) article, "On the Minimum Audible Angle," and J. D. Harris' (1972) monograph, "A Florilegium of Experiments on Directional Hearing," provide thorough studies of the locating ability of the auditory system. Stevens and Newman published their work concerning the duplex theory of sound localization in 1936. A good explanation of the ambiguity of sound location at high frequencies is provided in *Woodworth and Schlosburg's Experimental Psychology* (edited by Kling and Riggs, 1972). Wallach, Newman, and Rosenzweig studied the precedence offert and click lateralization in 1949. In addition to Yost's (1974) study, Mills (1960) also studied lateralization involving interaural time. Elfner and Perrott (1967) and Mills (1960) studied lateralization involving interaural intensity. Jeffress and Taylor (1961) studied the relationship between lateralization and localization.

Green and Henning (1969) and Green and Yost (1975) completely summarize the work in binaural masking. Licklider and Hirsh both made their observations concerning the masking level difference in 1948. The models proposed by Jeffress (1972), Durlach (1972), Hafter and Carrier (1969), and Osman (1971) indicate the type of theory that has been used to account for the MLD.

In recent years some investigators (Yost, Wightman, and Green, 1971; Henning, 1974; McFadden and Pasanen, 1975) have shown that signals with only high-frequency spectral content but with regular low-frequency fluctuations of amplitude in the time domain (such as high-frequency beating tone) can be lateralized on the basis of an interaural temporal difference. Thus it appears that *any* stimulus with a low-frequency amplitude change might be localized using interaural time. This again implies that some aspect other than the place of excitation might provide the neural substrate for the processing of interaural temporal differences.

CHAPTER 13
Loudness and Pitch

Loudness
Pitch
Difference Tones
Other Subjective Attributes of Sound

In Chapters 10 through 12 we have discussed measures of the auditory system's sensitivity to the frequency, intensity, and phase composition of acoustic events. This chapter deals with observer's descriptions and evaluations of frequency and intensity. As we stated briefly in Chapter 1, we most often refer to intensity as loudness and to frequency as pitch. Chapter 12 described those changes in phase that can result in the perception of a stimulus' location in space when the phase is presented as an *interaural phase difference*. Since the subjective effect of phase has already been discussed, this chapter will be concerned with loudness and pitch, the *subjective* aspects of intensity and frequency.

LOUDNESS

In order to study loudness we must use such psychophysical procedures as scaling and matching. Figure 13.1 displays the results of a loudness matching experiment by Fletcher and Munson. The data are plotted as the intensity in decibels of SPL of a comparison tone, required by the observer to match (equate) the comparison tone in *loudness* to the standard tone, as a function of the frequency of the comparison tone. The standard tone was a 1000-Hz sinusoid presented at various intensities expressed in decibels of SL. The various curves in Figure 13.1 represent the intensities of the standard used by Fletcher and Munson. For instance, for the curve labeled 40 dB the standard was a 40-dB SL, 1000-Hz tone, and the observer varied the intensity of the comparison tones presented at other frequencies until the comparison and standard tones sounded equally *loud*. Each contour (curve) is called an *equal-loudness contour* since every frequency presented at the intensity described by the curve sounds the same in loudness. For

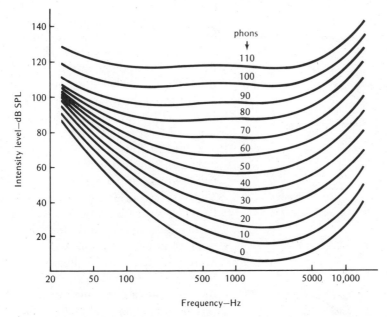

Figure 13.1 Intensity in dB SPL of comparison tones judged equally loud as a 1000-Hz standard tone as a function of frequency of the comparison tones. The curves represent intensity levels of the 1000-Hz standard tone expressed in phons. Each curve is called an equal-loudness contour. *(Adapted from Fletcher and Munson, 1933, by permission)*

instance, the tones presented at 200 Hz, 60 dB SPL; at 1000 Hz, 47 dB SPL; and at 5000 Hz, 57 dB SPL are all judged to be equal in loudness although they are different in intensity (the 40-dB equal-loudness contour).

Two terms are used to describe or measure the *loudness* of a stimulus. *Loudness level* is measured in *phons;* a phon is the intensity in decibels of SPL of an equally loud 1000-Hz tone. All tones judged equal in loudness to a 40-dB SPL, 1000-Hz tone have a loudness level of 40 phons. The tones presented at intensities such that they are equal in loudness to a 70-dB SPL, 1000-Hz tone all have a loudness level of 70 phons. Another way to measure loudness is with the *sone;* a *sone* is the loudness of a 1000-Hz tone presented at 40 dB SPL. Thus, 1 sone equals 40 phons. Any stimulus that is *n* sones loud is judged to be *n* times as loud as 1 sone, that is, *n* times as loud as the 1000-Hz,

40-dB SPL standard. Figure 13.2a is a plot of the loudness in sones of a 1000-Hz tone versus its intensity in dB SPL (at 1000 Hz, dB SPL is the same as dB in phons, thus the horizontal axis could also be phons). The sone scale in this figure, like the intensity scale, is logarithmic. The data are fit by approximately a straight line from about 30 phons. From the slope of this line we find that for approximately every 10-dB increase in intensity there is a doubling of loudness. An observer, therefore, must increase a tone's intensity by 10 dB before he judges its loudness to have doubled. The sone scale was obtained by a ratio scaling technique in which the observer is asked to adjust the intensity of a comparison tone so that it appears half as loud or twice as loud as the 1-sone standard (1000-Hz, 40-dB SL tone). This adjusted comparison tone becomes a new standard and a new comparison tone is pre-

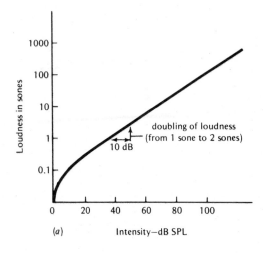

(a) Intensity—dB SPL

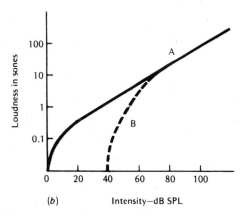

(b) Intensity—dB SPL

dBA measure is the total amount of noise, measured in decibels, that is passed through a filter with attenuation rates that match the 40-dB equal-loudness contour. That is, those frequency components in the noise that are in the 500-Hz to 5000-Hz region receive the most weight when the total noise power is computed in dBA. dBA is usually measured by a *sound pressure level meter,* with an A scale.

Figure 13.2b is also a plot of loudness versus intensity, but in this case curve B represents the loudness of a tone that was masked by a 30-dB spectrum level (N_0) wide-band noise. Curve A is the same as the one in Figure 13.2a. Notice that the threshold for the masked tone is 40 dB above the unmasked tone's threshold. Since both tones are at threshold (one at absolute threshold, the other at masked threshold), the two tones are of equal loudness when their actual intensities are 40 dB apart. However, when the actual intensity of both tones is 80 dB SPL, they are judged equally loud. This, in turn, means that the loudness of the masked tone (curve B) increased faster (steeper slope) than the unmasked tone. This increase in loudness (or the steep loudness slope) is sometimes called *loudness recruitment.* The loudness of the masked tone changes much more for each 10-dB increase in intensity than does the loudness of the unmasked tone. Curve B might represent the data from a patient whose *threshold* of hearing was 40 dB below normal threshold but who judges an 80-dB SPL tone the same in loudness as a normal subject would. The fact that the patient's loudness function shows loudness recruitment indicates certain hearing abnormalities.

Most of the interactions that have been studied using threshold as a psychoacoustical measure can also be investigated using loudness. For instance, the duration of a tone can be varied, and the subject can adjust the tone's power so that it remains equally loud. In so doing, the observer is helping in the measure-

Figure 13.2 13.2a: Loudness in sones of a 1000-Hz tone as a function of the intensity of the tone in dB SPL. The slope of the function indicates that approximately a 10-dB change in intensity is required to double loudness. **13.2b:** Curve A is the loudness curve in 13.2a; curve B is the curve from a 1000-Hz tone masked by a wide-band noise. Curve B shows loudness recruitment. *(Based on similar diagrams by Steinberg and Gardner, 1937)*

sented; this procedure is repeated several times in order to obtain a scale.

The 40-dB equal loudness contour is also used to calculate a measure of intensity called the decibel weighted by the A scale, or the *dBA.* The measure dBA is often used to decide when noise becomes a pollutant. The

ment of temporal integration. That is, a short sound will not be as loud as a long sound if their powers are equal and their durations are less than approximately 250 ms. The loudness of a sound can also be maintained at a constant sone or phon level as the bandwidth of a stimulus is narrowed in order to measure a critical band. In this case narrowing the bandwidth of a stimulus will decrease the loudness once the bandwidth is less than a critical band. *Loudness adaptation* (or perstimulatory fatigue) occurs during exposure to an adapting stimulus much in the same way TTS occurs following exposure to a fatiguing stimulus. The change in loudness adaptation, however, takes place while the adapting stimulus is being presented. That is, a stimulus appears softer if it is kept on for a very long time. The loudness of a stimulus is usually measured by having the subject match a comparison stimulus to the adapting stimulus in terms of loudness. As the adapting stimulus remains on for longer and longer periods of time, the intensity of the matching stimulus must be decreased, indicating that the loudness of the adapting stimulus has decreased. In these and other cases the data from threshold experiments are not substantially different from those obtained in loudness studies. That is not to say, however, that there are not differences the understanding of which is important for a more complete knowledge of auditory function.

As we mentioned in Chapter 1, although changes in intensity are highly correlated with loudness changes, the relationship is not perfect. That is, changes in frequency, duration, intensity and bandwidth can all affect the perceived loudness of a stimulus even though the intensity of the stimulus remains fixed. Thus, one should remember that loudness is a subjective evaluation of sound, whereas intensity is an objective measure of vibratory amplitude, including the amplitude of sound.

PITCH

The subjective label of pitch has come to represent different aspects of an auditory stimulus. Generally, pitch is highly correlated with frequency. However, in many instances *observers report perceiving a pitch in the absence of any energy at the frequency that corresponds to the reported pitch.* The often-discussed relation of frequency to pitch is predictable on the basis of the encoding of frequency performed by the cochlea and VIIIth nerve fibers or, more generally, by the tonotopic or place organization of the auditory system. The fact that observers report pitches for stimuli that contain no energy at the frequency of the pitch means that pitch is probably encoded by mechanisms in addition to those involved with the place theory of hearing. Hence experiments on pitch perception are very important to our understanding of the auditory system's ability to process frequency information.

Experiments on pitch are usually performed with the matching procedure in which a standard tone (sometimes a sinusoid) is used as the basis for pitch matches of comparison stimuli. Scaling procedures have been attempted in the measurement of pitch, but they yield graphs that look very different from those obtained in the measurement of loudness. This difference stems from the *qualitative aspects of pitch.* That is, as the pitch of a stimulus changes, it does not appear to vary along a dimension of greater to smaller or more to less. The change appears to occur along many dimensions at once, whereas the changes in loudness are *quantitative,* in that they can be scaled along a single dimension. One tone can be said to be greater in loudness than another tone, but one pitch may not be *greater* than another pitch.

Many attempts have been made to scale pitch, such as the seven-tone musical scale

(A, B, C, D, E, F, G). The data in Figure 13.3 represent an attempt by Stevens and Volkman to scale the pitches associated with sinusoids according to the *mel scale,* in which a standard 1000-Hz, 40-dB SPL tone is assigned an arbitrary pitch of 1000 mels. The observer, using the ratio scaling technique, then adjusts the frequency of a comparison tone until it sounds twice the pitch of the standard; the observer then adjusts the frequency again until it is twice the pitch of the preceding stimulus, and so on. From this the mel scale is developed in much the same way the sone scale was calculated.

The intensity of a tone can often influence its pitch. The data in Figure 13.4 represent equal pitch contours. The horizontal axis shows how much the observer had to change the frequency of a tone that had the intensity shown on the vertical axis in order to match the pitch associated with a certain standard frequency. The various curves represent different standard frequencies. Notice, for instance, that over a 40-dB range (30 to 70 dB SL on the vertical axis) the observer had to vary the frequency of a comparison tone 120 Hz (horizontal axis) in order for it to maintain the same pitch (equal pitch contour A) as the 7000-Hz standard. These matches are often difficult to obtain because there is a

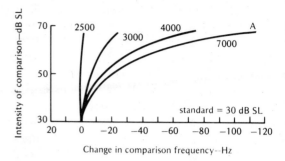

Figure 13.4 Intensity in dB SL of comparison tones as a function of the change in frequency of a 30-dB SL standard comparison tone necessary to make the comparison tones sound equal in pitch to the standard tone. The standard tone was presented at the frequencies shown on the various curves. *(Adapted from Stevens, 1935, by permission)*

great deal of variability associated with the results.

In discussing the threshold of audibility we mentioned that observers might be asked to detect the presence of a tonal-sounding stimulus instead of just detecting any sound. Tonality implies that the observer is detecting the presence of pitch. Von Bekesy found that a tone whose frequency was less than 1000 Hz must have a duration equal to 3 to 9 periods if the tone was to have a definite pitch. Above 1000 Hz this critical duration for the perception of tonality or pitch was 10 ms regardless of the frequency of the tone.

These experiments demonstrate the relationship between sinusoidal frequency and pitch. Broadband stimuli like noises will also have a pitchlike quality if their energies are concentrated in bands of frequency. The perceived pitch is associated with the frequency region where the energy is concentrated.

Thus there is a strong correlation between the pitch of a stimulus and the spectral location of its frequencies. Fletcher, however, replicated a startling observation when he demonstrated that observers hear a 100-Hz pitch associated with a stimulus consisting of a sum

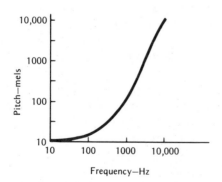

Figure 13.3 Pitch in mels as a function of frequency for a 50-dB SL tone. *(Adapted from Stevens and Volkman, 1940, by permission)*

of the frequencies of 700, 800, 900, and 1000 Hz. Since there is absolutely no energy at 100 Hz, the question remained as to what led to the reporting of this pitch. These four tones are all harmonics of 100 Hz (in fact 100 Hz is the highest frequency for which the tones could be harmonically related). The observation that a pitch could be associated with the fundamental of a complex stimulus even when the fundamental was absent in the spectrum of the complex stimulus is called the *case of the missing fundamental.*

Figure 13.5 demonstrates the amplitude spectrum and the time waveform (assuming all the tones had the same phase) associated with the tonal complex (700, 800, 900, and 1000 Hz). Notice that there is a 10-ms spacing between the major peaks in the complex time waveform. Since the frequency associated with a 10-ms period is 100 Hz, it may be assumed that the auditory system perceived the 100-Hz

pitch because of the 10 ms periodicity of the time waveform. In fact, any stimulus that has a periodic time waveform will have a perceived pitch equal to the reciprocal of the period, called periodicity pitch. For instance, since the time waveform shown in Figure 13.6 consists of a periodically occurring square wave whose period is 2 ms, this waveform will have a 500-Hz periodicity pitch. In this case, as can be seen from Figure 1.12, there is also energy at 500 Hz in the amplitude spectrum. Thus we can perceive a periodicity pitch when the complex stimulus has energy at the frequency of the pitch (the square wave) or when there is no energy at the frequency of the pitch (the missing fundamental tonal complex).

Although the periodicity concept appears to account for the data of the missing fundamental, there is a counterexample. If we add together the four tones (700, 800, 900, and 1000 Hz) when the phase of each tone is a

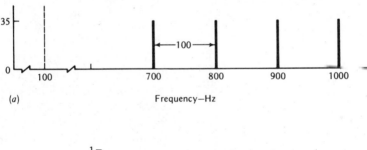

(a)   Frequency—Hz

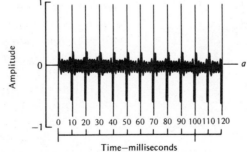

(b)   Time—milliseconds

Figure 13.5 Amplitude spectrum (**13.5a**) and time domain (**13.5b**) descriptions of a complex stimulus of tones of 700, 800, 900, and 1000 Hz added together with the same starting phase. The dotted line represents the pitch perceived at 100 Hz, though there is no power at 100 Hz. The time between the major peaks in 13.5b is 10 ms on the period of 100 Hz.

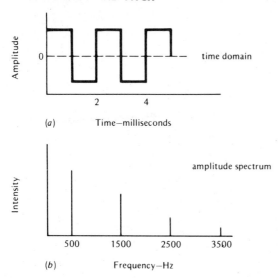

(a)

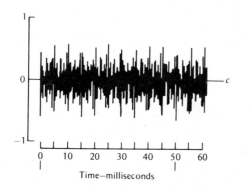

(b)

Figure 13.6 Time domain (**13.6a**) and amplitude spectrum (**13.6b**) descriptions of a 2-ms square wave. The square wave has a spectrum with the greatest intensity at 500 Hz, as well as a 2-ms period.

random variable, we obtain the time waveform in Figure 13.7. Patterson has shown that in this case the observer also perceives a 100-Hz pitch. This is confusing since it is impossible to determine any periodicity in the peaks of the randomlike time waveform shown in

Figure 13.7 Time domain description of the same stimuli (700, 800, 900, 1000 Hz) shown in Figure 13.5, but with the four sinusoids added together with random starting phases. Note the absence of any periodically occurring peaks, but the stimulus still has a 100-Hz pitch.

Figure 13.7. These and other data indicate that although the periodicity theory might be correct in some cases, there is other processing taking place in addition to period analysis.

When the pitch of a stimulus can be determined on the basis of periodicity in the time-domain waveform, hearing scientists believe that some aspect of the auditory nerve's ability to be phase-locked to the periodicity of low-frequency stimuli accounts for the way in which the auditory system processes these pitches. But since some stimuli that do not have this type of periodicity are still perceived as having pitches, theories based on phase locking cannot account for all of the pitch results. Thus the area of pitch perception still poses a real challenge for auditory theorists who attempt to describe the frequency-processing abilities of the auditory system.

DIFFERENCE TONES

In Chapter 11 we described the aural harmonics and difference tones produced by the nonlinearity of the auditory system. The first and second aural harmonics, difference tone $(f_1 - f_2)$, and a cubic difference tone $(2f_1 - f_2)$ are those nonlinear tones most often heard (see Appendix B for a discussion of nonlinear sinusoids). In recent years many investigators have studied the cubic difference tone, since in many conditions it is the most noticeable nonlinear tone. For instance, if a 1400- and 1680-Hz tone are summed, a cubic difference tone of 1120 Hz is perceived; that is, $(2 \times 1400) - 1680 = 1120$. This cubic difference tone can be heard when the intensities of the 1400 Hz and 1680 Hz are less than 40 dB SL, whereas the difference tone of 280 Hz ($1680 - 1400 = 280$) cannot be detected at these low intensities.

In order to describe the nonlinear tones we must specify their intensities and phases as well as their frequencies. The *cancellation method* is often used to obtain estimates of the intensity and phase of nonlinear tones. In the cancellation method one stimulus is used to elicit the nonlinear tone, for instance an 840-Hz and a 1000-Hz tone which produce a 680-Hz cubic difference tone; that is $(2 \times 840) - 1000 = 680$. Another stimulus is used to cancel the pitch of the nonlinear tone, in this case a 680-Hz cancellation tone. That is, if a 680-Hz cancellation tone is added to the nonlinear 680-Hz cubic difference tone 180° out of phase, then the two tones should cancel and no pitch at 680 Hz should be heard. This cancellation will occur only when the two tones are at equal intensity and 180° out of phase. The subject is presented the 840- and 1000-Hz tones (tones used to elicit the 680-Hz cubic difference tone) and the 680-Hz cancellation tone. The subject is instructed to adjust the intensity and phase of the 680-Hz cancellation tone until he cancels (no longer hears the 680-Hz pitch) the cubic difference tone.

Figure 13.8 displays the results from a cancellation experiment performed by Hall. The upper curve shows the intensity of the 680-Hz tone required to cancel the cubic difference tone as a function of the overall level of the two tones (840 and 1000 Hz) used to elicit the cubic difference tone. The lower curve shows the phase of the 680-Hz tone required to cancel the cubic difference tone.

The intensities and phases of the nonlinearities of the auditory system are crucial values to be determined if we are to describe how the system produces these nonlinearities. The cubic difference tone has been of special interest since it appears at low intensities, and the intensity and phase of the cubic difference tone changes in a complex way as a function of its pitch (that is, as a function of the separation in frequency between f_1 and f_2). Because of these relations, most scientists believe that the source of the cubic difference tone is in the inner ear; it probably results either from the nonlinear motion of the basilar membrane or from some nonlinearities that exist

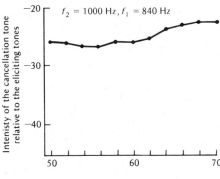

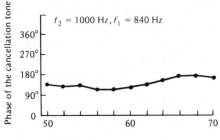

Figure 13.8   Intensity (**13.8a**) and phase (**13.8b**) of cubic difference tone (680 Hz) produced by 1000-Hz and 840-Hz eliciting tones as a function of the overall level of the eliciting tones. Note that intensity of the cubic difference tone is plotted in relation to the overall level of the eliciting tones. The results were obtained with the cancellation method. *(Adapted from Hall, 1975, by permission)*

when the hair cells stimulate the VIIIth nerve fibers. Our knowledge about aural nonlinearities is far from complete, since the perception of cubic difference tones is different from that of either aural harmonics or other difference tones.

OTHER SUBJECTIVE ATTRIBUTES OF SOUND

Complex stimuli have subjective attributes in addition to pitch and loudness, one of which is *timbre*. Timbre appears to be related to the bandwidth of the complex stimulus, especially for complex waveforms consisting of harmonically related sinusoids. In addition to timbre, musicians often refer to the consonance and dissonance of complex stimuli, such as notes of music. The scales of Western music are organized in octave relations, with each octave being divided into seven intervals (A, B, C, D, E, F, G). The interval between an octave is 2 to 1; if A is 440 Hz, then the next highest A is 880. The intervals within the octave, however, are in ratios of less than 2 to 1; for instance, the interval between G and C is in the ratio of 3 to 2. *Consonant* pairs are those notes played at intervals that result in a pleasant sound. *Dissonant* pairs are played at intervals that sound unpleasant to many musicians.

We have already discussed the *beats* (Chapter 10) associated with mixing two sinusoids whose frequencies differ by a few hertz. The sensation of beats gives way to *flutter* and then to *roughness* as the frequency difference between the two tones is increased.

S. S. Stevens determined that sounds also have attributes of *density* and *volume*. The density of a tone increases as its frequency or intensity increases. Increases in volume are generally associated with decreases in frequency and intensity. Thus volume and density are approximate opposites.

The fact that different sounds elicit different subjective descriptions is not surprising. To what extent these subjective labels are an integral part of auditory processing is not known at this time. Many scientists believe that the labeling is more a function of culture and experience than of just auditory processing. For instance, many modern composers are writing music with dissonant intervals. Since some of this music is becoming popular, these intervals might not be labeled unpleasant in a few years.

Summary From equal-loudness contours and loudness scaling experiments we can construct the phon and sone scales of loudness. These scales enable us to relate the subjective description of loudness to the physical descriptions of frequency and intensity. The mel scale is constructed from a pitch-scaling experiment. Scales of pitch are more qualitative in nature than are loudness scales. Pitch and loudness are not perfectly correlated with their physical counterparts, frequency and intensity. The concept of the missing fundamental illustrates that pitch processing is sometimes dependent neither on spectral information at the frequency of the pitch nor on periodicity information associated with the period of the pitch. The intensities and phases of nonlinear tones (especially the cubic difference tone) are measured by the cancellation technique. Complex stimuli have additional subjective attributes such as timbre, consonance, dissonance, beats, flutter, roughness, density, and volume.

Supplement Loudness and pitch as subjective attributes of sound have been studied extensively by S. S. Stevens. His book *Psychophysics* (1975) and his article in *Science* (1970), "Neural Events and the Psychophysical Law," provide an insight into his work. Fletcher and Munson (1933) used the loudness matching technique to obtain the equal-loudness contours. Loudness is often measured in an alternating binaural loudness balance (ABLB) technique. In this procedure the standard tone is presented to one ear and the comparison tone to the other ear. The tones are alternated in time, and the subject adjusts the comparison tone until it appears as loud as the standard. Steinberg and Gardner (1937) provided insights about the relationship between masking and loudness that led to the concept of recruitment. A review of loudness adaptation can be found in Elliott and Fraser's (1970) chapter in *Foundations of Modern Auditory Theory.*

Stevens and Volkman (1940) studied the mel scale and Stevens (1935) explored the relationship of pitch to intensity. Stevens' (1961) article, "The Psychophysics of Sensory Function," explains the difference between qualitative and quantitative scales. Von Bekesy (1960) showed the relationship between duration and tonal pitch.

Wightman and Green (1974) and Plomp and Smoorenburg's (1970) book, *Frequency Analysis and Periodicity Detection in Hearing*, provide excellent reviews of periodicity pitch and the missing fundamental. Fletcher made his observations at Bell Laboratories in 1924. This area of research is important in indicating that neither the place theory nor the temporally based theory alone is sufficient to explain our perceptions of pitch. The student might have noted for the missing fundamental pitch (frequencies added together at 700, 800, 900, and 1000 Hz) that a *difference tone* exists at 100 Hz. Thus, the 100-Hz pitch might be due to the nonlinearity of the ear. This, however, does not seem to be the case. Licklider (1954), for instance, showed that the difference tone due to nonlinearity could be masked by a noise with frequencies near 100 Hz. Licklider then showed, however, that the pitch of the missing fundamental stimulus was unaffected by a masking noise with a frequency of 100 Hz. Since the nonlinear tone at 100 Hz was masked and the pitch was still perceived, nonlinearity did not yield the pitch. Patterson (1973) studied the pitch of the missing fundamental when tones were added together with random starting phases.

S. S. Stevens (1934) has studied the many subjective attributes of sounds. The study of music (see Ward's chapter in *Foundations of Modern Auditory Theory*) involves many of the subjective attributes assigned to sounds. Roederer's (1973) book, *Introduction to the Physics and Psychophysics of Music*, also provides an excellent review of the physics of sound and music.

A review of the cubic difference tone can be found in Smoorenberg's 1972 article. In addition, J. L. Hall's (1975) article displays some of the complexities of the intensity and phase of the cubic difference tone as a function of the overall level of the eliciting tones and their frequency separation. Appendix A shows how one could obtain difference tones and summation tones from a nonlinear equation ($y = x + x^2$). The cubic difference tone ($2f_1 - f_2$) is obtained if we write the nonlinear equation in the form $y = x + x^2 + x^3$. Thus the name *cubic* difference tone occurs because the tone is obtained by including the cubic (x^3) term in the nonlinear equation.

The equal-loudness contours of Figure 13.1 might be considered the curves used to defined loudness level in phons. This is not strictly the case since the standard stimulus for this figure was expressed in dB SL and phons are defined in terms of sound pressure level (SPL). However, the equal-loudness contours obtained by Fletcher and Munson (1933) are often used to describe loudness level in phons (Fig. 13.1).

CHAPTER 14
The Disciplines of Audition

Medicine
Speech
Engineering
Psychology
Noise Pollution

This book has attempted to describe the fundamentals of the structure and function of the auditory system. Our knowledge of this system has been obtained by scientists whose interests include medicine, psychology, electrical and mechanical engineering, music, education, physics, physiology, speech, and anatomy. Thus the study of auditory function, or audition, requires a multidisciplinary approach.

This last chapter describes some of the auditory research in these related fields. Scientists in these areas both use and add to the basic information described in all of the preceding chapters.

MEDICINE

The application of basic auditory knowledge aids those with auditory problems or abnormalities. The general area of medicine devoted to the study of auditory problems is called *otology*, which is part of a larger area called *otorhinolaryngology* or *otolaryngology*. "Oto" refers to the ear, "rhino" to the nose, and "laryngology" to the throat; thus this area of medicine is often referred to as the ear, nose, and throat (ENT) specialty. In addition to persons with an M.D. degree, those trained in the field of *clinical audiology* with either an M.A. or Ph.D. degree work with patients having auditory problems. The otologist receives his specialty training following his medical degree, whereas the audiologist receives his training as part of his M.A. or Ph.D. degree by meeting the requirements for certification set by the American Speech and Hearing Association.

The otologist and audiologist often work together in aiding someone with an auditory problem. The audiologist provides the diagnostic testing and rehabilitation, while the otologist may provide additional diagnostics and any necessary medical treatment. A type of auditory problem that illustrates the interrelationship between otologists and audiologists is malfunction of the middle ear. If a problem occurs in the middle ear of a patient, then the help that can be provided by otologists may include surgery.

Loss of hearing due to a middle ear dysfunction is usually called a *conductive* loss, whereas inner ear problems are referred to as *sensory* or *cochlear* losses, and central nervous system problems as *retrocochlear* (usually VIIIth nerve) or *neural* losses. The audiologist uses two types of hearing tests to determine when a hearing loss is conductive. He measures the patient's threshold for hearing when tones are presented to the ear via headphones and when the tonal vibrations are presented directly to the skull (measuring the bone-conducted threshold).

In the latter test the tonal vibrator, placed directly to the skull, vibrates the skull and in turn the inner ear and its fluids, in which the normal hearing processes begin in the inner ear. Presenting the tones via headphones excites the inner ear by the "normal" means of the tympanic membrane-ossicular chain-oval window mode of operation. This is often referred to as an air-conduction measure of hearing threshold. If the air- and bone-conduction thresholds are normal and the patient still reports auditory problems, then the malfunction is probably neural. If the bone threshold is normal but the air threshold is not, then the problem is probably in the middle ear (tympanic membrane-ossicular chain-oval window). That is, if the inner ear is excited via vibration of the skull and the patient's hearing is normal, the implication is that the inner ear is working normally. Since in this case the air threshold is abnormal and the inner ear is normal, the problem must be in

the transduction from the headphones to the inner ear, that is, in the middle ear. It is unusual for a patient to have an abnormal bone threshold and a normal air threshold. If both thresholds are abnormal, then the loss is probably in the inner ear or in the central nervous system.

The audiologist has another tool to determine the health of the middle ear. The *impedance audiometer* is used to test the function of the structures in the middle ear. As we learned in Chapters 4 and 5, the middle ear amplifies sound pressure so that air pressure can more efficiently drive fluid pressure in the inner ear. These structures of the middle ear move against some resistance in order to perform this task. As was mentioned in Chapter 4, the middle ear is often said to perform an impedance matching function between the two media of air and fluid. The *impedance audiometer* enables the audiologist to measure the amount and the nature of the movement of the middle ear structures. This is accomplished by generating a small pressure in the external auditory canal and then presenting a tone to the ear. The pressure in the canal should change in a specified way due to the movement of the tympanic membrane-ossicular chain-oval window structures when the tone is presented. If these structures are not functioning normally, then the pressure change in the external canal will be different from the normal specified pressure. This indicates directly a mechanical problem with the function of the middle ear structures.

When the audiologist determines by means of the air- and bone-conduction threshold tests or with impedance audiometry that a patient has a middle-ear problem, the otologist can quite often help. In many cases the ossicular chain might move because of some disease, so that sounds are not being properly transferred to the oval window. In such cases the otologist might perform an operation called a *stapedectomy*. This is a microsurgical operation in which the otologist separates the tympanic membrane from the wall of the external auditory canal and either repairs the damaged ossicular chain or replaces the stapes with a piece of material that forms an artificial stapes. In most cases this restores the patient's hearing threshold to within 10 dB of his bone-conduction threshold. There are many other services that the audiologist and otologist can provide (for instance, audiologists often recommend hearing aids), but correction of middle-ear problems represents the area of greatest success.

SPEECH

Often an inability to use the auditory system results in poor speech. Thus, the *speech pathologist* and clinical audiologist often work together in helping to correct a patient's speaking problems. Since humans rely to such a great extent on speech for communication, there are large areas of mutual interest among scientists working in audition and those investigating speech.

Much work has been devoted to understanding our ability to perceive speech, but unfortunately the speech waveform is extremely complex, and hence our knowledge about speech perception is incomplete.

However, a variety of ways are used to describe and analyze the speech waveform. We can divide spoken language into small units. Words and letters are small units of speech, but they do not relate directly to our auditory perception of speech. From the auditory point of view we are interested in the "sound" of words or letters; hence, the unit of speech is the *phoneme*. Phonemes allow us to describe the differences among, e.g., "had, head, heed, and hid." These four words sound different because of the middle sound or middle phoneme. Another means of describing the speech waveform is in terms of the *speech production mechanisms*. English consonants can be described in terms of *place of articulation* and

manner of articulation. Places of articulation are the glottis, the palate, the gums, the teeth, and the lips. The major manners of articulation, which are plosive, fricative, and nasal, refer to the way in which the air pressure coming from the voice mechanisms is changed to produce certain sounds. Plosives are created by a blockage followed by a sudden release of air pressure; fricatives are created by a turbulent flow of air from the mouth, and nasals by allowing the nasal cavities to participate as a place of articulation. We can relate the type of phoneme to the place and manner of articulation.

We also know that the speech waveform is a complex stimulus, which may be viewed as a sum of sinusoids. There are, therefore, temporal and spectral units of the speech waveform. These units are perhaps the most crucial for the auditory processing of speech. We shall refer to the spectral and temporal properties of the speech waveform as the *acoustic properties of speech*. In order to describe the acoustic properties of speech it is useful to consider the speech signal as coming from a *resonator (vocal tract)* being driven by a *pulsating sound pressure wave (vocal folds)*. That is, the vocal folds vibrate air, which is forced through the vocal tract, and the vocal tract *resonates* or *filters* the sound caused by the vocal folds. Thus the speech waveform has acoustic properties associated with both the vocal folds and the vocal tract. The frequency at which the vocal folds vibrate is referred to as the *fundamental frequency* of a voice. The frequencies at which the vocal tract resonates are called *formant frequencies*. Most speech sounds (phonemes) differ in the frequencies of the various formants, that is, the way in which the vocal tract resonates. Figure 14.1 shows the time-domain waveform and frequency-domain spectrum of a speech sound. The spectrum of the repeated pulses (the vocal fold vibration) is a line spectrum. This spectrum is then changed by the vocal tract, creating peaks that are the formant frequencies (labeled F_1,

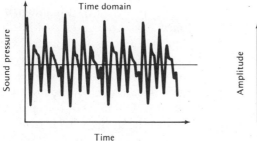
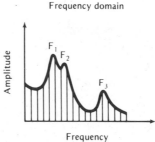

Figure 14.1 Time-domain and amplitude spectrum of a speech waveform. The vocal fold vibration is the repetition in the time domain that yields the line spectrum. The vocal tract produces resonant peaks in the spectrum at the formant frequencies F_1, F_2, and F_3. These are the acoustic properties of speech.

F_2, and F_3 in Fig. 14.1). These spectral properties are the acoustic properties of speech.

Speech scientists are studying how we perceive speech and the relationships of acoustic, phonetic, and speech production mechanism properties of speech to our recognition of speech. In general, our knowledge about the perception of such simple stimuli as sinusoids provides some, but not much, assistance in understanding speech perception. Although we can determine the spectrum for a speech waveform or we can manipulate the waveform in the time domain, there are subtle changes that are crucial in affecting speech recognition. That is, some spectra of speech sounds can be altered drastically (by changing the spectral location of the formant frequencies) without a great loss in recognition, whereas other waveforms are extremely sensitive to spectral changes. That is, the intelligibility of speech is related in a complex way to the spectrum of the sound. The same is true for changes in the time-domain structure of speech. Such diversity of variation is not often predicted on the basis of our present knowledge of the perception of simple stimuli. Undoubtedly, our experience with speech and its linguistic structure is crucial to our ability to recognize speech. Thus an understanding of speech perception will involve scientists with

interests in speech, language, and psychology, as well as in audition.

ENGINEERING

Models of the auditory system are often designed to understand various properties of auditory function in addition to speech production and recognition. For instance, electrical models are often developed by electrical engineers in order to understand the complex electrophysiology of the auditory system. Sometimes these models refer to a specific anatomical structure, such as a hair cell. Other models are more general in nature and might be used to describe an entire range of results. Filter models are often used to describe results of critical band experiments as cited in Chapter 11. The models may be in the form of a set of equations or they may be computer simulations. In some cases actual physical models might be built, such as those of von Bekesy, to study the actions of the cochlear partition.

When the middle ear or the fluids of motion in the inner ear are studied, mechanical engineers often provide the needed insights. The dynamic properties of these very small structures are of great interest to mechanical engineers. Quite often their inquiry into the function of the motion of these structures reveals a fundamental relationship of auditory processing.

PSYCHOLOGY

Chapters 8 and 9 described some of the problems associated with obtaining behavioral measures of auditory function. Classically, the field of experimental psychology has included the area of sensory psychology. Scientists who have been interested in the relationship between sensory processing and behavior have provided much of our knowledge of audition. Since the auditory system is not independent of the rest of an organism's sensory, motor, and cognitive systems, quite often scientists interested in other systems provide insights into auditory processing.

For years psychologists have studied selective attention, which is the inability of humans to monitor accurately more than one event at a time. One means of studying selective attention is to present two different messages, one to each ear. In studying a subject's ability to understand both messages some investigators have concluded that messages coming into the right ear (for right-handed subjects) are slightly easier to detect than those coming into the left ear. They hypothesize that the right ear messages are being processed primarily by the left hemisphere of the brain. Since the right ear advantage seems largest for messages with a language content (for example, speech) versus discriminations involving pure tones, the investigators conclude that the left hemisphere acts as a center for speech or language processing. Such claims have strong implications for auditory function. Thus many scientists from other fields are trying to test the assumptions associated with a left hemisphere speech center. At present there are investigations concerning the extent to which this phenomenon involves auditory processing.

In addition to the problems of understanding speech, many psychologists and musicologists have been interested in the perception of music. Chapter 13 described the perception of pitch, pointing out that it is not fully understood. The perceptions of time, consonance, and dissonance are also not clearly understood. The fact that there is a wide range of ability shown by subjects in their recognition of pitch is of interest to the auditory scientist. That is, does the person with "absolute pitch" have a different auditory system from someone without it, or is the ability to recognize pitches a learned trait? Answers to these types of questions will provide a greater understanding of the auditory system.

NOISE POLLUTION

In recent years psychologists, audiologists, otolaryngologists, and engineers have combined their efforts to try to decrease the noise in our environment. In Chapter 11 we defined noise as a stimulus whose amplitude varied randomly in time. A more general definition of *noise* is *unwanted sound*. The sound levels in our communities and places of work have in recent years reached such a level that some sound has become noise, or unwanted sound. As such, noise has presented a pollution problem to many people. Intense noise seems to be unwanted for at least the following reasons. Noise can cause:

1. Permanent hearing loss and/or physiological damage
2. Temporary threshold shifts
3. Work interference
4. Speech interference
5. Sleep interference
6. Annoyance

We have already discussed the area of temporary hearing loss due to intense noise and have mentioned problems of permanent damage (PTS, Chap. 11). The federal government has developed the "damage risk table," which indicates the intensity and duration of noise that can cause PTS in individuals who are repeatedly exposed to noise. The data of Table 14.1 show that there is a trade between the intensity of noise as measured in dBA (see Chap. 12) and the noise's continuous duration. The table simply implies that people should avoid repeated exposure to these levels and durations of sound. Auditory scientists are continuing to study noise pollution and ways it can be controlled or stopped.

The list of scientists who have shown interest from time to time in the auditory system would probably be endless. The point of this chapter is to acquaint you with a few of the areas related to audition and to indicate some of the questions investigators in these areas are probing.

The fundamentals of auditory processing have been covered in this book. We hope that those who find audition or its related areas interesting will be stimulated by this book to explore this broad field of science further. The investigation of how we hear is a dynamic pursuit.

Table 14.1   Permissible Noise Exposures

Table showing the allowable intensity of sound in dBA for various durations. When the daily noise exposure is composed of two or more periods of noise exposure at different levels, their combined effect should be considered, rather than the individual effect of each. If the sum of

$$\frac{C_1}{T_1} + \frac{C_2}{T_2} + \cdots + C_n/T_n$$

exceeds unity, then the mixed exposure should be considered to exceed the limit value. C_n indicates the total time of exposure at a specified noise level, and T_n indicates the total time of exposure permitted at that level.

T_n, Duration per Day (hours)	Sound Level (dBA)
8	90
6	92
4	95
3	97
2	100
1½	102
1	105
½	110
¼ or less	115

Summary   The areas of medicine, including otolaryngology and audiology, speech science, engineering, and psychology have provided valuable information concerning audition. The speech sound can be described by its phonetic units, speech production mechanisms (manner and place of articulation), or acoustic properties (fundamental frequency and formant frequencies). In recent years many of these disciplines have combined to study noise pollution.

Supplement   *The Speech Chain: The Physics and Biology of Spoken Language* by Denes and Pinson (1966) provides an excellent textbook for a low-level coverage of speech.

The research in audition can be found in such journals as *Acoustica, Acta Otolaryngology, Archives of Otolaryngology, Audiology, Brain Research, Brain and Language, Experimental Neurology, Journal of the American Audiology*

Society, The Journal of the Acoustical Society of America, Journal of Neuro-physiology, Journal of Experimental Psychology, Journal of Speech and Hearing Disorders, Journal of Speech and Hearing Research, Perception and Psychophysics, Physiological Psychology, and *Sound and Vibration.*

Comprehensive coverage of audition can be found in the following texts or reference books: *Woodworth's and Schlosberg's Experimental Psychology,* Volume I: *Sensation and Perception,* edited by Kling and Riggs (1972); *Handbook of Experimental Psychology,* edited by S. S. Stevens (1951); and *The Human Senses* by F. A. Geldard (1972). Excellent review articles are also found in the *Annual Review of Psychology* and the *Annual Review of Physiology.*

Advanced topics in audition are covered in the two volumes of *Foundations of Modern Auditory Theory,* edited by J. V. Tobias (1970, 1972); *The Auditory Periphery: Biophysics and Physiology,* by P. Dallos (1973); *Basic Mechanisms in Hearing,* edited by A. R. Moller (1973a); *Frequency Analysis and Periodicity Detection in Hearing,* edited by R. Plomp and G. F. Smoorenburg (1970); *Experiments in Hearing,* by G. von Bekesy (1960); *Facts and Models in Hearing,* edited by E. Zwicker and E. Terhardt (1974), and in the three parts of Volume 5 of the *Handbook of Physiology* (1, 2: 1974, 1975), edited by W. D. Keidel and W. D. Neff.

APPENDIX A
Sinusoids

The sinusoidal function plays an important role in describing the physics of sound. The theorems developed by Joseph Fourier describe the sinusoid as the basic building block for analyzing sound. The sinusoidal function is:

$$y = \sin x \qquad (A.1)$$

When speaking in terms of vibration, the function is

$$y = A \sin (2\pi f t + \theta) \qquad (A.2)$$

where A is peak amplitude, f frequency in cycles per second (or hertz) t time in seconds, and θ the starting phase angle in radians.

The rolling circle shown in Figure A.1 illustrates the relationship among these variables. As the circle rolls, the projection of the point P will be traced on the plane shown at the right. This projection of the point P describes the sinusoidal function, as given by equation (A.2). Notice that the total height that P's projection can travel in the vertical direction is the diameter of the circle. Half

of this total distance is the radius of the circle, which corresponds to A in equation (A.2). The speed at which the circle rolls will determine how often the projection of the point P repeats itself, corresponding to f in equation (A.2). Notice that as soon as the circle rolls one full turn or 360° (2π radians), the projection has completed one cycle and will now repeat itself on the next roll. Finally, if the point is moved from P_0 to P_1, it has been moved on the circle by an angle θ. This angle will alter the sinusoid at the moment the circle begins rolling. θ thus becomes the starting phase angle in equation (A.2). P_1 can be moved anywhere around the circle; thus the angle θ (or the phase angle) has a value between 0° and 360° or between 0 and 2π radians.

Sinusoidal motion is often referred to as *simple harmonic motion;* it can be described as a swinging pendulum like that shown in Figure A.2, where D is the amplitude of the sinusoidal motion, the rate of swing is the frequency, and the starting point P_0 relative to

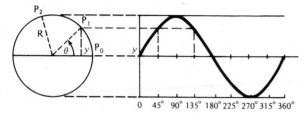

Figure A.1 As a circle rolls, a projection of a point on the circle, P, plots out a sinusoidal function. Radius R is the amplitude of the sinusoid; the frequency is the rate at which the circle rolls; the starting phase angle is angle θ, at which point P is relative to P_0; y represents an instantaneous amplitude.

the point P_1 is the starting phase of the simple harmonic motion.

Sinusoids can also describe the relationship between sides and angles of triangles. In this context the sinusoidal function is one of many *trigonometric functions*. Figure A.3 is a triangle with sides A, B, C and angles a (opposite side A), b (opposite side B), and c (opposite side C). The following equations describe

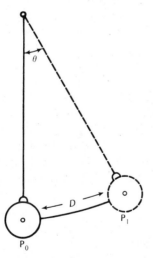

Figure A.2 As a pendulum swings from P_0 to P_1 and back, it plots out a sinusoidal function. D is the amplitude of the sinusoid.

some of the trigonometric relationships among sides and angles,

$$\sin a = \frac{A}{B}, \quad \cos a = \frac{C}{B}, \quad \tan a = \frac{A}{C} \quad \text{(A.3)}$$

where sin is the sine function, cos the cosine function, and tan the tangent function.

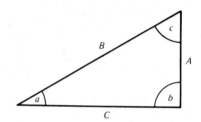

Figure A.3 Trigonometric functions are derived from the relationships among the sides, A, B, C, and the angles, a, b, c, of a right triangle.

Another way to view these three trigonometric relationships is seen in Figure A.4. The circle is a unit circle (radius of 1); "sin a" describes how far the point P has moved *along* the unit circle from the zero (or starting) position in the vertical direction, and "cos a" describes how far point P has moved along the unit circle from the zero (or starting) point in the horizontal direction. Notice, therefore, that the sine function starts at 0, goes to 1, back through 0 to –1, then to 0 again as angle a increases from 0° to 360°. The cosine function, however, starts at 1, goes to 0, then to –1, back to 0, and then to 1 as angle a increases from 0° to 360°. The projection of point P may be viewed as the same projection P described in Figure A.1.

The tangent function is formed from the sin and cos functions:

$$\tan a = \frac{\sin a}{\cos a} \quad \text{(A.4)}$$

This can easily be seen from equation (A.3) and the relations of equation (A.3),

$$A = B \sin a \quad \text{and} \quad C = B \cos a \quad \text{(A.5)}$$

Given equation (A.4), we see that the tangent can take on values from minus infinity to positive infinity as the angle a is varied. Table A.1 lists the numerical values of the sin, cos, and tan functions for angles between 0° and 360° in 5° steps.

Some of the relationships among the trigonometric functions that provide powerful tools in analyzing acoustical signals are as follows:

$$\sin a = \cos (90° - a) \quad \text{or} \quad \cos a = \sin (90° - a)$$
(A.6)

$$\sin^2 a + \cos^2 a = 1$$
(A.7)

Equations (A.6) and (A.7) can be derived directly from the unit circle shown in Figure A.4.

$$\sin (a \pm b) = \sin a \cos b \pm \cos a \sin b \quad \text{(A.8)}$$
$$\cos (a \pm b) = \cos a \cos b \mp \sin a \sin b \quad \text{(A.9)}$$
$$\sin a + \sin b = 2 [\sin \tfrac{1}{2}(a + b) \times \cos \tfrac{1}{2}(a - b)]$$
(A.10)

$$\sin 2a = 2 \sin a \cos a \quad \text{(A.11)}$$
$$\sin a \sin b = \tfrac{1}{2} [\cos (a - b) - \cos (a + b)] \quad \text{(A.12)}$$

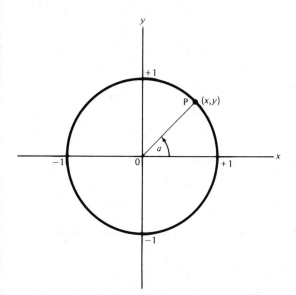

Figure A.4 The sine and cosine functions can be viewed as the distance point P moves along a circle.

Many more relationships can be derived from those listed above. For instance, we may derive $\cos 2a$ from equation (A.9):

$$\cos 2a = \cos (a + a) = \cos a \cos a - \sin a \sin a$$
$$= \cos^2 a - \sin^2 a$$

Let us now rearrange equation (A.7) to read $\sin^2 a = 1 - \cos^2 a$ and substitute for $\sin^2 a$ in the equation above for $\cos 2a$. We then obtain

$$\cos 2a = \cos^2 a - (1 - \cos^2 a) = 2 \cos^2 a - 1$$
(A.13)

Using Sinusoids to Describe Acoustic Events

These few ideas concerning sinusoids and trigonometry can help solve and describe a great variety of acoustic situations. Two examples of the use of these concepts are: (1) to determine the instantaneous amplitude of a sinusoid at different times and for different frequencies and starting phases, and (2) to investigate nonlinearities.

Suppose that there is a 100-Hz sinusoid with a peak amplitude A and a starting phase of 0°, and we would like to know the instantaneous amplitude one-thousandth of a second (1 millisecond) after the sinusoidal vibration begins. We can use equation (A.2) and Table A.1 to obtain this result. Equation (A.2), or $y = A \sin (2\pi ft + \theta)$, is the definition of a sinusoid when the sinusoidal terms are expressed in radians. We can change the equation for terms expressed in degrees by using the following:

$$y = A \sin (360° \frac{1}{T} t + \theta)$$
(A.14)

where T is the period of the sinusoid in seconds ($1/T$, of course, equals f), θ the starting phase, A the peak amplitude, and y the instantaneous amplitude. In our example $T = 1/100$ second (10 ms), $t = 1/1000$ second (1 ms), and $\theta = 0°$. So

Table A.1 Sine, Cosine, and Tangent Values for Angles from 0 to 360 Degrees, in 5-Degree Steps

Angle (degrees)	sin	cos	tan	Angle (degrees)	sin	cos	tan
0.0	0.0000	1.0000	0.0000	180.0	0.0000	−1.0000	0.0000
5.0	0.0872	0.9962	0.0875	185.0	−0.0872	−0.9962	0.0875
10.0	0.1736	0.9848	0.1763	190.0	−0.1736	−0.9848	0.1763
15.0	0.2588	0.9659	0.2679	195.0	−0.2588	−0.9659	0.2679
20.0	0.3420	0.9397	0.3640	200.0	−0.3420	−0.9397	0.3640
25.0	0.4226	0.9063	0.4663	205.0	−0.4226	−0.9063	0.4663
30.0	0.5000	0.8660	0.5774	210.0	−0.5000	−0.8660	0.5774
35.0	0.5736	0.8192	0.7002	215.0	−0.5736	−0.8192	0.7002
40.0	0.6428	0.7660	0.8391	220.0	−0.6428	−0.7660	0.8391
45.0	0.7071	0.7071	1.0000	225.0	−0.7071	−0.7071	1.0000
50.0	0.7660	0.6428	1.1918	230.0	−0.7660	−0.6428	1.1918
55.0	0.8192	0.5736	1.4281	235.0	−0.8192	−0.5736	1.4281
60.0	0.8660	0.5000	1.7321	240.0	−0.8660	−0.5000	1.7321
65.0	0.9063	0.4226	2.1445	245.0	−0.9063	−0.4226	2.1445
70.0	0.9397	0.3420	2.7475	250.0	−0.9397	−0.3420	2.7475
75.0	0.9659	0.2588	3.7321	255.0	−0.9659	−0.2588	3.7321
80.0	0.9848	0.1736	5.6713	260.0	−0.9848	−0.1736	5.6713
85.0	0.9962	0.0872	11.4300	265.0	−0.9962	−0.0872	11.4300
90.0	1.0000	0.0000	∞	270.0	−1.0000	0.0000	∞
95.0	0.9962	−0.0872	−11.4300	275.0	−0.9962	0.0872	−11.4300
100.0	0.9848	−0.1736	−5.6713	280.0	−0.9848	0.1736	−5.6713
105.0	0.9659	−0.2588	−3.7321	285.0	−0.9659	0.2588	−3.7321
110.0	0.9397	−0.3420	−2.7475	290.0	−0.9397	0.3420	−2.7475
115.0	0.9063	−0.4226	−2.1445	295.0	−0.9063	0.4226	−2.1445
120.0	0.8660	−0.5000	−1.7321	300.0	−0.8660	0.5000	−1.7321
125.0	0.8192	−0.5736	−1.4281	305.0	−0.8192	0.5736	−1.4281
130.0	0.7660	−0.6428	−1.1918	310.0	−0.7660	0.6428	−1.1918
135.0	0.7071	−0.7071	−1.0000	315.0	−0.7071	0.7071	−1.0000
140.0	0.6428	−0.7660	−0.8391	320.0	−0.6428	0.7660	−0.8391
145.0	0.5736	−0.8192	−0.7002	325.0	−0.5736	0.8192	−0.7002
150.0	0.5000	−0.8660	−0.5774	330.0	−0.5000	0.8660	−0.5774
155.0	0.4226	−0.9063	−0.4663	335.0	−0.4226	0.9063	−0.4663
160.0	0.3420	−0.9397	−0.3640	340.0	−0.3420	0.9397	−0.3640
165.0	0.2588	−0.9659	−0.2679	345.0	−0.2588	0.9659	−0.2679
170.0	0.1736	−0.9848	−0.1763	350.0	−0.1736	0.9848	−0.1763
175.0	0.0872	−0.9962	−0.0875	355.0	−0.0872	0.9962	−0.0875
				360.0	0.0000	1.0000	0.0000

$$y = A \sin\left(360° \times \frac{1}{1/100} \times \frac{1}{1000} + 0\right)$$

$$= A \sin\left(\frac{360° \times 100}{1000}\right)$$

$$= A \sin\left(360° \times \frac{1}{10}\right) = A \sin 36°$$

From Table A.1 we see that the sine of 35° is 0.57, so $A \sin 36°$ is approximately $A \times 0.57$. That is, 1 ms after a 100-Hz vibration begins, the instantaneous amplitude is $0.57A$ in magnitude. Thus, if the peak amplitude was 100 dynes/cm² of pressure, the instantaneous amplitude at 1 ms would be 57 dynes/cm².

If θ were $44°$ instead of $0°$, then the equation would be

$$A \sin (36° + \theta) = A \sin (36° + 44°) = A \sin (80°)$$
$$= A \times 0.98$$

or in our example, where A is 100 dynes/cm², the instantaneous amplitude of a 100-Hz vibration with starting phase of $44°$ would be 98 dynes/cm² at 1 ms after it started.

Nonlinearity

A linear system, as we stated in Chapter 3, is one that can be described by a straight-line relationship between the input to the system and its output. The general equation for a straight line is:

$$y = mx + b \qquad (A.15)$$

where m is a slope constant, b an intercept constant, x the input, and y the output. Thus the simplest linear system is

$$y = x \qquad (A.16)$$

where $m = 1$ and $b = 0$.

A nonlinear system is one that can be described by a relationship between an input and output that is not represented by a straight line. One such simple nonlinear equation is

$$y = x + x^2 \qquad (A.17)$$

If we assume that the input to the system is the sum of two sinusoids, $A \sin (2\pi f_1 t)$ and $A \sin (2\pi f_2 t)$, then

$$x = A \sin (2\pi f_1 t) + A \sin (2\pi f_2 t)$$

according to equation (A.17). (Throughout this discussion we shall assume that all phase angles, θ, are zero.) Since $y = x + x^2$, the value of y is as follows:

$$y = A \sin (2\pi f_1 t) + A \sin (2\pi f_2 t) +$$
$$[A \sin (2\pi f_1 t) + A \sin (2\pi f_2 t)]^2$$
$$= A \sin (2\pi f_1 t) + A \sin (2\pi f_2 t) +$$
$$[A^2 \sin^2 (2\pi f_1 t) + 2A^2 \sin (2\pi f_1 t)$$
$$\sin (2\pi f_2 t) + A^2 \sin^2 (2\pi f_2 t)] \qquad (A.18)$$

Let us look at the last three terms of equation (A.18) and use trigonometric identities.

First, using equation (A.12),

$$A^2 \sin^2 (2\pi f_1 t) = A^2 [\sin (2\pi f_1 t) \sin (2\pi f_1 t)]$$
$$= \frac{A^2}{2} [-\cos (2\pi(2f_1)t) +$$
$$\cos (2\pi(0)t)]$$
$$= \frac{A^2}{2} [-\cos (2\pi(2f_1)t) + 1]$$
$$= \frac{-A^2}{2} \cos (2\pi(2f_1)t) + \frac{A^2}{2}$$
$$= \frac{A^2}{2} - \frac{A^2}{2} \cos (2\pi(2f_1)t) \qquad (A.19)$$

Second, using equation (A.12),

$$2A^2 \sin (2\pi f_1 t) \sin (2\pi f_2 t) =$$
$$A^2 \cos (2\pi(f_1 - f_2)t) - A^2 \cos (2\pi(f_1 + f_2)t) \qquad (A.20)$$

Third, using equation (A.19) but substituting f_2 for f_1,

$$A^2 \sin^2 (2\pi f_2 t) = \frac{-A^2}{2} \cos (2\pi(2f_2)t) + \frac{A^2}{2}$$
$$= \frac{A^2}{2} - \frac{A^2}{2} \cos (2\pi(2f_2)t) \qquad (A.21)$$

By combining these three parts with the results of equation (A.18), we have

$$y = A \sin (2\pi f_1 t) + A \sin (2\pi f_2 t) -$$
$$\frac{A^2}{2} \cos (2\pi(2f_1)t) -$$
$$\frac{A^2}{2} \cos (2\pi 2f_2)t) + A^2 \cos (2\pi(f_1 - f_2)t) -$$
$$A^2 \cos (2\pi(f_1 + f_2)t) + A^2 \qquad (A.22)$$

This in turn means that when f_1 and f_2 are the input frequencies of x, the following frequencies described in equation (A.22) constitute the output y if the output y is from the nonlinear system described in equation (A.17). These frequencies are: $f_1, f_2, 2f_1, 2f_2, f_1 - f_2$, and $f_1 + f_2$. These may be the aural harmonics $(2f_1, 2f_2)$ and combination tones $(f_1 - f_2, f_1 + f_2)$ described in Chapters 3, 11, and 13.

APPENDIX B
Logarithms

The logarithm may be viewed as a way to solve the following equation for x; that is, if

$$y = 10^x \qquad \text{(B.1)}$$

then

$$x = \log_{10} y \qquad \text{(B.2)}$$

In other words, $\log_{10} y$ (or, for simplicity, $\log y$) is the logarithm to the base 10 of the number y. Thus x is the number to which 10 must be raised in order to obtain the answer y. A set of simple relationships between x and $\log y$ can be demonstrated as follows:

$0 = \log 1$, since $1 = 10^0$
$1 = \log 10$, since $10 = 10^1$
$2 = \log 100$, since $100 = 10^2$
$3 = \log 1000$, since $1000 = 10^3$

or, in general,

$$n = \log 10^n, \text{ since } 10^n = 10^n \qquad \text{(B.3)}$$

So, for instance, $\log 1,000,000$ is $\log 10^6 = 6$.

There are two simple rules concerning logarithms which are used to solve most problems.
Rule 1:

$$\log (x \cdot y) = \log x + \log y \qquad \text{(B.4)}$$

Rule 2:

$$\log (x/y) = \log x - \log y$$

A special case of rule 1 is rule 1a:

$$\log x^n = n \log x$$

since

$\log x^n = \log (x \cdot x \cdot x \ldots, n \text{ times})$
$\qquad = \log x + \log x + \ldots, n \text{ times}$
$\qquad = n \log x$

These two rules are useful in dealing with problems in which x is not a whole number or y is not some integer multiple of 10. For instance, what is the log of 412 or what is $10^{0.63}$?

Tables of logarithms are available that have the logarithms of numbers between 1 and 10;

so if you use these tables to find log 412, you are really looking up log 4.12, which is 0.615. Any answer such as 0.615, when found in the logarithm tables, is called a *mantissa*. The two rules can help determine logarithms of other numbers besides those from 1 to 10, such as 412: log 412 = log (4.12 × 100) = log 4.12 + log 100 = 0.615 + 2 = 2.615 (remember from equation (B.3), log 100 = 2). The number 2 is called the *characteristic* of the logarithm. Additional examples are as follows:

> log 2.16 = 0.335 (obtained directly from a logarithm table)
> log 2165 = log (2.165 × 1000) = log 2.165 + log 1000 = 0.335 + 3 = 3.335
> log 0.31 = log 3.1/10 (using rule 2) = log 3.1 − log 10 = 0.491 − 1 = −0.509
> log 0.0031 = log 3.1/1000 = log 3.1 − log 1000 = 0.491 − 3 = −2.509

To solve the equation $y = 10^{0.63}$, we simply go backward through the table. That is, log 4.26 is 0.63, so $10^{0.63}$ equals 4.26, thus $y = 4.26$.

The primary use for logarithms in audition is in working with the decibel. Table B.1 displays decibels as either energy (power) or pressure ratios. That is, the middle column of the table represents either:

$$dB = 10 \log \text{(energy ratio)} = 10 \log \frac{E}{E_{\text{ref}}}$$

or

$$dB = 20 \log \text{(pressure ratio)} = 20 \log \frac{p}{p_{\text{ref}}} \quad \text{(B.5)}$$

The numbers in Table B.1 to the right of the dB column are for power and pressure ratios greater than one; thus these decibels are positive. The two columns to the left of the dB column are for power and pressure ratios less than one; thus these decibels are negative. That is, a pressure ratio of 1.122 equals +1.0 dB, and a pressure ratio of 0.8913 equals −1.0 dB.

Table B.1 is the same as a logarithm table, provided that the dB values are divided by 10 when the ratio is power and by 20 when the ratio is pressure. For example, log 1.122 is 0.05, since Table B.1 shows 1.112 is 1 dB in pressure (thus 1 dB/20 = 0.05) or 0.5 dB in power (thus 0.05 dB/10 = 0.05).

Notice that the values in the table range from 0.1 to 10 in pressure ratios, from 0.01 to 100 in power ratios, and from −20 to +20 in dB.

Rules 1 and 2 can then be used to obtain values of power or pressure ratio of values of decibels outside the range shown in the table. Six examples are given here.

1. A pressure ratio of 15 equals how many dB? That is, 20 log 15 = ?. 20 log 15 = 20 log (10 × 1.5) = 20 log 10 + 20 log 1.5 = 20 dB + 3.6 dB = 23.6 dB, since 20 log 10 is 20 dB and 20 log 1.5 is 3.6 dB. Thus, 20 log 15 = 23.6 dB.

2. A power ratio of 2500 equals how many dB? That is, 10 log 2500 = ?. 10 log 2500 = 10 log (100 × 10 × 2.5) = 10 log 100 + 10 log 10 + 10 log 2.5 = 20 dB + 10 dB + 4 dB = 34 dB.

3. A power ratio of 0.008 equals how many dB? That is, 10 log 0.008 = ?. 10 log 0.008 = 10 log [8/(10 × 100)] = 10 log 8 − (10 log 10 + 10 log 100) = 9 dB − (10 dB + 20 dB) = 9 dB − 30 dB = −21 dB.

4. What is 31 dB in a pressure ratio? That is, 31 dB = 20 log ?. 31 dB = 20 dB + 11 dB; 20 dB = 20 log 10, obtained from the pressure column in Table B.1 and 11 dB = 20 log 3.548, also obtained from the pressure column in the table. Thus 20 dB + 11 dB = 20 log 10 + 20 log 3.548 = 20 log (10 × 3.548) = 20 log (35.48). Therefore the answer is 35.48.

5. What is 115 dB in a power ratio? That is, 115 dB = 10 log ?. 115 dB = (20 dB) × 5 + 15 dB; thus (20 dB) × 5 + 15 dB = 10 log (100^5) + 10 log 31.62 = 10 log (100^5 × 31.62) = 10 log 316,200,000,000. So the answer is 316,200,000,000.

6. What is −42 dB in a pressure ratio? −42 dB = −20 dB − 20 dB − 2 dB = 10 log 0.1 + 10 log 0.1 + 10 log 0.794 = 10 log (0.1 × 0.1 × 0.794) = 10 log 0.00794. So the answer is 0.00794.

Table B.1 Table of Decibel Values

The value of decibels (dB), shown in the middle column, corresponds to the pressure ratios (p_2/p_1), that is $20 \log p_2/p_1$ and the energy or power ratios (E_2/E_1), that is, $10 \log E_2/E_1$. Values on the left are for ratios of less than 1.0, and the decibels should be read as negative dB. The values on the right are for ratios greater than 1.0, and the decibels should be read as positive dB.

p_2/p_1	E_2/E_1	$-$ dB $+$	p_2/p_1	E_2/E_1	p_2/p_1	E_2/E_1	$-$ dB $+$	p_2/p_1	E_2/E_1
1.0000	1.0000	0.0	1.0000	1.0000	0.5623	0.3162	5.0	1.7783	3.1623
0.9772	0.9550	0.2	1.0233	1.0471	0.5495	0.3020	5.2	1.8197	3.3113
0.9550	0.9120	0.4	1.0471	1.0965	0.5370	0.2884	5.4	1.8621	3.4674
0.9333	0.8710	0.6	1.0715	1.1483	0.5248	0.2754	5.6	1.9055	3.6308
0.9120	0.8318	0.8	1.0965	1.2023	0.5129	0.2630	5.8	1.9498	3.8019
0.8913	0.7943	1.0	1.1220	1.2589	0.5012	0.2512	6.0	1.9953	3.9811
0.8710	0.7586	1.2	1.1482	1.3183	0.4898	0.2399	6.2	2.0417	4.1687
0.8511	0.7244	1.4	1.1749	1.3804	0.4786	0.2291	6.4	2.0893	4.3652
0.8318	0.6918	1.6	1.2023	1.4454	0.4677	0.2188	6.6	2.1380	4.5709
0.8128	0.6607	1.8	1.2303	1.5136	0.4571	0.2089	6.8	2.1878	4.7863
0.7943	0.6310	2.0	1.2589	1.5849	0.4467	0.1995	7.0	2.2387	5.0119
0.7762	0.6026	2.2	1.2883	1.6596	0.4365	0.1905	7.2	2.2909	5.2481
0.7586	0.5754	2.4	1.3183	1.7378	0.4266	0.1820	7.4	2.3442	5.4954
0.7413	0.5495	2.6	1.3490	1.8197	0.4169	0.1738	7.6	2.3988	5.7544
0.7244	0.5248	2.8	1.3804	1.9055	0.4074	0.1660	7.8	2.4547	6.0256
0.7079	0.5012	3.0	1.4125	1.9953	0.3981	0.1585	8.0	2.5119	6.3096
0.6918	0.4786	3.2	1.4454	2.0893	0.3890	0.1514	8.2	2.5704	6.6070
0.6761	0.4571	3.4	1.4791	2.1878	0.3802	0.1445	8.4	2.6303	6.9183
0.6607	0.4365	3.6	1.5136	2.2909	0.3715	0.1380	8.6	2.6915	7.2444
0.6457	0.4169	3.8	1.5488	2.3988	0.3631	0.1318	8.8	2.7542	7.5858
0.6310	0.3981	4.0	1.5849	2.5119	0.3548	0.1259	9.0	2.8184	7.9433
0.6166	0.3802	4.2	1.6218	2.6303	0.3467	0.1202	9.2	2.8840	8.3177
0.6026	0.3631	4.4	1.6596	2.7542	0.3388	0.1148	9.4	2.9512	8.7097
0.5888	0.3467	4.6	1.6982	2.8840	0.3311	0.1096	9.6	3.0200	9.1202
0.5754	0.3311	4.8	1.7378	3.0200	0.3236	0.1047	9.8	3.0903	9.5500

In general, to find the dB value for some pressure or power ratio, we divide the ratio value by 10 as many times as necessary to leave a remainder of less than 10 for pressure or less than 100 for power. Next, we look in the correct column for the dB value of this final remaining ratio. Then for each division by 10 we must add 20 dB for pressure or 10 dB for power to this dB value. (If the ratio is less than 1.0, the process is similar except that for each division by 10, we *subtract* either 10 or 20 dB.)

To calculate the power or pressure ratio from a given dB value the process is reversed.

p_2/p_1	E_2/E_1	$-$ dB $+$	p_2/p_1	E_2/E_1	p_2/p_1	E_2/E_1	$-$dB $+$	p_2/p_1	E_2/E_1
0.3162	0.1000	10.0	3.1623	10.0000	0.1778	0.0316	15.0	5.6234	31.6230
0.3090	0.0955	10.2	3.2359	10.4713	0.1738	0.0302	15.2	5.7544	33.1134
0.3020	0.0912	10.4	3.3113	10.9648	0.1698	0.0288	15.4	5.8885	34.6740
0.2951	0.0871	10.6	3.3885	11.4816	0.1660	0.0275	15.6	6.0256	36.3081
0.2884	0.0832	10.8	3.4674	12.0227	0.1622	0.0263	15.8	6.1660	38.0192
0.2818	0.0794	11.0	3.5481	12.5893	0.1585	0.0251	16.0	6.3096	39.8110
0.2754	0.0759	11.2	3.6308	13.1826	0.1549	0.0240	16.2	6.4566	41.6873
0.2692	0.0724	11.4	3.7154	13.8039	0.1514	0.0229	16.4	6.6070	43.6519
0.2630	0.0692	11.6	3.8019	14.4545	0.1479	0.0219	16.6	6.7609	45.7092
0.2570	0.0661	11.8	3.8905	15.1357	0.1445	0.0209	16.8	6.9183	47.8634
0.2512	0.0631	12.0	3.9811	15.8490	0.1413	0.0200	17.0	7.0795	50.1192
0.2455	0.0603	12.2	4.0738	16.5960	0.1380	0.0191	17.2	7.2444	52.4812
0.2399	0.0575	12.4	4.1687	17.3781	0.1349	0.0182	17.4	7.4131	54.9546
0.2344	0.0550	12.6	4.2658	18.1971	0.1318	0.0174	17.6	7.5858	57.5445
0.2291	0.0525	12.8	4.3652	19.0547	0.1288	0.0166	17.8	7.7625	60.2565
0.2239	0.0501	13.0	4.4669	19.9528	0.1259	0.0158	18.0	7.9433	63.0963
0.2188	0.0479	13.2	4.5709	20.8931	0.1234	0.0151	18.2	8.1283	66.0700
0.2138	0.0457	13.4	4.6774	21.8778	0.1202	0.0145	18.4	8.3177	69.1837
0.2089	0.0437	13.6	4.7863	22.9988	0.1175	0.0138	18.6	8.5114	72.4443
0.2042	0.0417	13.8	4.8978	23.9833	0.1148	0.0132	18.8	8.7097	75.8585
0.1995	0.0398	14.0	5.0119	25.1190	0.1122	0.0126	19.0	8.9126	79.4336
0.1950	0.0380	14.2	5.1286	26.3029	0.1096	0.0120	19.2	9.1202	83.1772
0.1905	0.0363	14.4	5.2481	27.5425	0.1072	0.0115	19.4	9.3326	87.0972
0.1862	0.0347	14.6	5.3703	28.8405	0.1047	0.0110	19.6	9.5500	91.2020
0.1820	0.0331	14.8	5.4954	30.1997	0.1023	0.0105	19.8	9.7724	95.5002
					0.1000	0.0100	20.0	10.0000	100.0000

That is, we subtract the dB value by 20 dB as many times as necessary to leave a remainder of less than 20 dB. Next, we look up the appropriate ratio value for this remaining dB value. Then, for each subtraction of 20 dB, we multiply this ratio by 10 for pressure or by 100 for power to calculate the final answer. (For negative values of dB, we divide by either 10 or 100 for each subtraction by 20 dB.) Using the table of decibel values and rules 1 and 2, we can solve any problem involving decibels or logarithms.

APPENDIX C
Anatomy and Histology

Anatomy is the science that studies the structure of the animal body and the relation of its parts. In order to discuss the relationship among various parts of the body it is necessary to develop an appropriate vocabulary. For instance, terms like "upper" and "lower" are relative and hence meaningless unless you know in what position the animal is placed. Figure C.1 illustrates how confusing this situation can be when one attempts to compare anatomy of an upright (that is, vertical) two-legged animal with that of a horizontally oriented four-legged animal. The anatomist has developed a vocabulary that differs for animals carried in the horizontal versus the vertical position. For illustrative purposes let us consider the humans and the dog shown in Figure C.1. The head of the human is the *superior* end whereas that of the dog is termed *anterior* end or *rostral* (which literally means having a beak). The terms *cephalic* and *cranial* may be applied to the head end of an animal carried in either position. The terms "superior" and "anterior" have additional meanings: *superior* is often used as a relative term meaning a structure occupying a higher

position than another structure. For example, if you are standing, your nose is superior to your mouth; but if you are lying on your back, your nose is superior to your ear. *Inferior* is the opposite of superior and thus is used to describe a structure occupying a lower position than another structure. *Anterior* refers to the forward part of an organ or body; thus for horizontally oriented animals it is the head end, but for vertically oriented animals it refers to the belly surface of the body. The more general use of the term *anterior* is to describe a structure that is situated in front of another structure. *Ventral* means toward the belly and is, therefore, synonomous with anterior for humans. *Posterior* is the opposite of anterior; thus, it is used to describe a structure situated behind another structure. Posterior can also refer to the tail end of a horizontally oriented animal. *Dorsal* refers to the back side and is, therefore, the upper side of horizontal animals and is the same as the posterior of humans.

Other anatomical terms do not have these dual meanings. In the text we have made an attempt to use these less ambiguous terms and

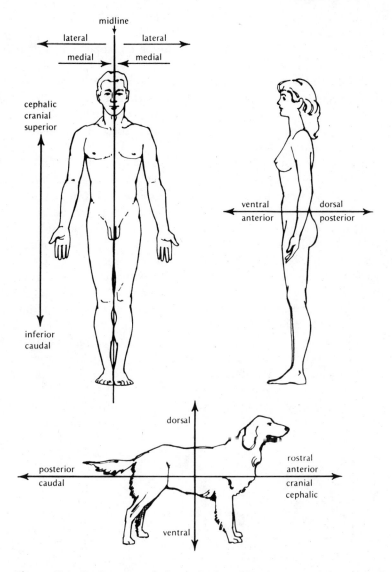

Figure C.1 Basic anatomical terminology. Terms as used in vertically and horizontally oriented animals.

to define them when they are used for the first time. For quick reference the following definitions should be helpful:

Medial means the middle, or toward a line drawn lengthwise through the middle of the body (midline).

Lateral means the sides of the body (right and left) or away from the midline.

Peripheral means at or near the surface.

Central means situated near the middle or center of the body. In this text it is often used to mean the part situated toward the center of the head or cortex.

Proximal means near and is, therefore, used with a particular structure as a reference.

Distal means away from some reference structure.

External means toward the outer surface.

Internal means toward the inner surface.

In discussions of anatomy the anatomist will often divide the body into various sections or planes. These divisions are not so important in the study of the ear's anatomy because much of the anatomy is so small that its relationship to the body as a whole is not nearly as important as the relationship of the various structures of the ear to each other. Thus the auditory anatomist can concern himself mainly with *microanatomy*—that is, the details of the structures as seen through the microscope—rather than the relationship of the structures to the body as a whole. When studying the structures of the ear with a microscope one often concentrates on the minute structure of tissue. This is called *histology*. The histologist may study normal or abnormal tissues with any of a number of microscopic techniques.

To assist the reader in interpreting many of the *photomicrographs* (photographs taken via the microscope) in this text and in other sources, we shall briefly explain a variety of microscopic techniques. There are two main types of microscopy, light and electron. The most widely used methods of light microscopy in the study of the anatomy of the auditory system are the *standard light transmission microscope* and the *phase contrast light* microscope. With the standard light microscope a thin slice or section of the specimen of interest is placed in the scope. A strong light is passed through it from one side, and on the opposite side the investigator observes the light that passes through the specimen with a magnification system of lenses. Figure C.2 shows a block diagram of the standard transmission light microscope and two of the other microscopes discussed later. Figure 5.5a in Chapter 5 shows a photomicrograph of the organ of Corti taken with a standard light microscope. In 5.5a the organ of Corti has been sectioned (sliced) in a plane that affords a view of the relative positions of the hair cells, the tectorial membrane, the tunnel of Corti, and various

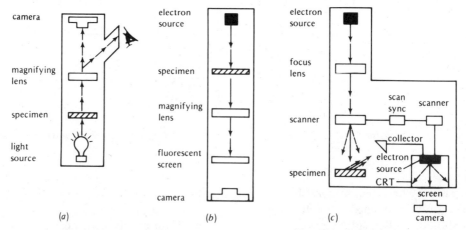

Figure C.2 Simple block diagrams of three types of microscopes. **C.2a:** Standard light transmission microscope. **C.2b:** Direct electron microscope. **C.2c:** Scanning electron microscope. The first two types are similar in that they both transmit the signal (either light or electrons) through the specimen. The scanning electron microscope reflects electrons off the surface of the specimen.

other structures. The plane in which a specimen is sectioned may be referred to by various terms such as "cross sectional" or "longitudinal." The exact meaning of such terms is relative to whatever the writer considers the "normal" orientation of the tissue of interest. The important point is that an investigator has an endless possible number of planes in which to section the specimen. It is therefore the responsibility of the investigator to section in the plane that gives the best view of the particular tissue under investigation. Photographs of the specimen are taken and important parts can be labeled for illustrative purposes. Following are the abbreviations used to label the photomicrographs in this text:

A—afferent nerve
BC—border cell
BM—basilar membrane
C—Claudius' cell
Cn—cochlear nerve
CP—cuticular plate
D—Deiters' cell
E—efferent nerve fibers
Fn—facial nerve
Gc—ganglion cell
H—Hensen's cell
HC—hair cell
HP—habenula perforata
HS—Hensen's stripe
IAM—internal auditory meatus
IHC—inner hair cell
IP—inner pillar
IS—inner spiral bundle
ISC—inner sulcus cell
m—microvilla
M—modiolus
Mc—mitochondria
MNF—myelinated nerve fibers
n—nerve
N—nucleus
OC—organ of Corti
OHC 1—outer hair cell, row 1
OHC 2—outer hair cell, row 2

OHC 3—outer hair cell, row 3
OP—outer pillar
OS—outer spiral fibers
OW—oval window
PC—pillar cell
PP—phalangeal process
R—radial fibers
Rm—Reissner's membrane
RW—round window
S—stapes
Sc—stereocilia
Sl—spiral ligament
SL—spiral lamina
Sm—scala media
SM—stapedial muscle
SN—space of Nuel
St—scala tympani
Sv—scala vestibuli
SV—stria vascularis
TB—temporal bone
TC—tunnel of Corti
TL—tympanic layer
Tm—tectorial membrane
TR—tunnel radial fibers
TSB—tunnel spiral bundle
tt—tensor tympani

Another method of light microscopy is phase contrast microscopy. The phase contrast microscope takes advantage of the fact that light passes through various tissues with different speeds, thus differentially affecting its phase. The phase contrast microscope changes these phase differences (which are not visible to the eye) into amplitude differences, which appear as differences in brightness (that is, light-dark contrast). The phase contrast microscope is often used in conjunction with the *whole mount* or *surface preparation technique*. With this technique whole portions of the organ of Corti and basilar membrane of 1 to 5 mm in length can be placed in the microscope for observation, and a sizable number of adjacent hair cells can be viewed. Another advantage of this technique is that we can focus at different levels within the specimen. For instance, Figure C.3 shows the same specimen with the microscope focused at three different levels. Thus by adjusting the microscope to be in focus at various levels within the specimen we can obtain a visual "slice" of the specimen without the inherent difficulties normally encountered in attempting mechanical slicing of the very delicate organ of Corti.

Since the 1950s the *transmission* or *direct electron microscope* has gained in popularity because of its remarkable resolving power. The specimen is sliced in sections and placed in the scope. Instead of passing light through the specimen, electrons are transmitted in a beam through the specimen. The electron beam is diffracted by the specimen in a manner similar to the way the light beam is diffracted in the light microscope. The electron beam is magnified by electromagnetic lenses and then directed toward a fluorescent screen, where the image is produced and photographed. By comparing the transmission electron micrographs in Figure 5.7 with the light micrograph of Figure 5.5a (Chapter 5) we can obtain an idea of the resolving capabilities of this instrument. Figure 5.7 shows a great deal more detail than Figure 5.5a, and Figure C.4 demonstrates an even higher magnification of the base of one outer hair cell. Figures C.5 and C.6 show similar comparisons of a transmission electron micrograph and a micrograph taken with a scanning electron microscope.

The *scanning electron microscope* (SEM) has a better resolving power than the light microscope, but it does not have the same level of capability as the electron microscope just described. The SEM has the advantage of having a greater depth of field. This means that a larger portion of the viewed specimen will be in focus. The SEM does not use a beam of electrons transmitted through the specimen. Instead it uses an electron beam

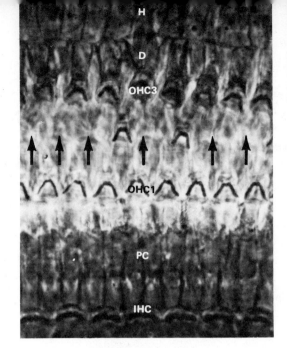

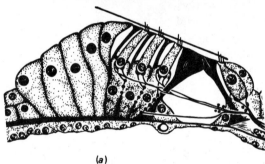

(a)

Figure C.3 Phase contrast micrographs focused at three different levels of the monkey organ of Corti. **C.3a:** Focused on the stereocilia. The typical W pattern of the outer hair cells' stereocilia is clearly seen. After the ear was exposed to noise, only two of the hair cells' stereocilia remain (W patterns) in the second row of outer hair cells; the missing stereocilia are indicated by arrows. **C.3b:** Focused at the level of the cuticular plate. Scarring is shown in the area of the missing hair cells (arrows). **C.3c:** Focused at the level of the body of the hair cells. The drawing below each micrograph shows, with a line, the level at which the microscope was focused. (*Photographs courtesy of Dr. Ivan Hunter-Duvar, Hospital for Sick Children, Toronto*)

that is focused on the specimen and loosens electrons from the surface of the specimen. These loosened electrons and the reflected electron beam are collected and used to form

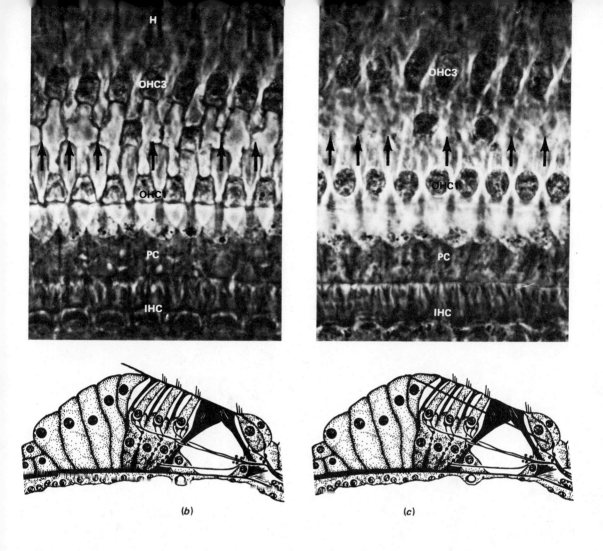

(b)

(c)

an image on a screen that resembles a television set. This process allows one to view only the surface of the specimen. The SEM derives its name from the fact that the electron beam scans over the specimen in a systematic fashion. The specimen is usually prepared to emit electrons by prior coating with a very thin layer of gold or other soft metals. The scan of the microscope's electron beam is synchronized with the scan of the electron beam in the cathode-ray tube (similar to a TV picture tube). The collected electrons that are loosened from the specimen, or reflected by it, modulate the electron beam of the picture tube to create the image. Figures C.5, C.6, C.7,

and C.8 show various SEM photographs taken from the cathode-ray tube and illustrate the great depth of field and resulting three-dimensional quality of this technique as compared to other techniques.

The various types of microscopes have their advantages and disadvantages. A complete laboratory interested in the anatomy of the inner ear will have the ability to use each of these types of instruments, matching the advantages of a particular microscope to their particular need. The foregoing discussion of the various microscopic and histological techniques is very superficial. The reader who is interested in more information will find the

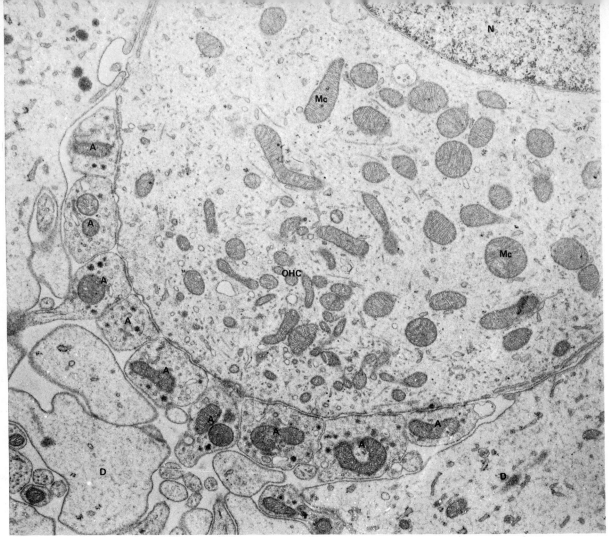

Figure C.4 Transmission electron micrograph showing the synapse of the afferent nerve fibers (A) at the base of an outer hair cell (OHC). Detailed structures such as the mitochondria (Mc) can be clearly seen. *(Chinchilla photograph courtesy of Dr. Ivan Hunter-Duvar, Hospital for Sick Children, Toronto)*

following sources useful: Bohne (1972), Engstrom et al. (1966), Hayat (1970), Hearle et al. (1973), Kuhn et al. (1971), Lipscomb (1974), Meek (1970), Pease (1964), and Schuknecht (1974). Also highly recommended are chapters in the book edited by Smith and Vernon (1976).

The anatomy of the auditory system central to the cochlea consists of neurons. The branch of anatomy which investigates the nervous system and nerve tissue is *neuroanat-*

omy. There are many kinds of neurons: *receptor neurons*, which receive stimulation from sensory receptor cells (such as the hair cell in the ear) and in turn excite other neurons; *interneurons*, which receive stimulation from one neuron and pass it to the next; *motorneurons*, which receive stimulation from a neuron and in turn stimulate a muscle; and various other neurons depending upon one's method of classification. For our present purposes it will suffice to consider the receptor

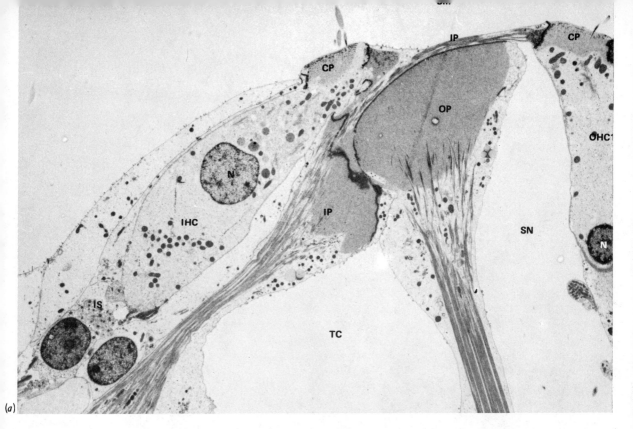

(a)

Figure C.5 **C.5a:** Transmission electron micrograph showing the structure of part of the organ of Corti in detail not achievable with other methods of microscopy. **C.5b:** Scanning electron micrograph of the same area for comparison. Note the lack of detailed structure of the hair cells. *(Chinchilla photographs courtesy of Dr. Ivan Hunter-Duvar, Hospital for Sick Children, Toronto)*

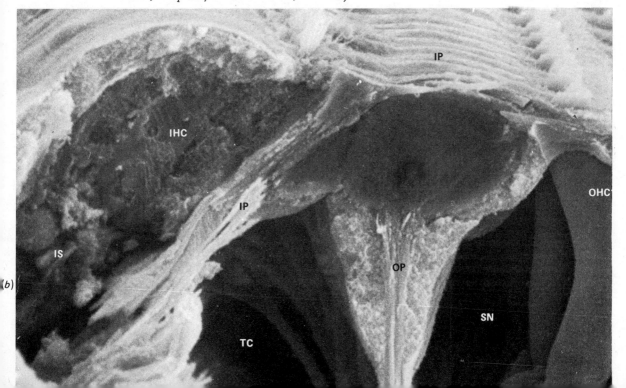

(b)

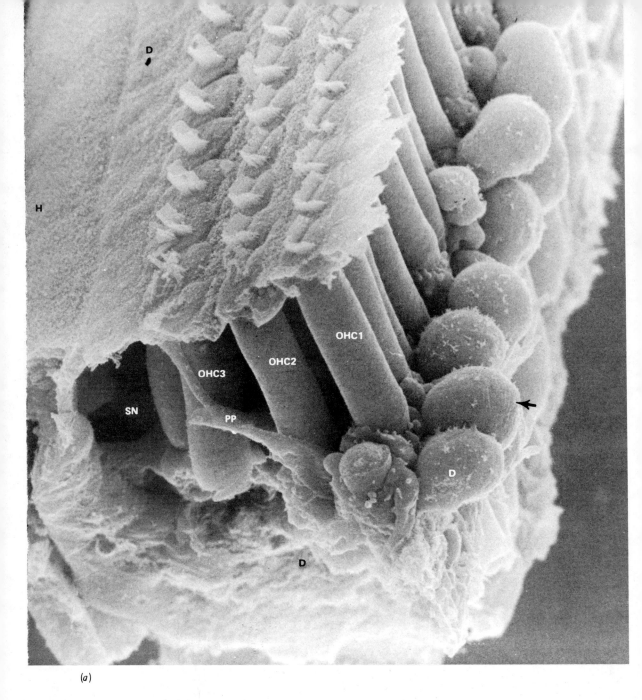

(a)

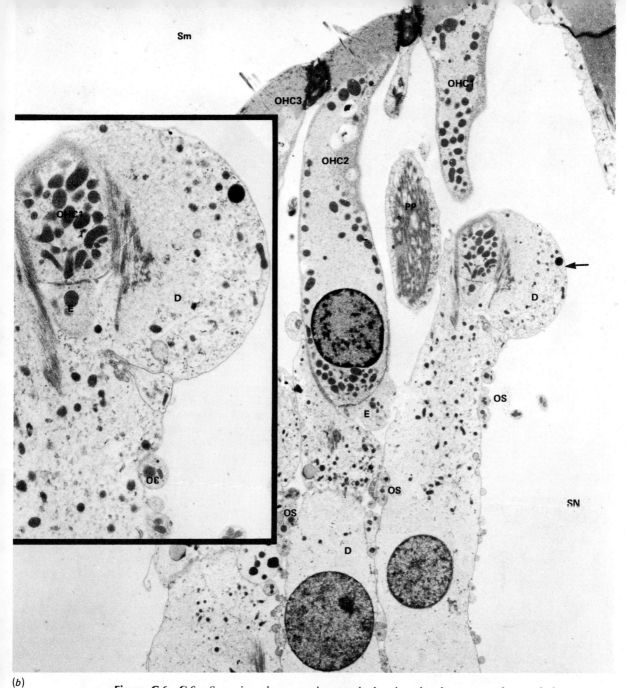

(b)

Figure C.6 **C.6a:** Scanning electron micrograph showing the three rows of outer hair cells and their supporting structures. The great depth of field adds a three-dimensional quality not achievable with other methods. **C.6b:** Transmission electron micrograph of the same area for comparison. Note the complete lack of depth but great detail. The resolving power of the transmission electron microscope is emphasized in the insert, which shows the detailed structure of the Deiters' cell bulge at the base of the first row of outer hair cells (located with an arrow in each large photograph). *(Chinchilla photographs courtesy of Dr. Ivan Hunter-Duvar, Hospital for Sick Children, Toronto)*

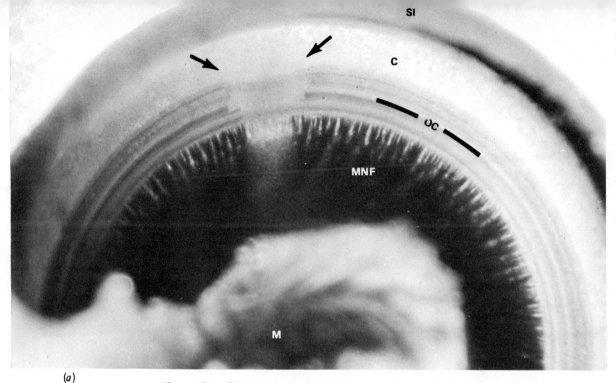

(a)

Figure C.7 **C.7a:** Low-power light micrograph of a large portion of the cochlea. The curvature of the cochlea is obvious. The innervation of the organ of Corti (OC) by the myelinated nerve fibers (MNF) leaving the modiolus (M) is clearly seen. The arrows indicate an area where the organ of Corti is missing due to a lesion or disruption caused by acoustic overstimulation, that is, a loud sound. **C.7b:** Scanning electron micrograph of the organ of Corti at the edge of the lesion. The outer hair cells are extremely distorted and appear to have sealed the tunnel of Corti. *(Chinchilla photographs courtesy of Dr. Ivan Hunter-Duvar, Hospital for Sick Children, Toronto)*

(b)

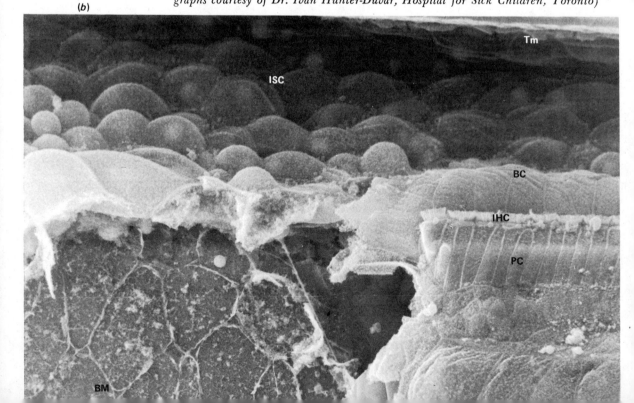

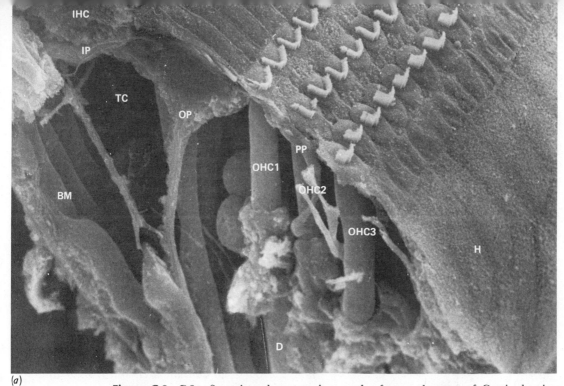

(a)

Figure C.8 **C.8a:** Scanning electron micrograph of normal organ of Corti, showing normal ultrastructure. **C.8b:** Scanning electron micrograph of organ of Corti that has been damaged by acoustic overstimulation. The effects of sound damage on the outer hair cells are clearly shown by the fact that they are now absent (except for some remnants of OHC2). *(Chinchilla photographs courtesy of Dr. Ivan Hunter-Duvar, Hospital for Sick Children, Toronto)*

(b)

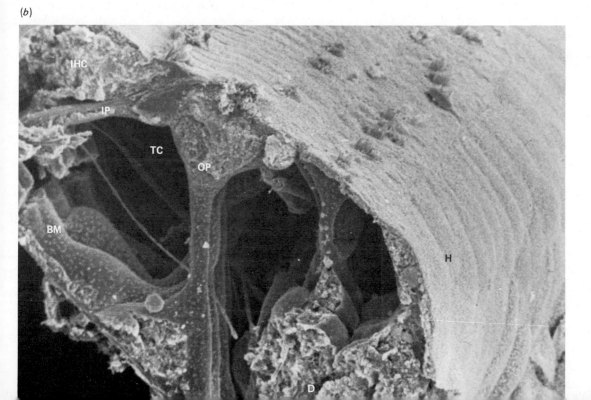

neuron in Figure C.9 to illustrate the general anatomy of a neuron. The neuron consists of three main parts: the *cell body* or *soma,* the *dendrites,* and the *axon.* The wall of the cell body is called the cell membrane. Inside the cell body is the nucleus. The nucleus is surrounded by intracellular fluids called cyto-

Figure C.9 Basic structure of a receptor neuron such as those found in the auditory nerve.

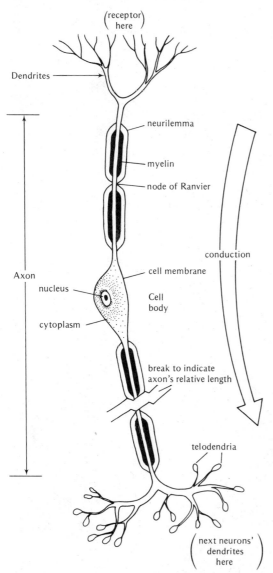

plasm and is responsible for the metabolic activities of the cell. The dendrites are specialized for receiving excitation from another cell, receptor cell, or nerve. The axon is usually elongated and is specialized for transmitting the excitation out of the cell. Most neurons have several dendrites to receive stimulation and only one axon to deliver neural impulses. Axons may, however, have several branches called *collaterals* and they may also have many endings called *telodendria.* Transmission of stimulation from one neuron to another takes place across an interspace called a *synapse.* When observed by direct electron microscopy the axon can be shown to contain *vesicles* at a synapse and a thickened cell membrane. These synaptic vesicles, which appear as little round sacs, are thought to contain a chemical used in transmitting stimulation across the synaptic gap or junction. Axons may be covered with two coverings or sheaths: the *neurilemma* and the *myelin sheath.* The neurilemma is a very thin sheath found on the outside of the peripheral nerve fibers, which aids the axon in regeneration when it is injured. Neurons in the central nervous system generally do not have a neurilemma. Myelin sheath is relatively thick fatty substance that surrounds the axon and serves as sort of an insulator. This myelin sheath is interrupted at regular intervals called the *nodes of Ranvier.* These nodes are thought to assist the neuron in the transmission of neural impulses called action potentials. The myelin sheath does not cover the cell body. Groups of neuron cell bodies in the central nervous system are called ganglia. A similar grouping of cell bodies in the central nervous system is referred to as *nucleus.* A bundle of nerve fibers or axons in the periphery is usually referred to as a *nerve.* In the central system such a bundle may be called a *tract.* A further discussion of how neurons transmit information can be found in Appendix **D.**

APPENDIX D
Physiology

The study of the *function* of body structure is called *physiology*. This appendix deals primarily with *neurophysiology* or *neurology*, the physiology of nerves and nuclei, and will explain how a nerve discharge begins in a nerve cell and how it is propagated down the nerve's axon to the next nerve.

The cell's membrane separates the *intracellular* and *extracellular fluids*. The intracellular and extracellular fluids contain water and chemicals whose mixture causes *ions* to be formed. Ions take on positive or negative electric charges; the charges of the ions differ between the intracellular and extracellular fluids.

An electrical difference in charge between two ions produces an *electric potential*. That is, the potential exists for the flow of electric current. For instance, the two poles of a battery are of opposite charge since each pole consists of different chemicals with opposite ionic charges. Thus a potential difference exists between the poles of the battery. Electric current will flow between the poles if a conductor, such as a metal wire, is connected between the poles of the battery.

Since there is a difference in the charge of the ions between the intracellular and extracellular fluids, a potential difference exists across the cell membrane. This potential difference always exists whether or not the nerve is excited, and so this permanent potential difference is called a *resting potential*.

The intracellular fluid consists primarily of *potassium* and has a *negatively charged ionic field;* the extracellular fluid is primarily *sodium* and has a *positively charged ionic field*. The resting potential difference between the two fluids ·(across the cell membrane) is between 50 and 90 millivolts (mV). See Figure D.1.

The nervous system thus possesses the potential for the flow of electric current. The most widely accepted theory of how this flow is initiated concerns a change in the permeability of the cell membrane to potassium and sodium as a function of excitation of the nerve. The chain reaction is outlined below: first, some *adequate stimulus* (such as the shearing of the hair cell cilia) changes the permeability of the cell membrane that allows for sodium to flow into the cell and potassium

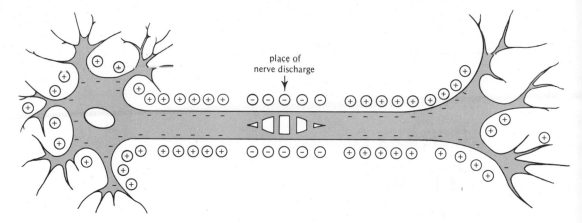

Figure D.1 Positive (outside the cell) and negative (inside the cell) ions and their charges as a function of stimulation of a nerve. The ions are transported through the cell wall at the point of the nerve discharge.

to flow from it. This exchange of chemicals, and hence of ions, changes the potential difference from a negative value to a positive one. When the potential difference reaches *a critical potential difference,* then the cell membrane immediately in front of the initial point of change in cell permeability also changes in permeability. An ion exchange occurs at this point along the nerve. Meanwhile, the ions move toward the resting state back at the initial region of excitation. At this initial place of excitation the sodium begins to flow from the cell and the potassium begins to flow into it until the resting potential is reached at this point along the cell. An ion exchange is propagated down the nerve. Meanwhile the membrane behind the propagated chemical exchange is being restored to its initial state.

This change in the transfer of ions can be measured by noting the electric potential change at *one point* along the nerve (see Figure D.2). The resting potential is approximately –45mV. Next a positive increase (A) in the potential occurs when the critical voltage is reached. The increase to +40mV at B is a result of the flow of sodium into the cell and potassium out of the cell. Then as the

cell membrane goes back to its resting state and the ions flow the other way, there is a decrease in the potential with some overshoot to –70 mV at point C. Finally, at point D the potential difference is back at its resting state. The time between B and C is called the *absolute refractory period* of the nerve impulse. During this time no new discharge can occur since the flow of ions must reach a resting state before they can move again. The time be-

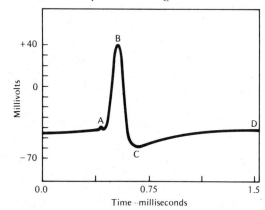

Figure D.2 Voltage changes during stimulation of a nerve. From the resting potential there is an increase, A, to a positive voltage, B, then a negative overshoot, C, and back to the resting potential, D. This is the voltage change that exists at the point of nerve discharge shown in Figure D.1.

tween C and D is the *relative refractory period,* since it is difficult (but not impossible) for a new discharge to occur then. The refractory periods indicate the limit as to how often a nerve impulse can be propagated down the nerve (the limit is about 1000 times a second, although this rate is rarely achieved).

Once the propagated discharge has reached the end foot of the axon, the discharge must cross the synapse before it can begin the chain of propagation down the next nerve fiber. There is even less known about the transfer across the synapse than about the details of the initial discharge. The best guess is that small chemical packets called vesicles (they rest at the synapse) aid in transferring the chemical action across the synapse.

One important point concerning the nerve discharge should be emphasized. Once a discharge begins, it remains the same amplitude and travels at the same speed independent of the parameters of the stimulus that initially excited the nerve. This is referred to as the *all-or-none law of nerve conduction.* The all-or none law poses a real challenge for understanding how the nervous system encodes the multitude of events occurring in the complex world.

ELECTROPHYSIOLOGY

Electrophysiology is the study of the electrochemical changes in the nervous system. Its main technique involves implanting an electrode into neural tissue and measuring the potential difference between the change in the tissue and some other point. The other point (reference electrode) might be another part of the nervous system or some neutral location. Each time a spike discharge is propagated down the nerve, the electrode will respond to the potential difference. This potential difference is then amplified and fed to some recording instrument.

The auditory electrophysiologist is concerned with the potential differences existing not only in nerves but also in the structures of the inner ear. No matter where these differences exist, the electrode always measures the differences in electric charge between two points. As described earlier, this difference has the potential for electric current flow.

OTHER AUDITORY PHYSIOLOGICAL TECHNIQUES

The auditory physiologist is interested in the mechanical function of the middle and inner ears as well as in the electrophysiological changes in the auditory nerves and nuclei. The extremely small size of the vibrating objects in the ear presents a problem for measurement.

The physiological measures most often used are electrical. Sometimes electric signals such as the cochlear microphonic (CM) can be recorded at a great distance from the ear. However, since the distance is great the CM amplitude is very small relative to the other background electrical activity associated with bodily functions. Presumably, most of this background activity is uncorrelated with the presentation of a signal to the ear and is thus considered noise. The CM, of course, is perfectly correlated with the occurrence of the acoustic signal since the CM always occurs. Thus, if the signal is presented many times and the electrical responses of the distant electrode following each stimulus presentation are summed, the uncorrelated background noise should tend to be canceled and the CM associated with the signal presentation enhanced. This technique is called *signal averaging.* A computer is required for the addition and has been used to study many different types of weak electric potentials, especially those associated with auditory-evoked changes in the EEG or brain waves recorded from the top of the head.

Since such membranes as the tympanic membrane, oval and round window membranes, and basilar membrane all vibrate, techniques have been developed to study their vibrations. However, since the amplitude of vibration is so incredibly small, only recently has modern technology provided the means of measurement. Four of these tools are: *realtime holography, the Mössbauer technique, optical heterodyne spectroscopy,* and *laser interferometry.* Holography, laser interferometry, and spectroscopy take advantage of the laser beam to produce a light source that reflects off the membranes so that the vibrations can be measured. The Mössbauer technique involves radioactivity. Thus our knowledge of audition is dependent on technology from other areas of science and engineering.

References and Index of Names

Boldface page numbers after authors' names denote pages on which adaptations of their figures appear. Also, the sources of adapted figures are identified by italicized figure and page numbers in parentheses following the appropriate reference citations.

Abel, S. M., 138, **138**, 140

Abel, S. M. (1972). Duration discrimination of noise and tone bursts. *J. Acoust. Soc. Amer.* 51: 1219–1224. *(Fig. 10.9, 138)*

Abeles, M., 107; *see Goldstein*

Ades, H. W., 33, 62, 63, **92**, 108, 192; *see Engstrom*

Ades, H. W. (1959). Central auditory mechanisms. *Handbook of physiology*, Sec. 1, Vol. 1, *Neurophysiology*, Field, J., Magoun, H. W., Hall, V. E. (eds.). Washington, D.C.: American Physiological Society. *(Fig. 7.1, 92)*

Ades, H. W., and Engstrom, H. (1972). Inner ear studies. *Acta Otolaryng. (Stockholm)*, Suppl. 301.

Ades, H. W., and Engstrom, H. (1974). Anatomy of the inner ear. *Handbook of sensory physiology*, Vol V(1), Keidel, W. D., and Neff, W. D. (eds.). New York: Springer. *(Fig. 4.1, 33)*

Adrian, E. D., 89

Adrian, E. D. (1931). The microphonic action of the cochlea in relation to theories of hearing. *Report of a discussion on audition*. London: Physical Society, pp. 5–9.

Anderson, A., 192; *see Engstrom*

Anderson, D. J., 83, 86, 90; *see Hind; see Rose*

Anderson, D. J., Rose, J. E., Hind, J. E., and Brugge, J. F. (1971). Temporal position of discharges in single auditory nerve fibers within the cycle of a sine-wave stimulus: frequency and intensity effects. *J. Acoust. Soc. Amer.* 49:1131–1139.

Angelborg, C., 62, 63

Angelborg, C., and Engstrom, H. (1973). The normal organ of Corti. *Basic mechanisms in hearing*, Moller, A. (ed.). New York and London: Academic.

Balogh, K., 90; *see Ishii*

Bekesy, G. von 34, **35**, **37**, **39**, 41, 42, 43, 47, 56, **59**, **60**, 62, 71, 72, 89, 113, 120, **131**, 140, 175, 179, 182

Bekesy, G. von (1936a). Zur Physik des Mittelohres und uber das Horen bei fehlerhaftem Trommelfell. *Akust. Z.* 1:13–23 (104–115). *(Fig. 4.8, 41)*

Bekesy, G. von (1936b). Uber die Hörschwelle und Fühlgreuze lungsamer sinusförmiger Luftruch schwankuger. *Ann. Phys.* 26:554–566.

Bekesy, G. von (1941). Uber die Messung der Schwingungsamplitude der Gehorknochelchen mittels einer kapazitiven Sonde. *Akust. Z.* 6:1–16 (20–23, 30–31, 53–57, 95–104). *(Fig. 4.6, 37; Fig. 4.7, 39)*

Bekesy, G. von (1943). Uber die Resonanzkurve und die Abklingzeif der verschiedenen Stellen der Schneckentrennwand. *Akust. Z.* 8:66–76. *(Fig. 5.14, 59)*

Bekesy, G. von (1947a). A new audiometer. *Acta Otolaryng. (Stockholm)* 35:411–422.

Bekesy, G. von (1947b). The variation of phase along the basilar membrane with sinusoidal vibrations. *J. Acoust. Soc. Amer.* 19:452–460. *(Fig. 5.15, 60)*

Bekesy, G. von (1949). On the resonance curve and the decay period at various points on the cochlear partition. *J. Acoust. Soc. Amer.* 21:245–254.

Bekesy, G. von (1951). Microphonics produced by touching the cochlear partition with a vibrating electrode. *J. Acoust. Soc. Amer.* 23:29–35 (672–684).

Bekesy, G. von (1960). *Experiments in hearing*. New York: McGraw-Hill. *(Fig. 4.2, 34; Fig. 4.6, 37; Fig. 10.2, 131)*

Bekesy, G. von, and Rosenblith, W. A. (1951). The mechanical properties of the ear. *Handbook of experimental psychology*, Stevens, S. S. (ed.). New York: Wiley.

Benson, D. A., 107

Benson, D. A., and Teas, D. C. (1972). Human auditory evoked response: Specific effects of signal strength and performance criterion. *Percept. Psychophys.* 11:203–208.

Beranek, L. L., 22

Beranek, L. L. (1954). *Acoustics.* New York: Mc-Graw-Hill.

Berlin, C. L., 90; *see* Cullen

Biddulph, R., 135, **136**, 140; *see* Shower

Bilger, R. C., 140; *see* Jesteadt

Billone, M., 63, 89; *see* Dallos

Billone, M., and Raynor, S. (1973). Transmission of radial shear forces to cochlear hair cells. *J. Acoust. Soc. Amer.* 54:1143–1156.

Birdsall, T. G., 140; *see* Green

Bogert, B., 62; *see* Peterson

Bohne, B. A., 198

Bohne, B. A. (1972). Location of small cochlear lesions by phase contrast microscopy prior to thin sectioning. *Laryngoscope* 82(4):1–16.

Boring, E. C., 128

Boring, E. C. (1942). *Sensation and perception in the history of experimental psychology.* New York: Appleton.

Boudreau, J. C., 108; *see* Tsuchitani

Boyle, A. J. F., 62; *see* Johnstone

Bray, C., 89; *see* Wever

Bredberg, G., 62, 63; *see* Engstrom; *see* Lindeman

Bredberg, G. (1968). Cellular pattern and nerve supply of the human organ of Corti. *Acta Otolaryng. (Stockholm),* Suppl. 236.

Brown, P. B., 108; *see* Goldberg, J. M.

Brugge, J. F., **86**, 90, **103**, 108, *see* Anderson, D. J.; *see* Hind; *see* Rose

Brugge, J. F., and Merzenich, M. M. (1973). Patterns of activity of single neurons of the auditory cortex in monkey. *Basic mechanisms in hearing,* Moller, A. G. (ed.). New York: Academic, pp. 754–772. *(Fig. 7.10, 103)*

Buchwald, J. S., 107

Buchwald, J. S., and Huang, C. M. (1975). *Far field* acoustic responses: Origins in the cat. *Science* 189:382–384.

Carrier, S. C., 165; *see* Hafter

Casseday, J. H., 107; *see* Neff

Cheatham, M. A., 89; *see* Dallos

Clark, L. F., **85**, 90; *see* Kiang

Clarke, F. R., 120; *see* Egan

Cohen, L., 107; *see* Donchin

Coombs, C. H., 128

Coombs, C. H., Dawes, R. M., and Tversky, A. (1970). *Mathematical psychology: An elementary introduction.* Englewood Cliffs, N.J.: Prentice-Hall.

Cross, P. M., 198; *see* Hearle

Cudahay, E., 154; *see* Leshowitz

Cullen, J. K., 90

Cullen, J. K., Jr., Ellis, M. S., and Berlin, C. L. (1972). Human acoustic nerve action potential recordings from the tympanic membrane without anesthesia. *Acta Otolaryng. (Stockholm)* 74: 15–22.

Dallos, P., **33**, 42, 62, 89, 91, 182

Dallos, P. (1969). Comments on the differential electrode technique. *J. Acoust. Soc. Amer.* 45: 999–1007.

Dallos, P. (1970). Low-frequency auditory characteristics: species dependence. *J. Acoust. Soc. Amer.* 48:489–499.

Dallos, P. (1973). *The auditory periphery: Biophysics and physiology.* New York: Academic. *(Fig. 4.1, 33)*

Dallos, P., Billone, M. C., Durrant, J. D., Wang, C. Y., and Raynor, S. (1972). Cochlear inner and outer hair cells: functional differences. *Science* 177: 356–358.

Dallos, P., and Cheatham, M. A. (1971). Travel time in cochlea and its determination from CM data. *J. Acoust. Soc. Amer.* 49:1140–1143.

Darshan, S. D., 154; *see* Henderson

Davis, H., 63, **67**, **69**, **72**, 89, 90, 91, 107; *see* Pestalozza; *see* Saul; *see* Tasaki; *see* Teas

Davis, H. (1956). Initiation of nerve impulses in the cochlea and other mechanoreceptors. *Physiological triggers and discontinuous rate processes,* Bullock, T. H. (ed.). Washington, D.C.: American Physiological Society, pp. 60–71. *(Fig. 6.1, 67)*

Davis, H. (1960). Mechanism of excitation of auditory nerve impulses. *Neural mechanisms of the auditory and vestibular systems,* Rasmussen, T., and Windle, W. F. (eds.). Springfield, Ill.: Thomas, pp. 21–39. *(Fig. 6.6, 72)*

Davis, H. (1968). Auditory responses evoked in the human cortex. *Hearing mechanisms in vertebrates,* De Reuck, A. V. S., and Knight, J. (eds.). London: Churchill, pp. 259–269.

Davis, H. (1976). Principles of electric response audiometry, *Ann. Otol.,* Suppl. 28:3.

Davis, H., and Eldredge, D. H. (1959). An interpretation of the mechanical detector action of the cochlea. *Ann. Otol.* 68:665–674.

Davis, H., Fernandez, C., and McAuliffe, D. R. (1950). The excitatory process in the cochlea. *Proc. Nat. Acad. Sci. USA* 36:580–587.

Dawes R. M., 128; *see* Coombs

Denes, P. B., 181

Denes, P. B. and Pinson, E. N. (1966). *The speech chain: The physics and biology of spoken lan-*

guage. Murray Hill N.J.: Bell Telephone Laboratories.

Diamond, I. T., **92**, 107; *see* Neff

Diamond, I. T. (1973). Neuroanatomy of the auditory system: Report on a workshop. *Arch. Otolaryng. (Chicago)* 98:397–413. *(Fig. 7.1, 92)*

Donchin, E., 107

Donchin, E., and Cohen, L. (1967). Averaged evoked potentials and intramodality selective attention. *Electroenceph. Clin. Neurophysiol.* 22: 537–546.

Dorland, A., **46**

Dorland, A. (1965). *Dorland's illustrated medical dictionary*. Philadelphia: Saunders. *(Fig. 5.1, 46)*

Durlach, N. I., 165

Durlach, N. I. (1972). Binaural signal detection: Equalization and cancellation theory. *Foundations of modern auditory theory*, Vol. II, Tobias, J. V. (ed.). New York: Academic.

Durrant, J. D., 63; *see* Dallos

Duvall, A. J., 63; *see* Tonndorf

Egan, J. P., 120, 122, **152**, 154; *see* Postman

Egan, J. P. (1975). *Signal detection theory and ROC analysis*. New York: Academic.

Egan, J. P., and Clarke, F. R. (1966). Psychophysics and signal detection. *Experimental methods and instrumentation in psychology*, Sidowski, J. B. (ed.). New York: McGraw-Hill.

Egan, J. P. and Hake, H. W. (1950). On the masking pattern of a simple auditory stimulus. *J. Acoust. Soc. Amer.* 22:622–630.

Eggermont, J. J., 90

Eggermont, J. J., Odenthal, D. W., Schmidt, P. H., and Spoor, A. (1974). Electrocochleography basic principles and clinical applications. *Acta Otolaryng (Stockholm)*, Suppl. 316:1–84.

Eldredge, D. H., 62, 89, 90, 91; *see* Davis; *see* Tasaki; *see* Teas

Eldredge, D. H. (1974). Inner ear: Cochlear mechanics and cochlear potentials. *Handbook of sensory physiology*, Vol. V(1), Keidel, W. D., and Neff, W. D. (eds.). New York: Springer.

Eldredge, D. H., and Miller, J. D. (1971). Physiology of hearing. *Ann. Rev. Physiol.* 33:281–310.

Elfner, L., 165

Elfner, L., and Perrott, D. (1967). Lateralization and intensity discrimination. *J. Acoust. Soc. Amer.* 42:441–445.

Elliot, L. L., 154

Elliot, L. L. (1962). Backward and forward masking of probe tones of different frequencies. *J. Acoust. Amer.* 34:728.

Elliott, D. N., **102**, 108, 154, 175; *see* Trahiotis

Elliott, D. N., and Fraser, W. R. (1970). Fatigue and adaptation. *Foundations of modern auditory theory*, Vol. 1, Tobias, J. V. (ed.). New York: Academic.

Elliott, D. N., and Trahiotis, C. (1972). Cortical lesions and auditory discrimination. *Psychol. Bull.* 77:198–222. *(Fig. 7.9, 102)*

Ellis, M. S., 90; *see* Cullen

Engen, Trygg, 119, 128

Engen, Trygg (1972). *Woodworth and Schlosberg's experimental psychology*, 3rd ed., Vol. 1, Chaps. 2 and 3, Kling, J. W., and Riggs, L. A. (eds.). New York: Holt, Rinehart and Winston.

Engstrom, H., **33**, 62, 63, 90, 198; *see* Ades; *see* Angelborg

Engstrom, H. (1958). On the double innervation of the sensory epithelia of the inner ear. *Acta Otolaryng. (Stockholm)*, 49:109–118.

Engstrom, H., and Ades, H. W. (1975). Inner ear studies—II. *Acta Otolaryng. (Stockholm)*, Suppl. 319.

Engstrom, H., Ades, H. W., and Anderson, A. (1966). *Structural pattern of the organ of Corti*. Baltimore: Williams & Wilkins.

Engstrom, H., Ades, H. W., and Bredberg, G. (1970). Normal structure of the organ of Corti and the effect of noise-induced cochlear damage. *Sensorineural hearing loss, a Ciba Foundation symposium*, Wolstenholme, G. E. W., and Knight, J. (eds.). London: Churchill, pp. 127–156.

Engstrom, H., Ades, H. W., and Hawkins, J. E., Jr. (1962). Structure and functions of the sensory hairs of the inner ear. *J. Acoust. Soc. Amer.* 34: 1356–1363.

Erulkar, S. D., 108.

Erulkar, S. D. (1975). Physiological studies of the inferior colliculus and medial geniculate complex. *Handbook of sensory physiology*, Vol. V(2), Keidel, W. D., and Neff, W. D. (eds.). New York: Springer.

Evans, E. F., 90, 91, 108; *see* Whitfield

Evans, E. F. (1968). Cortical representation. *Hearing mechanisms in vertebrates*, De Reuck, A. V. S., and Knight, J. (eds.). London: Churchill, pp. 272–287.

Evans, E. F. (1970a). Narrow "tuning" of cochlear nerve fiber responses in the guinea pig. *J. Physiol. (London)* 206:14–15.

Evans, E. F. (1970b). Narrow tuning of the responses of cochlear nerve fibers emanating from the exposed basilar membrane. *J. Physiol. (London)* 208:75–76.

Evans, E. F. (1972a). Does frequency sharpening occur in the cochlea? *Hearing theory*. Eindhoven: IPO, pp. 27–34.

Evans, E. F. (1972b). "The frequency response and other properties of single fibers in the guinea pig cochlear nerve." *J. Physiol. (London)* 226:263–287.

Evans, E. F. (1975). Cochlear nerve and cochlear nucleus. *Handbook of sensory physiology*, Vol. V(2), Keidel, W. D., and Neff, W. D. (eds.). New York: Springer, pp. 2–108.

Evans, E. F., and Wilson, J. P. (1973). Frequency selectivity of the cochlea. *Basic mechanisms in hearing*, Moller, A. (ed.). New York: Academic, pp. 519–551.

Fechner, G., 110, 124
Feddersen, W. E., **157**, 165
Feddersen, W. E., Sandel, T. T., Teas, D. C., and Jeffress, L. A. (1957). Localization of high-frequency tones. *J. Acoust. Soc. Amer.* 29:988–991. *(Fig. 12.2, 157)*
Fernandez, C., 63, 89; *see* Davis; *see* Tasaki
Fex, J., 90, 91
Fex, J. (1968). Efferent inhibition in the cochlea by the olivocochlear bundle. *Hearing mechanisms in vertebrates, a Ciba Foundation symposium*. London: Churchill, pp. 169–181.
Fex, J. (1974). Neural excitatory processes of the inner ear. *Handbook of sensory physiology*, Vol. V(1), Keidel, W. D., and Neff, W. D. (eds.). New York: Springer, pp. 585–646.
Fletcher, H., **50**, 62, 149, 150, 154, 166, **167**, 174, 175
Fletcher, H. (1924). The physical criterion for determining the pitch of a musical tone. *Phys. Rev.* 23:427–437.
Fletcher, H. (1940). Auditory patterns. *Rev. Mod. Phys.* 12:47–65.
Fletcher, H. (1953). *Speech and hearing in communication*. New York: Van Nostrand. *(Fig. 5.4, 50)*
Fletcher, H., and Munson, W. A. (1933). Loudness: Its definition, measurement, and calculation. *J. Acoust. Soc. Amer.* 5:82–108. *(Fig. 13.1, 167)*
Flock, A., 91
Flock, A. (1974). Sensory transduction in hair cells. *Handbook of sensory physiology*, Vol. V(1), Keidel, W. D., and Neff, W. D. (eds.). New York: Springer, pp. 396–441.
Franks, J. R., **130**, **131**, 140; *see* Watson
Fraser, W. R., 154, 175; *see* Elliott, D. N.

Gacek, R. R., 90; *see* Spoendlin

Galambos, R., 96; *see* Rose
Gardner, M. B., 175; *see* Steinberg
Garner, W. R., 140
Garner, W. R. (1947). The effect of frequency spectrum on temporal integration of energy in the ear. *J. Acoust. Soc. Amer.* 19:808–811.
Geisler, C. D., 107; *see* Rose
Geldard, F. A., 182
Geldard, F. A. (1972). *The human senses*. New York: Wiley.
Gengel, R. W., **133**, 140; *see* Watson
Gersuni, G. V., 108
Gersuni, G. V. (ed.) (1971). *Sensory processes at the neuronal and behavioral levels*. New York: Academic.
Gersuni, G. V., and Vartanian, I. A. (1973). Time-dependent features of adequate sound stimuli and the functional organization of central auditory neurons. *Basic mechanisms in hearing*, Moller, A. R., (ed.). New York: Academic.
Glattke, T. J., 90; *see* Simmons
Godfrey, D. A., 108; *see* Kiang; *see* Morest
Goldberg, J. M., 108; *see* Hind
Goldberg, J. M., and Brown, P. B. (1968). Functional organization of the dog superior olivary complex: An anatomical and electrophysiological study. *J. Neurophysiol.* 31:639–656.
Goldberg, J. M., and Greenwood, D. D. (1966). Response of neurons of the dorsal and posteroventral cochlear nuclei of the cat to acoustic stimuli of long duration. *J. Neurophysiol.* 29:72.
Goldberg, J. M., and Neff, W. D. (1961a). Frequency discrimination after bilateral ablation of cortical auditory areas. *J. Neurophysiol.* 24:119–128.
Goldberg, J. M., and Neff, W. D. (1961b). Frequency discrimination after bilateral section of the brachium of the inferior colliculus. *J. Comp. Neurol.* 116:265–290.
Goldberg, J. P., 140, 154; *see* McGill
Goldstein, M. H., Jr., 91, 107
Goldstein, M. H., Jr. (1968). The auditory periphery. *Medical Physiology*, Vol. 2, Mountcastle, C. V. (ed.). St. Louis: Mosby, pp. 1499–1531.
Goldstein, M. H., Jr., and Abeles, M. (1975). Single unit activity of the auditory cortex. *Handbook of sensory physiology*, Vol. V(2), Keidel W. D., and Neff, W. D. (eds.). New York: Springer, pp. 199–218.
Grayson, R. L., 62
Green, D. M., 120, 140, 154, 165, 175; *see* Wightman; *see* Yost
Green, D. M. (1969). Masking with continuous and pulsed sinusoids. *J. Acoust. Soc. Amer.* 46:939–946.

Green, D. M. (1971). Temporal auditory acuity. *Psychol. Rev.* 78(6):542–551.

Green, D. M., Birdsall, T. G., and Tanner, W. P. (1957). Signal detection as a function of signal intensity and duration. *J. Acoust. Soc. Amer.* 29:523–541.

Green, D. M., and Henning, G. B. (1969). Audition. *Annual Rev. Psychol.* 20:105–128.

Green, D. M., and Swets, J. A. (1974). *Signal detection theory and psychophysics.* New York: Robert E. Krieger Publishing Company.

Green, D. M., and Yost, W. A. (1975). Binaural analysis. *Handbook of sensory physiology,* Vol. V(2), Neff, W. D., and Keidel, W. D. (eds.). New York: Springer.

Greenwood, D. D., **150**, 150, 154; *see* Goldberg, J. M.; *see* Hind

Greenwood, D. D. (1961). Auditory masking and the critical band. *J. Acoust. Soc. Amer.* 33:484–502. *(Fig. 11.7, 150)*

Greenwood, D. D. (1972). Masking by combination bands: Estimation of the levels of the combination bands $(n + 1)f_L - nf_h$. *J. Acoust. Soc. Amer.* 52:1144–1155.

Gross, N. B., 107; *see* Rose

Guinan, J. J., 43, 108; *see* Kiang; *see* Morest

Guinan, J. J., and Peake, W. T. (1967). Middle ear characteristics of anesthetized cats. *J. Acoust. Soc. Amer.* 41:1237–1261.

Hafter, E. R., 165

Hafter, E. R., and Carrier, S. C. (1969). Masking level differences obtained with pulsed tonal maskers. *J. Acoust. Soc. Amer.* 47:1041–1048.

Hake, H. W., 154; *see* Egan

Hall, J. L., 154, 173, **173**, 175

Hall, J. L. (1975). Non monotic behavior of distortion product $2f_1 - f_2$: Psychophysical observations. *J. Acoust. Soc. Amer.* 58:1046–1050. *(Fig. 13.8, 173)*

Hamernik, R. P., 154; *see* Henderson

Harris, J. D., 165

Harris, J. D. (1972). A florilegium of experiments on directional hearing. *Acta Otolaryng. (Stockholm),*Suppl. 298.

Harrison, J. M., **92**, **101**, 107, 108

Harrison, J. M., and Howe, M. E. (1974a). Anatomy of the afferent auditory nervous system of mammals. *Handbook of sensory physiology,* Vol. V(1), Keidel, W. D., and Neff, W. D. (eds.). New York: Springer. *(Fig. 7.1, 92)*

Harrison, J. M., and Howe, M. E. (1974b). Anatomy of the descending auditory system (mammalian). *Handbook of sensory physiology,* Vol.

V(1), Keidel, W. D., and Neff, W. D. (eds.). New York: Springer. *(Fig. 7.8, 101)*

Hawkins, J. E., 63, 147, **148**, **150**, 154

Hawkins, J. E., and Stevens, S. S. (1950). The masking of pure tones and of speech by white noise. *J. Acoust. Soc. Amer.* 22:6–13. *(Fig. 11.5, 148; Fig. 11.7, 150)*

Hayat, A., 198

Hayat, A. (1970). *Principles and techniques of electron microscopy,* Vol. 1. New York: Van Nostrand.

Hearle, J. W. S., 198

Hearle, J. W. S., Sparrow, J. T., and Cross, P. M. (1973). *The use of the scanning electron microscope.* New York: Pergamon.

Helle, R., 63

Helle, R. (1974). Enlarged hydromechanical cochlear model with basilar membrane and tectorial membrane. *Facts and models in hearing.* Zwicker, E., and Terhardt, E. (eds.). New York: Springer.

Helmholtz, H., 36, 37, 42

Helmholtz, H. (1868). Die Mechanik der Gehorknochelchen und des Trommelfelk. *Pflueger Arch.* 1:1–60. (Translated as *The mechanism of the ossicles of the ear and the membrana tympani.* Baltimore: William Wood & Company, 1873.)

Henderson, D., 154

Henderson, D., Hamernik, R. P., Darshan, S. D., and Mills, J. H. (eds.) (1976). *Effects of noise on hearing.* New York: Raven Press.

Henning, G. B., 165; *see* Green

Henning, G. B. (1974). Detectability of interaural delay in high-frequency complex waveforms. *J. Acoust. Soc. Amer.* 55:84–90.

Hilding, A. C., 63

Hilding, A. C. (1952). Studies on the otic labyrinth. *Ann. Otol.* 61:354–370.

Hillyard, S. A., 107; *see* Squires, K. C.

Hind, J. E., 83, **86**, 90, 107, 108; *see* Anderson, D. J.; *see* Rose

Hind, J. E. (1972). Physiological correlates of auditory stimulus periodicity. *Audiology* 11:42–57.

Hind, J., Anderson, D., Brugge, J., and Rose, J. (1967). Coding of information pertaining to paired low-frequency tones in single auditory nerve fibers of the squirrel monkey. *J. Neurophysiol.* 30:794–816. *(Fig. 6.13, 83)*

Hind, J. E., Goldberg, J. M., Greenwood, D. D., and Rose, J. E. (1963). Some discharge characteristics of single neurons in the inferior colliculus of the cat. II. Timing of the discharges and observations on binaural stimulation. *J. Neurophysiol.* 26:321–341.

Hirsh, I. J., 163, 165

Hirsh, I. J. (1948). The influence of interaural phase on interaural summation and inhibition. *J. Acoust. Soc. Amer.* 20:536–544.

Hood, D. C., **130**, **131**, 140; *see* Watson

Howe, M. E., 92, 101, 107, 108; *see* Harrison

Huang, C. M., 107; *see* Buchwald

Hughes, J. R., **96**; *see* Rose

Hughes, J. W., 140

Hughes, J. W. (1946). The threshold of audition for short periods of stimulation. *Proc. Roy. Soc.* 133B:486–490.

Ishii, D., 90

Ishii, D., and Balogh, K., Jr. (1968). Distribution of efferent nerve endings in the organ of Corti. Their graphic reconstruction in cochlea by localization of acetylcholinesterase activity. *Acta Otolaryngol. (Stockholm)*, 66:282–288.

Iurato, S., 62, 63, 90

Iurato, S. (1962). Functional implications of the nature and submicroscopic structure of the tectorial and basilar membranes. *J. Acoust. Soc. Amer.* 34:1386–1395.

Iurato, S. (1964). Fibre efferenti dirette e crociate alle cellule acustiche dell'organo del Corti. *Monit. Zool. It., Suppl.* 72:62–63.

Iurato, S. (1967). *Submicroscopic structure of the inner ear.* New York: Pergamon.

Iurato, S. (1974). Efferent innervation of the cochlea. *Handbook of sensory physiology*, Vol. V(1), Keidel, W. D., and Neff, W. D. (eds.), New York: Springer.

Jeffress, L. A., 154, **157**, 160, 165; *see* Feddersen

Jeffress, L. A. (1964). Stimulus-oriented approach to detection theory. *J. Acoust. Soc. Amer.* 36: 760–774.

Jeffress, L. A. (1970). Masking. *Foundations of modern auditory theory*, Vol. 1, Tobias, J. V. (ed.). New York: Academic.

Jeffress, L. A. (1972). Binaural signal detection: Vector theory. *Foundations of modern auditory theory*, Vol. 2, Tobias, J. V. (ed.). New York: Academic.

Jeffress, L. A., and Taylor, R. W. (1961). Lateralization vs. localization. *J. Acoust. Soc. Amer.* 33: 482–483.

Jerger, J., 42

Jerger, J. (ed.) (1975). *Handbook of clinical impedance audiometry.* Dobbs Ferry, N.Y.: American Electromedics Corporation.

Jesteadt, W., 140

Jesteadt, W., and Bilger, R. C. (1974). Intensity and frequency discrimination. I. One- and two-interval paradigms. *J. Acoust. Soc. Amer.* 55: 1266–1279.

Jewett, D. L., **106**, 107

Jewett, D. L., Romano, M. N., and Williston, J. S. (1970). Human auditory-evoked potentials: possible brain stem components detected on the scalp. *Science* 167:1517–1518.

Jewett D. L., and Williston, J. S. (1971). Auditory-evoked far fields averaged from the scalp of humans. *Brain* 94:681–696. *(Fig. 7.12, 106)*

Johnstone, B. M., 62

Johnstone, B. M., Taylor, K. J., and Boyle, A. J. (1970). Mechanics of the guinea pig cochlea. *J. Acoust. Soc. Amer.* 47:504–509.

Johnstone B. M., and Boyle, A. J. (1967). Basilar membrane vibration examined with the Mössbauer techniques. *Science* 158:389–390.

Kane, E. C., 108; *see* Kiang; *see* Morest

Keidel, W. D., 107, 182

Keidel, W. D., and Neff, W. D. (eds.). (1974, 1975). *Handbook of sensory physiology*, Vols. V(1) and V(2). New York: Springer.

Keith, A., 50; *see* Wrightson

Khanna, S. M., **37**, 42; *see* Tonndorf

Kiang, N. Y-S. 82, 85, 90, 99, 107, 108; *see* Morest; *see* Peake

Kiang, N. Y-S. (1965). Stimulus coding in the auditory nerve and cochlear nucleus. *Acta Otolaryngol. (Stockholm)* 59:186–200. *(Fig. 7.6, 99)*

Kiang, N. Y-S. (1968). A survey of recent developments in the study of auditory physiology. *Ann. Otol.* 77:656–676.

Kiang, N. Y-S., Morest, D. K., Godfrey, D. A., Guinan, J. J., Jr., and Kane, E. C. (1973). Stimulus coding at caudal levels of the cat's auditory nervous system: I. Response characteristics of single units. *Basic mechanisms in hearing*, Moller, A. R. (ed.). New York: Academic, pp. 455–478.

Kiang, N. Y-S., and Moxon, E. C. (1972). Physiological considerations in artificial stimulation of the inner ear. *Ann. Otol.* 81:714–730. *(Fig. 6.17, 82)*

Kiang, N. Y-S., Moxon, E. C., and Levine, R. A. (1970). Auditory-nerve activity in cats with normal and abnormal cochleas. *Sensorineural hearing loss, a Ciba Foundation symposium*, Wolstenholme, G. E. W., and Knight, J. (eds.). London: Churchill, pp. 241–268.

Kiang, N. Y-S., Watanabe, T., Thomas, E. C., and Clark, L. F. (1965). *Discharge patterns of single fibers in the cat's auditory nerve.* Cambridge, Mass.: M.I.T. Press. *(Fig. 6.20, 85)*

Kimura, R. S., 63, 90

Kimura, R. S. (1966). Hairs of the cochlear sensory cells and their attachment to the tectorial membrane. *Acta Otolaryng. (Stockholm)* 61:55–72.

Kimura, R., and Wersall, J. (1962). Termination of the olivocochlear bundle in relation to the outer hair cells of the organ of Corti in guinea pig. *Acta Otolaryng. (Stockholm)* 55:11–32.

Kirikae, I., 42

Kirikae, I. (1960). *The structure and function of the middle ear.* Tokyo: University of Tokyo Press.

Kling, J. W., 120, 165, 182

Kling, J. W., and Riggs, L. A. (eds.) (1972). *Woodworth and Schlosberg's experimental psychology,* 3rd Ed., Vol. 1: *Sensation and perception.* New York: Holt, Rinehart and Winston.

Kobrak, H. G., 42

Kobrak, H. G. (1959). *The middle ear.* Chicago: University of Chicago Press.

Kohlloffel, L. U. E., 62

Kohlloffel, L. U. E. (1972a). A study of basilar membrane vibrations. II. The vibratory amplitude and phase pattern along the basilar membrane (post mortem). *Acoustica* 27:66–81.

Kohlloffel, L. U. E. (1972b). A study of basilar membrane vibrations. III. The basilar membrane frequency response curve in the living guinea pig. *Acoustica* 27:82–89.

Kohlloffel, L. U. E. (1972c). A study of basilar membrane vibrations. I. Fuzziness detection. A new method for the analysis of microvibrations with laser light. *Acoustica* 27:49–65.

Konishi, T., 87, 90; *see* Teas

Konishi, T., and Nielsen, D. W. (1973). The temporal relationship between motion of the basilar membrane and initiation of nerve impulses in the auditory nerve fibers. *J. Acoust. Soc. Amer.* 53:325.

Kryter, K. D., 154

Kryter, K. D. (1970). *The effects of noise on man.* New York: Academic.

Kuhn, F. A., 198

Kuhn, F. A., Thalmann, R., and Marovitz, W. F. (1971). Nomarski differential interference contrast of the normal and pathologic guinea pig organ of Corti. *Laryngoscope* 81(11):1787–1801.

Lane, C. E., 143, 144, 146, 150, 151, 154; *see* Wegel

Langford, T. L., 107; *see* Moushegian

Lawrence, M., 43–44, 62, 91; *see* Wever

Leshowitz, B., 140, 154

Leshowitz, B., and Cudahay, E. (1972). Masking with continuous and gated sinusoids. *J. Acoust. Soc. Amer.* 51:1921–1929.

Leshowitz, B., and Wightman, F. L. (1971). On frequency masking with continuous sinusoids. *J. Acoust. Soc. Amer.* 49:1180–1190.

Levine, R. A., 90; *see* Kiang

Levitt, H., 122

Levitt, H. (1971). Transformed up-down methods in psychoacoustics. *J. Acoust. Soc. Amer.* 49:467–477.

Licklider, J. C. R., 31, 163, 165, 175

Licklider, J. C. R. (1948). Influence of interaural phase relations upon the masking of speech by white noise. *J. Acoust. Soc. Amer.* 20:150–159.

Licklider, J. C. R. (1951). Basic correlates of the auditory stimulus, in *Handbook of Experimental Psychology,* Stevens, S. S. (ed.). New York: Wiley.

Licklider, J. C. R. (1954). Periodicity by "pitch" and place "pitch." *J. Acoust. Soc. Amer.* 26:945.

Lim, D. J., 62, 63

Lim, D. J. (1969). Three-dimensional observation of the inner ear with the scanning electron microscope. *Acta Otolaryng. (Stockholm),* Suppl. 255:1–38.

Lim, D. J. (1972). Fine morphology of the tectorial membrane: Its relationship to the organ of Corti. *Arch. Otolaryng. (Chicago)* 96:199–215.

Lindeman, H. H., 63

Lindeman, H. H., and Bredberg, G. (1972). Scanning electron microscopy of the organ of Corti after intense auditory stimulation. Effects of stereocilia and cuticular surface hair cells. *Arch. Klin. Exp. Ohr. Nas. Kehlkopfheilk.* 203:1.

Lindsay, P. H., 95

Lindsay, P. H., and Norman, D. A. (1972). *Human information processing: An introduction to psychology.* New York: Academic. *(Fig. 7.2, 95)*

Lipscomb, D. M., 198

Lipscomb, D. M. (1974). *An introduction to the laboratory study of the ear.* Springfield, Ill.: Thomas.

Marks, L. E., 128

Marks, L. E. (1974). *Sensory processes: The new psychophysics.* New York: Academic.

Marovitz. W. F., 198; *see* Kuhn

McAuliffe, D. R., 63; *see* Davis

McFadden, D., 122, 165

McFadden, D. (1970). Three computational versions of proportion correct for use in forced-choice experiments. *Percept. Psychophys.* 8:336–393.

McFadden, D., and Pasanen, E. G. (1975). Binaural beats at high frequencies. *Science* 190:394–397.

McGill, W. J., 140, 154

McGill, W. J., and Goldberg, J. P. (1968). A study of the near miss involving Weber's law and pure tone intensity discrimination. *Percept. Psychophys.* 2:91–100.

Meek, G. A., 198

Meek, G. A. (1970). *Practical electron microscopy for biologists.* New York: Wiley.

Merzenich, M. M., **103**, 108; *see* Brugge

Merzenich, M. M., Schindler, R. A., and Sooy, F. A. (eds.) (1974). *Proceedings of the First International Conference on Electrical Stimulation of Electrical Prosthesis Treatment of Profound Sensory Neural Deafness in Man.* San Francisco: Velo-Bind, Inc.

Miller, G. A., 154

Miller, G. A. (1947). Sensitivity to changes in the intensity of white noise and its relation to masking and loudness. *J. Acoust. Soc. Amer.* 19:609–619.

Miller, J. D. 90; *see* Eldredge

Miller, J. M., 108; *see* Snow

Mills, A. W., 156, **158**, **159**, **162**, 165

Mills, A. W. (1956). On the minimum audible angle. *J. Acoust. Soc. Amer.* 30:237–246.

Mills, A. W. (1960). Lateralization of high-frequency tones. *J. Acoust. Soc. Amer.* 32:132–134. *(Fig. 12.7, 162)*

Mills, A. W. (1972). Auditory localization. *Foundations of modern auditory theory,* Vol. 2, Tobias, J. V. (ed.). New York: Academic. *(Fig. 12.3, 158; Fig. 12.4, 159)*

Mills, J. H., 154; *see* Henderson

Moller, A. R., **36**, 42, 43, 91, 108, 182

Moller, A. R. (1970). The middle ear. *Foundations of modern auditory theory,* Vol. 2, Tobias, J. V. (ed.). New York: Academic, pp. 133–194. *(Fig. 4.4, 36)*

Moller, A. R. (ed.) (1973a). *Basic mechanisms in hearing.* New York: Academic.

Moller, A. R. (1973b). Coding of amplitude-modulated sounds in the cochlear nucleus of the rat. *Basic mechanisms in hearing,* Moller, A. R. (ed.). New York, Academic, pp. 593–622.

Moller, A. R. (1974). The acoustic middle ear muscle reflex. *Handbook of sensory physiology,* Vol. V(1), Keidel, W. D., and Neff, W. D. (eds.). New York: Springer.

Morest, D. K., 108; *see* Kiang

Morest, D. K., Kiang, N. Y-S., Kane, E. C., Guinan, J. J., Jr., and Godfrey, D. A. (1973). Stimulus coding at caudal levels of the cat's auditory nervous system: II. Patterns of synaptic organization. *Basic mechanisms in hearing,* Moller, A. R. (ed.). New York: Academic, pp. 479–510.

Mountcastle, V. B., 108

Mountcastle, V. B. (1968). Central neural mechanisms in hearing. *Medical physiology,* Mountcastle, V. B. (ed.). St. Louis: Mosby, pp. 1499–1531.

Moushegian, G., **100**, 107

Moushegian, G., Rupert, A., and Langford, T. L. (1967). Stimulus coding by medial superior olivary neurons. *J. Neurophysiol.* 30:1239–1261.

Moushegian, G., Rupert, A., and Whitcomb, M. (1972). Processing of auditory information by medial superior olivary neurons. *Foundations of modern auditory theory,* Tobias, Jerry (ed.). New York: Academic. *(Fig. 7.7, 100)*

Moxon, E. C., **82**, 90; *see* Kiang

Munson, W. A., 166, **167**, 174, 175; *see* Fletcher

Naftalin, L., 63

Naftalin, L., Spencer, H. M., and Stephens, A. (1964). The character of the tectorial membrane. *J. Laryng.* 78:1061–1078.

Neff, W. D., 107, 108, 182; *see* Goldberg, J. M.; *see* Keidel

Neff, W. D. (ed.) (1966–1974). *Contributions to sensory physiology.* New York: Academic. (Published approximately annually.)

Neff, W. D., Diamond, I. T., and Casseday, J. H. (1975). Behavioral studies of auditory discrimination central nervous system. *Handbook of sensory physiology,* Vol. V(2), Keidel, W. D., and Neff, W. D. (eds.). New York: Springer, pp. 307–400.

Newman, E. B., 157, 158, 159, 160, 165; *see* Stevens; *see* Wallach

Nielsen, D. W., **87**, 90; *see* Konishi; *see* Teas

Norman, D. A., **95**; *see* Lindsay

Odenthal, D. W., 90; *see* Eggermont

Osman, E., 165

Osman, E. (1971). A correlation model of binaural masking level differences. *J. Acoust. Soc. Amer.* 50:1414–1511.

Pasanen, E. G., 165; *see* McFadden

Patterson, R., 172, 175

Patterson, R. (1973). Physical variables determining residue pitch. *J. Acoust. Soc. Amer.* 53:1565–1572.

Peake, W. T., 43, **73**, 89, 90; *see* Guinan; *see* Weiss

Peake, W. T., and Kiang, N. Y-S. (1962). Cochlear responses to condensation and rarefaction clicks. *Biophys. J.* 2:23–34. *(Fig. 6.7, 73)*

Pease, D. C., 198

Pease, D. C. (1964). *Histological techniques for electron microscopy.* New York: Academic.

Perrott, D., 165; *see* Elfner

Pestalozza, G., **69**

Pestalozza, G., and Davis, H. (1956). Electric responses of the guinea pig ear to high audio frequencies. *Amer. J. Physiol.* 185:595–600. *(Fig. 6.3, 69)*

Peterson, L., 62

Peterson, L., and Bogert, B. (1950). A dynamical theory of the cochlea. *J. Acoust. Soc. Amer.* 22:369–381.

Pfalz, R., 108

Pfalz, R. (1973). Efferent-crossed inhibition in the ventral cochlear nuclei. *Basic mechanisms in hearing.* Moller, A. G. (ed.). New York: Academic.

Pinson, E. N., 181; *see* Denes

Plomp, R., 91, 175, 182

Plomp, R., and Smoorenburg, G. F. (eds.) (1970). *Frequency analysis and periodicity detection in hearing.* Leiden: A. W. Sythoff.

Postman, L. J., **152**

Postman, L. J., and Egan, J. P. (1949). *Experimental psychology: An introduction.* New York, Harper & Row. *(Fig. 11.10, 152)*

Preston, R. E., 91; *see* Wright

Ranke, O. F., **58**

Ranke, O. F. (1942). Das Massenverhaltnis Zwischen Membran und Flussigkut im Innenohn. *Akust. Z.* 7:1–11. *(Fig. 5.12, 58)*

Rasmussen, T., 90; *see* Smith

Rasmussen, T. (1943). *Outlines of neuro-anatomy.* Dubuque, Iowa: William C. Brown.

Rasmussen, T., and Windle, W. F. (eds.) (1960). *Neural mechanisms of the auditory and vestibular systems.* Springfield, Ill.: Thomas.

Rauch, I., 63; *see* Rauch, S.

Rauch, S., 63

Rauch, S., and Rauch, I. (1974). Physicochemical properties of the inner ear especially ironic transport. *Handbook of sensory physiology,* Vol. V(1), Keidel, W. D., and Neff, W. D. (eds.). New York: Springer, pp. 647–682.

Raynor, S., 63; *see* Billone; *see* Dallos

Reveau, J. P., 63; *see* Tonndorf

Rhode, W. S., 62

Rhode, W. S. (1971). Observations of the vibration of the basilar membrane in squirrel monkeys using the Mössbauer technique. *J. Acoust. Soc. Amer.* 49:1218–31.

Riesz, R. R., 135, **137**, 140, 154

Riesz, R. R. (1928). Differential intensity sensitivity of the ear for pure tones. *Phys. Rev.* 31:867–875. *(Fig. 10.7, 137)*

Riggs, L. A., 120, 165, 182; *see* Kling

Robinson, D. E., 122

Robinson, D. E., and Watson, C. S. (1972). Psychophysical methods in modern psychoacoustics. *Foundations of modern auditory theory,* Vol. 2, Tobias, J. V. (ed.). New York: Academic.

Roederer, J. G., 12, 22, 175

Roederer, J. G. (1973). *Introduction to the physics and psychophysics of music.* New York: Springer.

Romano, M. N., 107; *see* Jewett

Rose, J. E., **83**, **86**, 90, **97**, 107, 108; *see* Anderson, D. J.; *see* Hind

Rose, J. E., Brugge, J. F., Anderson, D. J., and Hind, J. E. (1967). Phase-locked response to low-frequency tones in single auditory nerve fibers of the squirrel monkey. *J. Neurophysiol.* 30:769–793. *(Fig. 6.21, 86)*

Rose, J. E., Galambos, R., and Hughes, J. R. (1959). Microelectrode studies of the cochlear nuclei of the cat. *Bull. Johns Hopkins Hosp.* 104:211–251. *(Fig. 7.4, 97)*

Rose, J. E., Gross, N. B., Geisler, C. D., and Hind, J. E. (1966). Some neural mechanisms in the inferior colliculus of the cat which may be relevant to localization of a sound source. *J. Neurophysiol.* 29:288–314.

Rose, J. E., Hind, J. E., Anderson, D. J., and Brugge, J. F. (1971). Some effects of stimulus intensity on response of auditory nerve fibers in the squirrel monkey. *J. Neurophysiol.* 34:685–699. *(Fig. 6.18, 83)*

Rosenblith, W. A., 108

Rosenblith, W. A. (ed.) (1959). *Sensory communication.* Cambridge, Mass.: M.I.T. Press.

Rosenzweig, M. R., 159, 165; *see* Wallach

Ross, D. A., 42; *see* Wiener

Rupert, A., **100**, 107; *see* Moushegian

Sandel, T. T., **157**, 165; *see* Feddersen

Sando, I., 108

Sando, I. (1965). The anatomical interrelationships of the cochlear nerve fibers. *Acta Otolaryng. (Stockholm)* 59:417–436.

Saul, L., 89

Saul, L., and Davis, H. (1932). Action currents in the central nervous system: I. Action currents of the auditory tracts. *Arch. Neurol. Psychiat.* 28:1104–1116.

Scharf, B., 150, 154

Scharf, B. (1970). Critical bands. *Foundations of modern auditory theory*, Vol. 1, Tobias, J. V. (ed.). New York: Academic, pp. 157–200. *(Fig. 11.7, 150)*

Schindler, R. A., 108; *see* Merzenich

Schmidt, P. H., 90; *see* Eggermont

Schuknecht, H. F., 96, 198

Schuknecht, H. F. (1974). *Pathology of the ear.* Cambridge, Mass.: Harvard University Press. *(Fig. 7.3, 96)*

Scott, R. E., 12, 31, 42

Scott, R. E. (1964). *Linear circuits.* Reading, Mass.: Addison-Wesley.

Shaw, E. A. G., 37

Shaw, E. A. G. (1974). The external ear. *Handbook of sensory physiology,* Vol. V(1), Keidel, W. D., and Neff, W. D. (eds.). New York: Springer. *(Fig. 4.5, 37)*

Shower, E. G., 135, 136, 140

Shower, E. G., and Biddulph, R. (1931). Differential pitch sensitivity of the ear. *J. Acoust. Soc. Amer.* 3:275–277. *(Fig. 10.6, 136)*

Sidowski, J. B., 120

Sidowski, J. B. (1966). *Experimental methods and instrumentation in psychology.* New York: McGraw-Hill.

Simmons, F. B., 90

Simmons, F. B., and Glattke, T. J. (1975). Electrocochleography. *Physiological measures of audiovestibular system,* Bradford, L. J. (ed.). New York: Academic, pp. 147–175.

Sivan, L. J., 131, 139

Sivan, L. J., and White, S. D. (1933). On minimum audible fields. *J. Acoust. Soc. Amer.* 4:288–321. *(Fig. 10.2, 131)*

Smith, C. A., 90, 91, 198

Smith, C. A. (1972). Preliminary observations on the terminal ramifications of nerve fibers in the cochlea. *Acta Otolaryng. (Stockholm)* 96:472–485.

Smith, C. A., and Rasmussen, T. (1963). Recent observations on the olivocochlear bundle. *Ann. Otol.* 78:489–506.

Smith, C. A., and Rasmussen, T. (1965). Degeneration in the efferent nerve endings in the cochlea after axonal section. *J. Cell Biol.* 26:63–77.

Smith, C. A., and Vernon, J. A. (eds.) (1976). *Handbook of auditory and vestibular research methods.* Springfield, Ill.: Thomas.

Smoorenburg, G. F., 91, 154, 175, 182; *see* Plomp

Smoorenburg, G. F. (1972). Combination tones and their origin. *J. Acoust. Soc. Amer.* 52:615–633.

Snow, J. B., Jr., 108

Snow, J. B., Jr., and Miller, J. M. (1975). *The central auditory pathways.* Course 355, Summary from American Academy of Ophthalmology and Otolaryngology. St. Louis: Annals Publishing Co.

Sohmer, H., 89; *see* Weiss

Sohmer, H., Feinmesser, M., Bauberger, T. L. (1972). Routine use of cochlear audiometry in infants with uncertain diagnosis, *Ann. Otol.* 81: 72–75.

Sokolich, W. G., 63; *see* Zwislocki

Sooy, F. A., 108; *see* Merzenich

Sparrow, J. T., 198; *see* Hearle

Spencer, H. M., 63; *see* Naftalin

Spoendlin, H., 63, 74, 75, 77, 90, 91

Spoendlin, H. (1966). *The organization of the cochlear receptor.* Basel: Karger, p. 227.

Spoendlin, H. (1970). Structural basis of peripheral frequency analysis. *Frequency analysis and periodicity detection in hearing.* Plomp, R., and Smoorenburg, G. F. (eds.). Leiden: A. W. Sythoff.

Spoendlin, H. (1973). The innervation of the cochlear receptor. *Proceedings of a symposium on basic mechanisms in hearing.* New York: Academic, pp. 185–234. *(Fig. 6.8, 74)*

Spoendlin, H. (1974). Neuroanatomy of the cochlea. *Facts and models in hearing.* Zwicker, E., and Terhardt, E. (eds.). New York: Springer, pp. 18–32. *(Fig. 6.9, 75), (Fig. 6.11, 77)*

Spoendlin, H. (1974). Neuroanatomy of the cochlea. *Proceedings of the first international conference on electrical stimulation of the acoustic nerve as a treatment for profound sensorineural deafness in man.* Merzenich, M. M., Schindler, R. A., and Sooy, F. A. (eds). Velo-Bind, Inc., pp. 7–23.

Spoendlin, H. II., and Gacek, R. R. (1963). Electronmicroscopic study of the efferent and afferent innervation of the organ of Corti in the cat. *Ann. Otol.* 72:660–686.

Spoor, A., 90; *see* Eggermont

Squires, K. C., 107

Squires, K. C., Squires, N. K., and Hillyard, S. A. (1975). Decision-related cortical potentials during an auditory signal detection task with cued observation interval. *J. Exp. Psychol.: Human Perception and Performance* 1:268–280.

Squires, N. K., 107; *see* Squires, K. C.

Steele, C. R., 63

Steele, C. R. (1973). A possibility for subtectorial membrane fluid motion. *Basic mechanisms in hearing,* Moller, A. (ed.). New York: Academic, pp. 69–90.

Steinberg, J. C., 168, 175

Steinberg, J. C., and Gardner, M. B. (1937). The dependence of hearing impairment on sound intensity. *J. Acoust. Soc. Amer.* 9:11–23.

Stephens, A., 63; *see* Naftalin

Stevens, S. S., 31, 110, 125, **126**, 128, 147, **148**, 150, 154, 157, 158, 160, 165, **170**, 174, 175, 182; *see* Hawkins

Stevens, S. S. (1934). Are tones spatial. *Amer. J. Psychol.* 46:145–147.

Stevens, S. S. (1935). The relation of pitch to intensity. *J. Acoust. Soc. Amer.* 6:150–154. *(Fig. 13.4, 170)*

Stevens, S. S. (ed.) (1951). *Handbook of experimental psychology.* New York: Wiley.

Stevens, S. S. (1961). The psychophysics of sensory function. *Sensory communication,* Rosenblith, W. A. (ed.). Cambridge, Mass.: M.I.T. Press.

Stevens, S. S. (1970). Neural events and the psychophysical law. *Science* 170:1043–1050.

Stevens, S. S. (1975). *Psychophysics,* Stevens, G. (ed.). New York: Wiley. *(Fig. 9.1, 126)*

Stevens, S. S., and Newman, E. B. (1936). The localization of actual sources of sound. *Amer. J. Psychol.* 48:297–306.

Stevens, S. S., and Volkman, J. (1940). The relation of pitch to frequency: A revised scale. *Amer. J. Psychol.* 53:329–353. *(Fig. 13.3, 170)*

Swets, J. A., 120, 122, 154; *see* Green

Swets, J. A. (ed.) (1964). *Signal detection and recognition by human observers· Contemporary readings.* New York: Wiley.

Tanner, W. P., 140; *see* Green

Tasaki, I., 68, **69**, 70, **71**, 89, 90

Tasaki, I. (1954). Nerve impulses in individual auditory nerve fibers of guinea pig. *J. Neurophysiol.* 17:97–122. *(Fig. 6.5, 71)*

Tasaki, I., Davis, H., and Eldredge, D. H. (1954). Exploration of cochlear potentials with a microelectrode. *J. Acoust. Soc. Amer.* 26:765–773. *(Fig. 6.2, 69)*

Tasaki, I., and Fernandez, C. (1952). Modification of cochlear microphonics and action potentials by KCl solution and by direct currents. *J. Neurophysiol.* 15:497–512.

Taylor, K. J., 62; *see* Johnstone

Taylor, R. W., 160, 165; *see* Jeffress

Teas, D. C., **87**, 89, 90, 91, 107, **157**, 165; *see* Benson; *see* Feddersen

Teas D. C. (1970). Cochlear processes. *Foundations of modern auditory theory,* Vol. 1, Tobias, J. V. (ed.). New York: Academic, pp. 255–304.

Teas, D. C., Eldredge, D. H., and Davis, H. (1962). Cochlear responses to acoustic transients: An interpretation of whole-nerve action potentials. *J. Acoust. Soc. Amer.* 34:1438–1459.

Teas, D. C., Konishi, T., and Nielsen, D. W. (1972). Electrophysiological studies on the spatial distribution of the crossed olivocochlear bundle along the guinea pig cochlea. *J. Acoust. Soc. Amer.* 51:1256–1264. *(Fig. 6.22, 87)*

Terhardt, E., 91, 182; *see* Zwicker

Thalmann, R., 198; *see* Kuhn

Thomas, E. C., **85**, 90; *see* Kiang

Titova, L. K., 62; *see* Vinnikov

Tobias, J. V., 154, 182

Tobias, J. V. (ed.) (1970, 1972). *Foundations of modern auditory theory,* Vols. 1 and 2. New York: Academic.

Tonndorf, J., **37**, 42, **57**, 62, 63

Tonndorf, J. (1959). Beats in cochlear models. *J. Acoust. Soc. Amer.* 31:608–619.

Tonndorf, J. (1960). Dimensional analysis of cochlear models. *J. Acoust. Soc. Amer.* 32:493–497. *(Fig. 5.11, 57)*

Tonndorf, J. (1970). Cochlear mechanics and hydrodynamics. *Foundations of modern auditory theory,* Vol. 1, Tobias, J. V. (ed.). New York: Academic.

Tonndorf, J., Duvall, A. J., III, and Reveau, J. P. (1962). Permeability of intracochlear membranes to various vital stains. *Ann. Otol.* 71:801–841.

Tonndorf, J., and Khanna, S. M. (1972). Tympanic membrane vibrations in human cadaver ears studied by time-averaged holography. *J. Acoust. Soc. Amer.* 52:1221–1233. *(Fig. 4.6, 37)*

Trahiotis, C., **102**, 108; *see* Elliott, D. N.

Trahiotis, C., and Elliott, D. N. (1970). Behavioral investigation of some possible effects of sectioning the crossed olivocochlear bundle. *J. Acoust. Soc. Amer.* 47:592–596.

Tsuchitani, C., 108

Tsuchitani, C., and Boudreau, J. C. (1966). Single unit analysis of cat superior olive S-segment with tonal stimuli. *J. Neurophysiol.* 29:684–697.

Tunturi, A. R., 108

Tunturi, A. R. (1955). Analysis of cortical auditory responses with the probability pulse. *Amer. J. Physiol.* 181:630.

Tunturi, A. R. (1960). Anatomy and physiology of the auditory cortex. *Neural mechanisms of auditory and vestibular systems,* Rasmussen, T., and Windle, W. F. (eds.). Springfield, Ill.: Thomas, pp. 181–200.

Tversky, A., 128; *see* Coombs

Van Bergeijk, W. A., 108

Van Bergeijk, W. A. (1962). Variation on a theme of Bekesy's: A model of binaural interaction. *J. Acoust. Soc. Amer.* 34:1431–1437.

Vartanian, I. A., 108; *see* Gersuni

Vernon, J. A , 198; *see* Smith

Vinnikov, Ya. A., 62

Vinnikov, Ya. A., and Titova, L. K. (1964). *The organ of Corti: Its histophysiology and histochemistry.* New York: Consultants Bureau.

Volkman, J., 175; *see* Stevens

Wallach, H., 159, 165

Wallach, H., Newman, E. B., and Rosenzweig, M. R. (1949). The precedence effect in sound localization. *Amer. J. Psychol.* 62:315–336.

Walzl, E. M., 108

Walzl, E. M. (1947). Representation of the cochlea in the cerebral cortex. *Laryngoscope* 57:778.

Wang, C. Y., 63; *see* Dallos

Ward, W. D., 154, 175

Ward, W. D. (1968). Susceptibility to auditory fatigue. *Contributions to sensory physiology,* Vol. 3, Neff, W. D. (ed.). New York: Academic.

Ward, W. D. (1970). Musical perception. *Foundations of modern auditory theory,* Vol. 1, Tobias, J. V. (ed.). New York: Academic.

Watanabe, T., 85, 90; *see* Kiang

Watson, C. S., 120, 122, 128, **130, 131, 133,** 140

Watson, C. S. (1974). Psychophysics. *Handbook of psychology,* Wohlman, B. (ed.). Englewood Cliffs, N.J.: Prentice-Hall.

Watson, C. S., Franks, J. R., and Hood, D. C. (1972). Detection of tones in the absence of external masking noise. I. Effects of signal intensity and signal frequency. *J. Acoust. Soc. Amer.* 52: 633–643. *(Fig. 10.1, 130; Fig. 10.2, 131)*

Watson, C. S., and Gengel, R. W. (1969). Signal duration and signal frequency in relation to auditory sensitivity. *J. Acoust. Soc. Amer.* 46: 989–997. *(Fig. 10.3, 133)*

Weber, 124

Webster, F. A., **164**

Webster, F. A. (1951). The influence of interaural phase on masked thresholds. I. The role of interaural time-deviation, *J. Acoust. Soc. Amer.* 23: 452–461. *(Fig. 12.8, 164)*

Wegel, R. L., **131,** 140, 143, 144, 146, 150, 151, 154

Wegel, R. L. (1932). Physical data and physiology of excitation of auditory nerve. *Ann. Otol.* 41: 740–779. *(Fig. 10.2, 131)*

Wegel, R. L., and Lane, C. E. (1924). The auditory masking of one sound by another and its probable relation to the dynamics of the inner ear. *Phys. Rev.* 23:266–285. *(Fig. 11.1, 144)*

Weiss, T. F., 89

Weiss, T. F., Peake, W. T., and Sohmer, H. S. (1971). Intracochlea potential recorded with micropipettes. II. Responses in the cochlear scalae to tones. *J. Acoust. Soc. Amer.* 50:587–601.

Wersall, J., 90; *see* Kimura

Wever, E. G., 43–44, 62, 63, 89, 91

Wever, E. G. (1949). *Theory of hearing.* New York: Wiley.

Wever, E. G. (1971). The mechanics of hair stimulation," *Trans. Amer. Otol. Soc.* 18:89–107.

Wever, E. G., and Bray, C. (1930). Action currents in the auditory nerve in response to acoustic stimulation. *Proc. Nat. Acad. Sci. USA* 16:344–350.

Wever, E. G., and Lawrence, M. (1954). *Physiological acoustics.* Princeton, N.J.: Princeton University Press.

Wever, E. G., Lawrence, M., and von Bekesy, G. (1954). A note on recent developments in auditory theory. *Proc. Nat. Acad. Sci. USA* 40:508–512.

Whitcomb, M., **100**; *see* Moushegian

White, S. D., **131**, 139; *see* Sivan

Whitfield, I. C., **92**, 108

Whitfield, I. C. (1967). *The auditory pathway.* Baltimore: Williams & Wilkins. *(Fig. 7.1, 92)*

Whitfield, I. C. (1968). Centrifugal control mechanisms of the auditory pathways. *Hearing mechanisms in vertebrates,* De Reuck, A. V. S., and Knight, J. (eds.). London: Churchill.

Whitfield, I. C., and Evans, E. F. (1965). Responses of auditory cortical neurons to stimuli of changing frequency. *J. Neurophysiol.* 28:655–672.

Whitfield, I. C., and Ross, H. F. (1965). Cochlear microphonic and summating potentials and the outputs of individual hair cell generators. *J. Acoust. Soc. Amer.* 38:126–131.

Wiener, F. M., 42

Wiener, F. M. (1947). Sound diffraction by rigid spheres and circular cylinders. *J. Acoust. Soc. Amer.* 19:444–451.

Wiener, F. M., and Ross, D. A. (1946). The pressure distribution in the auditory canal in a progressive sound field. *J. Acoust. Soc. Amer.* 18: 401–408.

Wightman, F. L., 140, 165, 175; *see* Leshowitz; *see* Yost

Wightman, F. L., and Green, D. M. (1974). The perception of pitch. *Amer. Sci.* 62:208–216.

Williston, J. S., **106**, 107; *see* Jewett

Wilson, J. P., 90; *see* Evans

Windle, W. F., 90; *see* Rasmussen

Worden, F. G., 108

Worden, F. G. (1966). Attention and auditory electrophysiology. *Progress in physiological psychology,* Vol. 1, Stellar, E., and Sprague, J. (eds.). New York: Academic.

Wright, C. G., 91

Wright, C. G., and Preston, R. E. (1975). Cochlear innervation in the guinea pig—II. *Acta Otolaryng. (Stockholm)* 80:335–342.

Wrightson, T., **50**

Wrightson, T., and Keith, A. (1918). *An enquiry into the analytical mechanism of the internal ear.* New York: Macmillan. *(Fig. 5.4, 50)*

Yost, W. A., **158**, 161, **161**, 165; *see* Green

Yost W. A. (1974). Discrimination of interaural phase differences. *J. Acoust. Soc. Amer.* 55:1299–1303. *(Fig. 12.3, 158; Fig. 12.6, 161)*

Yost, W. A., Wightman, F. L., and Green, D. M. (1971). Lateralization of filtered clicks. *J. Acoust. Soc. Amer.* 50:1526–1531.

Zemlin, W. R., 46, **58**, **61**

Zemlin, W. R. (1968). *Speech and hearing science: anatomy and physiology.* Englewood Cliffs, N.J.: Prentice-Hall. *(Fig. 5.1, 46; Fig. 5.13, 58; Fig. 5.16, 61)*

Zwicker, E., 91, 182

Zwicker, E., and Terhardt, E. (eds.) (1974). *Facts and models in hearing.* New York: Springer.

Zwislocki, J. J., 62, 63

Zwislocki, J. J. (1965). Analysis of some auditory characteristics. *Handbook of mathematical psychology,* Vol. 3, Luce, R. D., Bush, R. R., and Galanter, E., (eds.). New York: Wiley, pp. 1–97.

Zwislocki, J. J., and Sokolich, W. G. (1973). Velocity and displacement responses in auditory nerve fibers. *Science* 182:64–66.

Glossary and Index of Subjects

The glossary consists of the terms shown in **boldface** type. The definitions of these terms below are from the American National Standards Institute (ANSI). These definitions are reproduced with permission from American National Standard S.3.20–1974, copyright 1974 by the American National Standards Institute (copies of which may be purchased from the American National Standards Institute, 1430 Broadway, New York, N.Y. 10018).

Boldface page numbers indicate the pages where glossary and index terms are explained. Note that certain ANSI definitions below do not agree in detail with the uses of terms in this book.

Note 2: The use of the critical band to estimate masking should be limited to masking by noises having continuous spectra without excessive slopes or irregularities and to cases where masking exceeds 15 decibels.

Note 3: In order to be just masked in a wide-band continuous noise, the level of a pure tone in decibels must exceed the spectrum level of the continuous noise (at the same frequency) by 10 times the logarithm to the base 10 of the ratio of the critical bandwidth (for masking) to unit bandwidth. The antilogarithm to the base 10 of one-tenth of the "critical ratio" in decibels is equal to the bandwidth of the critical band (for masking).

critical ratio, 150, 154; *see* critical band

crossed olivocochlear bundle (COCB), **76–77,** 85–87, 100

    function of, 85–87

cross-modality matching, **126**

cross sectional, **195**

crura (crus), **34,** 34–36; *see* stapes

cubic difference tone, **145,** 172–173, 175

cuticular plate (CP), **50**

cutoff frequency, **25,** 25–27, 31

cycle, 4–5. A cycle is the complete sequence of values of a periodic quantity that occurs during one period.

damage risk criterion, 181. A damage risk criterion for hearing is the level of sound to which a population may be exposed for a specified time with a specified risk of hearing loss.

damage risk table, **181;** *see* damage risk criterion

decibel (dB), 17–19, **18,** 168, 188–191. The decibel is one-tenth of a bel. Thus, the decibel is a unit of level when the base of the logarithm is the tenth root of ten, and the quantities concerned are proportional to power.

Note 1: Examples of quantities that qualify are power (any form), sound pressure squared, particle velocity squared, sound intensity, sound-energy density, voltage squared. Thus the decibel is a unit of sound-pressure-squared level; it is common practice, however, to shorten this sound pressure level because ordinarily no ambiguity results from so doing.

Note 2: The logarithm to the base the tenth root of 10 is the same as ten times the logarithm to the base 10; e.g., for a number X^2, $\log_{10}^{1}/10X^2 = 10 \log_{10}X^2 = 20 \log_{10}X$. This last relationship is the one ordinarily used to simplify the language in definitions of sound pressure level, etc.

Note 3: One decibel is the level of a sound pressure, for example, that is equal to $10^{1/20}$ times the reference pressure; r decibels is the level corresponding to $10^{r/20}$ times the reference pressure.

dBA, **168,** 181

decibel of energy, **18**

decibel of power, **18**

decibel of pressure, **18**

    table of decibels, 190–191

Deiters' cells, 50; *see* cells of Deiters

Δf, 135–136, 164

ΔI, 136–137, 140–141, 142–143, 164

ΔT, 138, 140 .

dendrites, **204**

density of air (d_a), **16**

density (tonal), **174.** Density is that attribute of auditory sensation in terms of which sound may be ordered on a scale extending from diffuse to compact.

Note: The density of a tone increases with both intensity and frequency; thus, high-frequency tones will appear to be more compact (have greater density) than low-frequency tones.

descending pathways, **100**

descending series (method of limits), **111**

detectability index (d'), **120–122;** *see* normal detectability index

dichotic, **163.** Dichotic refers to the condition in which the sound stimulus presented at one ear differs from the sound stimulus presented at the other ear.

Note: The stimuli may differ in sound pressure, frequency, phase, time, duration, bandwidth, and so on.

difference limen, **110;** *see* differential threshold and difference threshold

difference threshold, **110,** 110–115, 119–120, 124, 135–138; *see* differential threshold ΔF and ΔI

difference tone, **29,** 145–146, 172–173, 175. A difference tone is a combination tone with a frequency equal to the difference between the frequencies of two primary tones or of their harmonics.

    cubic difference tone, **145;** *see* secondary difference tone

    primary difference tone, 145

differential electrode technique, **70,** 70–72

differential recording, **70–72**

differential threshold, 110; *see* difference threshold. The differential threshold, or difference limen, is the minimum change in stimulus that can be correctly judged as different from a reference stimulus in a specified fraction of the trials.

Note: Instead of the method of constant stimuli, which is implied by the phrase "a specified fraction of the trials," another psychophysical method (which should be specified) may be employed.

diotic, 163. Diotic refers to the condition in which the sound stimulus presented at each ear is **identical.**

direct scaling, **123,** 125–128

discharge rate, **82**

discrimination procedures, 109, 128

displacement, 2–3

dissonance, 174. Dissonance is the phenomenon in which tones presented together produce a harsh or unpleasant sensation.

distal, **194**

distortion, 30, 40. Distortion is an undesired change in waveform. Noise and certain desired changes in waveform, such as those resulting from modulation or detection, are not usually classed as distortion.

dorsal, **192**

dorsal cochlear nucleus (DCN), **96**

driving frequency, 24–25

duplex theory of localization, **165**

duration (*T*), 16, 132–135, 140

dynamic range, **17,** 88, 132; *see* auditory sensation area

ear canal, 33; *see* external acoustic meatus

eardrum, 33; *see* tympanic membrane

ear, nose, throat (ENT), **176;** *see* otolaryngology

efferent fibers (E), **74,** 85–87, 100

eighth cranial nerve, 73–78, 106, 238; *see* acoustic nerve

elasticity, **2**

electric potential, **205**

electrocochleography, **89–90,** 107

electrodes, 67

electroencephalogram (EEG), **104, 207**

electrophysiology, **207**

endocochlear potential (*syn.* endolymphatic potential) (EP), **67,** 87. The endocochlear potential is a resting electric polarization of the endolymph of the scala media, positive relative to the perilymph in the scala vestibuli and scala tympani and also to tissues outside of these canals.

Note: The endocochlear potential is about +80 millivolts with respect to the perilymph within the scala tympani, and about +75 millivolts with respect to the perilymph within the scala vestibuli.

endolymph, 47, 68. Endolymph is a watery fluid contained within the membranous labyrinth. It is thought to be secreted by the stria vascularis.

Note: The electric potential of the endolymph within the scala media is about +80 millivolts with respect to the perilymph within the scala tympani, and about +75 millivolts with respect to the perilymph within the scala vestibuli. This is called the endocochlear potential.

energy (E), **16,** 18–19, 23, 133. Energy is a measure of the capacity of a body to do work or of work that is done. The unit of measure is the erg, 1 erg being expended when a mass of 1 gm is accelerated 1 cm per second per second.

envelope, **144**

envelope of the traveling wave, **57,** 57–59

epitympanic recess, **34**

epitympanum, **34**

equal loudness contour, **166;** *see* loudness contour

eustachian tube, 34, 38; *see* auditory tube function of, 38

external, **194**

external acoustic meatus, 33, 36, 132. The external acoustic meatus, or ear canal, is the canal that conducts sound vibrations from the auricle to the tympanic membrane.

external auditory canal, **33,** 36 function of, 36

external auditory meatus, **33,** 132; *see* external acoustic meatus

external ear, 32; *see* outer ear. The external ear consists of the auricle and external acoustic meatus.

external hair cells, 49; *see* outer hair cells; hair cells

extracellular fluids, **205**

extratympanic electrocochleography, 90

facial nerve (Fn), 49

false alarm, 116. A false alarm is the event that occurs in a detection situation, during a specified observation interval, when a "signal-plus-noise" response (output) follows a "noise-alone" stimulus (input).

Note: A false dismissal and a correct detection are mutually exclusive for a "noise-alone" stimulus.

feeling threshold, **132;** *see* threshold of feeling

filter, 20, 4–28, **25,** 31, 56, 60, 149–150, 178; *see* wave filter in the cochlea, 56, 60

which the loudness values were determined must be stated explicitly.

beats, **144**

loudness adaptation, **169**

loudness contour, 166. A loudness contour is a curve that shows the related values of sound pressure and frequency required to produce a given loudness sensation for the typical subject for a stated manner of listening to the sound.

loudness level, 167, 175. (1) The (judged) loudness level of a sound, in phons, is numerically equal to the median sound pressure level, in decibels relative to 20 micronewtons per square meter, of a 1000-hertz reference tone presented to subjects as a frontally incident free sound field, and judged by the subjects in a number of trials to be as loud as the sound under test.

Note: The manner of listening to the unknown sound, which must be stated, may be considered as one of the characteristics of that sound.

(2) The (calculated) loudness level of a sound, in phons, is related to the loudness, in sones, by the equation

$$L = 40 + 10 \log_2 n_S$$

where L is the loudness level in phons and n_s is the loudness in sones.

Note: Since loudness levels obtained by subjective judgment may differ from those determined by other means, the conditions under which the loudness levels were determined must be stated explicitly.

loudness level contour, 175. A loudness level contour is a curve that shows the related values of sound pressure level and frequency required to produce a given loudness level for the typical subject for a stated manner of listening to the sound.

loudness recruitment, **168;** *see* recruitment

low-pass filter, 25, 25–28, 130. A low-pass filter is a wave filter having a single transmission band extending from zero frequency up to some critical or cutoff frequency, not infinite.

magnitude estimation, **125**

malleus, 34, 34–36. The malleus is the outermost of the three auditory ossicles that are located in the middle ear. Its shape resembles a club. The handle of the malleus (manubrium) is attached to the tympanic membrane, and the head of the malleus (capitulum) is attached to the body of the incus.

manner of articulation, **178**

mantissa, **189**

manubrium, 34, 34–36; *see* malleus

masked threshold, 143, 148, 154. The masked threshold is the threshold of audibility for a specified sound in the presence of another (masking) sound.

masker, **143, 154**

masking, 142–151, **142–144,** 147–151, 154, 163–165. (1) Masking is the process by which the threshold of audibility for one sound is raised by the presence of another (masking) sound.

(2) Masking is the amount by which the threshold of audibility of a sound is raised by the presence of another (masking) sound. The unit customarily used is the decibel.

binaural, **163–165**

critical band, 148–150, **149,** 154

masked threshold, **143,** 148, 154

noise, **147–151,** 154

temporal, **151,** 154

tonal, **142–144,** 150, 154

masking level difference (MLD), **163–164,** 165. Masking level difference is any decrease (improvement) in the masked threshold obtained when two ears are used instead of one. Masking level difference is expressed in decibels, as a function of the frequency of the masked tone.

matching procedure, 123, **127,** 166

medial geniculate body, **94**

medial plane, 193. The medial plane is a vertical plane that divides the body into left and right. It is perpendicular to the frontal plane.

mel, 170. The mel is a unit of pitch. One thousand mels is the pitch of a 1000-hertz pure tone for which the loudness level is 40 phons. The pitch of a sound that is judged by a subject to be n times that of a 1000-mel tone is n thousand mels; thus, the pitch of a sound subjectively judged to be n times that of a 1-mel tone is n mels.

membrane, **204–206**

method of adjustment, 111, 112, 127. The method of adjustment is a psychophysical method used primarily to determine thresholds; in this procedure the subject varies some dimension of a stimulus until that stimulus appears equal to or just noticeably different from a reference stimulus.

method, Bekesy, 112–113; *see* Bekesy method

method of constant stimuli, 111, 113. The method of constant stimuli is a psychophysical method used primarily to determine thresholds; in this procedure a number of stimuli, ranging from rarely to almost always perceivable (or rarely to almost always perceivably different from some reference stimulus), are presented one at a time. The subject responds to each presentation: "yes-no," "same-different," "greater than-equal to-less than," etc.

Note: A special case of the method of constant stimuli is the quantal method; here, fixed increments are added to a reference stimulus and the subject reports whether or not he perceives the increment.

method of cross-modality matching, 126. The method of cross-modality matching is a psychophysical method used primarily to scale sensations; in this procedure the subject adjusts a stimulus along some dimension until that stimulus appears equal to another stimulus received by a different sense modality.

method of limits, 111. The method of limits is a psychophysical method used primarily to determine thresholds; in this procedure some dimension of a stimulus, or of the difference between two stimuli, is varied incrementally until the subject changes his response.

method of magnitude estimation, 125. The method of magnitude estimation is a psychophysical method used primarily to scale sensations; in this procedure the subject assigns to a set of stimuli, numbers that are proportional to some subjective dimension of the stimuli.

method of paired comparisons, 124–125. The method of paired comparisons is a psychophysical method used primarily to scale sensations; in this procedure stimuli are presented in pairs to a subject who compares them along some dimension.

method of rank order, 125. The method of rank order is a psychophysical method used primarily to scale sensations; in this procedure stimuli are presented to a subject and he orders them along some dimension.

method of ratio production, 128. The method of ratio production is a psychophysical method used primarily to scale sensations; in this procedure the subject adjusts a stimulus along some dimension until that stimulus appears to be a specific fraction or multiple of a reference stimulus.

Note 1: When the variable stimulus is adjusted to some fraction of the reference, the procedure is called fractionation; when adjusted to some multiple, multiplication.

Note 2: When the variable stimulus is adjusted

to appear equal to the reference stimulus, the procedure is known as matching.

method of theory of signal detection, **115–119,** 120–122

methods (psychophysical), 110–115, 118–122, 125–128

adaptive procedure, **118–119,** 122

matching, **127**

microanatomy, **194**

microvilla (M), 54

middle ear, 32, 33–36, 38, 41, 43–44. The middle ear, or tympanic cavity, is the air-filled chamber within the mastoid portion of the temporal bone that contains the three auditory ossicles. It communicates with the auditory tube and the mastoid cells.

function of, 38, 41

middle ear reflex, 40–42; *see* stapedial and tensor tympani muscles

measures of, 43–44

midline, **161**

millisecond (ms), **5**

minimal audible angle (MAA), **156–157**

minimal audible field (MAF), 131–132, 139–140. The minimum audible field is the sound pressure level of a tone at the threshold of audibility measured in a free sound field for a subject facing the sound source. The value of the sound pressure level is determined after the subject is removed from the field.

minimal audible pressure (MAP), **130–131,** 139–140. The minimum audible pressure is the sound pressure of a tone at the threshold of audibility that is presented by an earphone and measured or inferred at the tympanic membrane.

miss, **116;** *see* false alarm

missing fundamental, **171–172,** 175

mitochondria (Mc), 198

modiolus (M), **47,** 78. The modiolus is the conically shaped central core of the cochlea. It contains the spiral ganglion of the cochlea and forms the inner wall of the scala vestibuli and the scala tympani.

monaural, 163; *see* monotic. Monaural pertains to the use of only one ear.

monotic, 163. Monotic refers to the condition in which a sound stimulus is presented at only one ear.

Mössbauer technique, 62, 72, **208**

motor neurons, **198**

music, **180**

musical scale, 170, 174–175. A musical scale is a series of notes (symbols, sensations, or stimuli) arranged from low to high by a specified scheme of intervals, suitable for musical purposes.

Note: The "interval" between two sounds is defined as their spacing in pitch or frequency, whichever is indicated by the context. The frequency interval is expressed by the ratio of the frequencies or by a logarithm of this ratio.

myelin sheath, **79, 204**

myelinated nerve fiber (MNF), **79, 204**

nasopharynx (nose cavity), **34, 38**

nerve (n), **208;** *see* acoustic nerve

nerve discharge, **80, 205–206**

neural loss, **177**

neurilemma, **204**

neuroanatomy, **198,** 204

neurology, **205**

neurophysiology, **205**

nodes of Ranvier, **204**

noise, **146–147, 180;** *see* random noise. (1) Noise is any undesired sound. By extension, noise is any unwanted disturbance within a useful frequency band, such as undesired electric waves in a transmission channel or device.

(2) Noise is an erratic, intermittent, or statistically random oscillation. The noise may be steady, nonsteady, or impulsive.

Note 1: If ambiguity exists as to the nature of the noise, a phrase such as "acoustic noise" or "electric noise" should be used.

Note 2: Since the above definitions are not mutually exclusive, it is usually necessary to depend upon context for the distinction.

noise pollution, **41, 154, 180–181**

noise power per unit band width (N_0), **146–147,** 150; *see* spectrum level

nominal scales, **128**

nonlinearity, **29–31, 40, 187**

nonlinear system, **29–31, 187**

normal detectability index (d'), **120–122**

Note 1: For a yes-no experiment, the value of the index can be computed from the conditional probability of a detection and the conditional probability of a false alarm. The equation is: $d' = -1$ (^{P}Detection) $- -1$ (^{P}False Alarm) where -1 is the inverse of the normal distribution function.

Note 2: For a balanced two-alternative forced-choice experiment $d' = 2 -1$ (^{P}Correct).

Note 3: Contours of constant normal detectability index are often plotted as curves on a receiver-operating-characteristic graph, and

this family is called the "normal receiver-operating-characteristic."

Note 4: A detector may be a subject or any other decision device.

nuclei-nucleus (N), **94, 204**

octave, **25–27,** 174. (1) An octave is the interval between two sounds having a basic frequency ratio of two.

(2) An octave is the pitch interval between two tones such that one tone may be regarded as duplicating the basic musical import of the other tone at the nearest possible higher pitch.

Note 1: The interval, in octaves, between any two frequencies, is the logarithm to the base 2 (or 3.322 times the logarithm to the base 10) of the frequency ratio.

Note 2: The frequency ratio corresponding to an octave pitch interval is approximately, but not always exactly, 2:1.

decibel per octave, **26–27**

off response, **99**

on-off response, **99**

on-response, **99**

optical heterodyne spectroscopy, **208**

ordinal scales, **128**

organ of Corti (OC), **49,** 49–56. The organ of Corti is a series of neuroepithelial hair cells (receptor cells for hearing) and their supporting structures lying against the osseous spiral lamina and the basilar membrane within the scala media of the cochlea. It extends from the base of the cochlea to its apex.

Note 1: In cross section, the inner and outer pillar cells (rods of Corti) of the organ of Corti form the triangular inner tunnel of Corti. The inner rods rest on the edge of the osseous spiral lamina and the outer rods rest upon the basilar membrane. A single row of sensory cells (inner hair cells) is found on the inward side of the inner rods (toward the modiolus), and three or four rows of sensory cells (outer hair cells) are located on the outer side of the outer rods. The upper ends of the hair cells form part of the reticular lamina that is supported by the rods of Corti and constitutes the upper surface of the organ of Corti. The tectorial membrane, in which the hairlike processes extending from the upper ends of the hair cells are imbedded, lies above the reticular lamina. Nerve fibers of the cochlear nerve make contact with the lower ends of the inner and outer hair cells.

level that is judged by subjects to produce the same pitch.

place of articulation, **178**

place theory, **87–88**, 97, 169, 172, 175

posterior, 192

posterior ligament of the incus, 34

posteroventral cochlear nucleus (PVCN), **96**

post-stimulus time histograms (PST), **84**, 84–85, 98, **99**

potassium (K), 205

power (*P*), **16**, 18–19, 133. Power is the rate at which energy is expended or work is done. The unit of measure is the watt.

power function, **126**, 126–128; *see* psychophysical power law

precedence effect, 159–160, 165

pressure (*p*), 1, **16**, 18–19, 38. Pressure is a measure of force divided by the area to which the force is applied. It is usually measured in dynes per square centimeter.

instantaneous pressure, **16**

primary difference tone, 145; *see* difference tone

probe tone, **151**

promontory, 90

propagate, 14–15, 22

proximal, 194

psychoacoustics, 2. Psychoacoustics is the science that deals with the psychological correlates of the physical parameters of acoustics. Psychoacoustics is a branch of psychophysics.

psychometric function, 113–114, 118, 130, 140. A psychometric function is a mathematical relationship in which the independent variable is a measure of a stimulus and the dependent variable is a measure of response.

psychophysical power law, 126; *see* power function. The psychophysical power law describes the relationship between stimulus magnitude and the resulting sensation magnitude. In mathematical terms $\psi = k(\phi - \phi_0)^n$ where ψ is sensation magnitude, ϕ is stimulus magnitude, ϕ_0 is the absolute threshold, n is a constant related to a given sense modality, and k is a proportionality constant.

Note: The psychophysical power law replaces the Weber-Fechner equation, which held that equal stimulus ratios corresponded to equal sensation differences. The psychophysical power law states that equal stimulus ratios correspond to equal sensation ratios.

psychophysics, 3, **109**, 119, 128. Psychophysics is the science that deals with the quantitative relationship between physical and psychological events. Psychophysics is a branch of psychology.

qualitative aspects of pitch, **169**

quantal theory of threshold, **120**

quantitative aspects of loudness, **169**

radial fibers (R), **74**

random noise, 146; *see* noise. Random noise is an oscillation for which the instantaneous magnitude is not specified for any given instant of time. The instantaneous magnitudes of a random noise are specified only by probability distribution functions giving the fraction of the total time that the magnitude, or some sequence of magnitudes, lies within a specified range.

Note 1: The joint behaviors of magnitudes at different instants of time are usually referred to as "higher order statistics" and are also given in terms of probabilities or certain mean values. Spectrum densities and autocorrelation functions are common examples of such higher order statistics.

Note 2: A random noise for which the instantaneous magnitudes occur according to the Gaussian distribution is called "Gaussian random noise."

range, **155**

ranking method, **125**

rarefaction, **14**

rarefaction click, **73**

ratio comparisons (method), **125–126**

ratio scale, **17**, 17–19, 128, 167

reactance (X), **20**, 23

real-time holography, **208**

receiver-operating-characteristic (ROC), **116**, 116–118. A receiver-operating-characteristic is a graphical summary of the performance of a detector. Detection probability is plotted on the ordinate, and false alarm probability is plotted on the abscissa. These are conditional probabilities, that is, the probability that the condition (signal present or signal absent) is true. A family of nonintersecting curves is often plotted with either constant detectability index or constant signal-to-noise ratio as the parameter. Each curve shows how detection probability and false-alarm probability vary monotonically as a function of the decision criteria (operating point) of the detector.

Note: A detector may be a subject or any other decision device.

receptor neurons, **198**

recruitment, 168, 175. Recruitment is the otological condition in which weak sounds are not heard while strong sounds are heard as loudly as by

for concept (2). Not all sound waves can evoke an auditory sensation; for example, ultrasound.

Note 2: The medium in which the sound exists is often indicated by an appropriate adjective; for example, airborne, waterborne, structure-borne.

sound analysis, 2, 24–31

sound intensity (I), 17, 20; *see* sound power level

sound level meter, 168. A sound level meter is an instrument including a microphone, an amplifier, an output meter, and frequency weighting networks for the measurement of noise and sound levels in a specified manner.

sound power level, 17, 20. Sound power level, in decibels, of a sound is 10 times the logarithm to the base 10 of the ratio of the power of this sound to the reference power. The reference power should be explicitly stated.

Note: The standard reference sound power is 1 picowatt.

sound pressure level (SPL), 19, 130. Sound pressure level, in decibels, of a sound is 20 times the logarithm to the base 10 of the ratio of the pressure of this sound to the reference pressure. The reference pressure should be explicitly stated.

Note 1: The standard reference pressure is 20 micronewtons per square meter for sound in gases and 1 micronewton per square meter for sound in liquids.

Note 2: Unless otherwise explicitly stated, it is to be understood that the sound pressure is the effective (root-mean-square) sound pressure.

Note 3: It is to be noted that in many sound fields the sound pressure ratios are not the square roots of the corresponding power ratios.

sound pressure level meter, 168; *see* sound level meter

sound production, 1–4, 9

sound shadow, 21, 21–22, 156, 158. A sound shadow is a region in which a sound field is reduced in magniture relative to the free field value as a result of its incidence on an obstacle.

Note 1: The reduction in magnitude may be due to reflection, refraction, absorption, or scattering of the sound field by the obstacle.

Note 2: The sound shadow produced by the auricle and/or the head may assist in the localization of sounds at frequencies of about 1500 Hz and above.

sound transmission, 2, 14–17

space of Nuel (SN), 53

spectrum, 9, 9–11. (1) The spectrum of a function

of time is a description of its resolution into components, each of different frequency and (usually) different amplitude and phase.

(2) "Spectrum" is also used to signify a continuous range of components, usually wide in extent, within which waves have some specified common characteristic; e.g., "audio-frequency spectrum."

Note: The term "spectrum" is also applied to functions of variables other than time, such as distance.

amplitude spectrum, 9, 9–11

continuous spectrum, 9, 9–11

line spectra, 9, 9–11

phase spectrum, 9, 9–11

spectrum level (N_0), 146, 146–147, 150; *see* noise power per band width. The spectrum level of a specified signal at a particular frequency is the level of that part of the signal contained within a band of unit width, centered at the particular frequency. Ordinarily this has significance only for a signal having a continuous distribution of components within the frequency range under consideration. The words "spectrum level" cannot be used alone but must appear in combination with a prefatory modifier; e.g., pressure, velocity, voltage, power.

Note: For illustration, if L_{ps} be a desired pressure spectrum level, p the effective pressure measured through the filter system, p_0 reference sound pressure, Δf the effective bandwidth of the filter system, and $\Delta_0 f$ the reference bandwidth (1 hertz), then

$$L_{ps} = 10 \log_{10} \frac{p^2/\Delta f}{p_0^2/\Delta_0 f}$$

For computational purposes, if L_p is the band pressure level observed through the filter, the above relation reduces to

$$L_{ps} = L_p - 10 \log_{10} \frac{\Delta f}{\Delta_0 f}$$

speech pathologist, **178**

speech production mechanism, **178**

speech recognition, 179, 181

speed of sound (c), **15**, 16

velocity of sound, 15

sphere (area of), **20**

spiral ganglion of the cochlea, 195. The spiral ganglion of the cochlea is composed of the cell bodies of the neurons of the cochlear nerve. It is located within the modiolus. The dendritic processes of these bipolar neurons make synaptic contact with the hair cells. The axons